D1369844

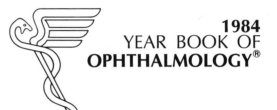

1984
YEAR BOOK OF
OPHTHALMOLOGY®

THE 1984 YEAR BOOKS

The YEAR BOOK series provides in condensed form the essence of the best of the recent international medical literature. The material is selected by distinguished editors who critically review more than 500,000 journal articles each year.

Anesthesia: *Drs. Kirby, Miller, Ostheimer, Saidman, and Stoelting.*

Cancer: *Drs. Clark, Cumley, and Hickey.*

Cardiology: *Drs. Harvey, Kirkendall, Kirklin, Nadas, Resnekov, and Sonnenblick.*

Critical Care Medicine: *Drs. Rogers, Booth, Dean, Gioia, McPherson, Michael, and Traystman.*

Dentistry: *Drs. Cohen, Hendler, Johnson, Jordan, Moyers, Robinson, and Silverman.*

Dermatology: *Drs. Sober and Fitzpatrick.*

Diagnostic Radiology: *Drs. Bragg, Keats, Kieffer, Kirkpatrick, Koehler, Sorenson, and White.*

Digestive Diseases: *Drs. Greenberger and Moody.*

Drug Therapy: *Drs. Hollister and Lasagna.*

Emergency Medicine: *Dr. Wagner.*

Endocrinology: *Drs. Schwartz and Ryan.*

Family Practice: *Dr. Rakel.*

Medicine: *Drs. Rogers, Des Prez, Cline, Braunwald, Greenberger, Bondy, Epstein, and Malawista.*

Neurology and Neurosurgery: *Drs. De Jong, Sugar, and Currier.*

Nuclear Medicine: *Drs. Hoffer, Gottschalk, and Zaret.*

Obstetrics and Gynecology: *Drs. Pitkin and Zlatnik.*

Ophthalmology: *Dr. Ernest.*

Orthopedics: *Dr. Coventry.*

Otolaryngology: *Drs. Paparella and Bailey.*

Pathology and Clinical Pathology: *Dr. Brinkhous.*

Pediatrics: *Drs. Oski and Stockman.*

Plastic and Reconstructive Surgery: *Drs. McCoy, Brauer, Haynes, Hoehn, Miller, and Whitaker.*

Psychiatry and Applied Mental Health: *Drs. Freedman, Lourie, Meltzer, Nemiah, Talbott, and Weiner.*

Sports Medicine: *Drs. Krakauer, Shephard, and Torg, Col. Anderson, and Mr. George.*

Surgery: *Drs. Schwartz, Najarian, Peacock, Shires, Silen, and Spencer.*

Urology: *Drs. Gillenwater and Howards.*

The YEAR BOOK of

Ophthalmology®
1984

Edited by

J. TERRY ERNEST, M.D., Ph.D.
Illinois Eye and Ear Infirmary,
Professor of Ophthalmology, Department of Ophthalmology,
University of Illinois, Chicago;
Research to Prevent Blindness, Inc., Eye Research Professor;
Adjunct Professor, Technological Institute,
Northwestern University

YEAR BOOK MEDICAL PUBLISHERS, INC.
CHICAGO

The editor for this book was Bonita Coors, and the production manager was H. E. Nielsen.

Table of Contents

The material covered in this volume represents literature reviewed up to January 1984.

Journals Represented 7
Introduction. 9

1. LIDS, LACRIMAL APPARATUS, AND ORBIT 11
   Treatment of Ocular Socket Problems,
   by ALLEN M. PUTTERMAN, M.D.. 11

2. MOTILITY 35
   Botulinum Toxin, *by* EUGENE R. FOLK, M.D., MARILYN T. MILLER,
   M.D., AND LAWRENCE I. CHAPMAN, M.D.. 35

3. VISION, REFRACTION, AND CONTACT LENSES. 55
   The Reliability of Retinal Visual Acuity Measurements
   Behind Cataracts, *by* DAVID L. GUYTON, M.D. 55

4. CONJUNCTIVA 71
   Blepharitis, *by* JOEL SUGAR, M.D. 71

5. CORNEA AND SCLERA 87
   Refractive Surgery, *by* RONALD E. SMITH, M.D. 87

6. GLAUCOMA 111
   Automated Perimetry, *by* JACOB T. WILENSKY, M.D.. 111

7. LENS 133
   Cataract Surgery, *by* EDWARD COTLIER, M.D.,
   AND WARREN FAGADAU, M.D.. 133

8. THE UVEA. 153
   The Promise of Cyclosporine, *by* HOWARD H. TESSLER, M.D.. . . 153

9. VITREOUS 169
   Intravitreal Antineoplastic Drugs,
   by GHOLAM A. PEYMAN, M.D.. 169

10. RETINA 189
    Pigmentary Photoreceptor Dystrophies: Progression as
    Monitored by Visual Field and Electroretinogram Testing,
    by GERALD A. FISHMAN, M.D.. 189

11. NEURO-OPHTHALMOLOGY 223
     Optic Neuritis—Current Status, *by* MARCEL FRENKEL, M.D. 223

12. MEDICAL OPHTHALMOLOGY AND DRUG THERAPY 243
     **Treatment of Ocular Inflammatory Disease With
     Nonsteroidal Antiinflammatory Drugs,**
     by LEE M. JAMPOL, M.D. 243

13. SURGERY 259
     Yag Laser Photodisruption, *by* MORTON F. GOLDBERG, M.D. . . . 259

14. BASIC SCIENCES, INJURIES AND MISCELLANEOUS 287
     Microcomputers for the Ophthalmologist,
     by JOHN S. READ, M.S. 287

Journals Represented

Acta Neurochirurgica
Acta Neurologica Scandinavica
Acta Ophthalmologica
Alabama Journal of Medical Sciences
American Journal of Epidemiology
American Journal of Medicine
American Journal of Neuroradiology
American Journal of Ophthalmology
American Journal of Roentgenology
Annales de Chirurgie Plastique
Annals of Allergy
Annals of Neurology
Annals of Plastic Surgery
Archives of Internal Medicine
Archives of Ophthalmology
Archives of Otolaryngology
British Journal of Ophthalmology
British Journal of Plastic Surgery
British Medical Journal
Canadian Journal of Ophthalmology
Cancer
Chest
Clinical Pediatrics
Cutis
Diabete et Metabolisme
European Journal of Applied Physiology and Occupational Physiology
Geriatrics
Graefes Archive for Clinical and Experimental Ophthalmology
Headache
Illinois Medical Journal
International Ophthalmology Clinics
Investigative Ophthalmology and Visual Science
Japanese Journal of Ophthalmology
Journal of the American Academy of Dermatology
Journal of the American Medical Association
Journal Francais d'Ophtalmologie
Journal of Gerontology
Journal of Neurosurgery
Journal of Occupational Medicine
Journal of Oral and Maxillofacial Surgery
Journal of Pediatric Ophthalmology and Strabismus
Journal of Prosthetic Dentistry
Klinische Monatsblätter für Augenheilkunde

Lancet
Mount Sinai Journal of Medicine (New York)
Neurology
Neuroradiology
New York State Journal of Medicine
Ocular Inflammation Therapy
Ophthalmic Surgery
Ophthalmologica
Ophthalmology
Postgraduate Medical Journal
Psychological Medicine
Schweizerische Medizinische Wochenschrift
Science
South African Medical Journal
Southern Medical Journal
Stroke
Transactions of the American Ophthalmological Society
Transactions of the Ophthalmological Societies of the United Kingdom
Wiener Klinische Wochenschrift

Introduction

This year the laser seems to have reached a new pinnacle with the demonstration of its efficacy in selected cases, such as senile macular degeneration, presumed ocular histoplasmosis syndrome, glaucoma, and posterior capsule opacity. There is another factor here, however, which may well turn out to be more important than the laser. We would not have the confidence to use this treatment modality in such a broad spectrum of eye diseases were it not for the randomized clinical trial. Clinical research in ophthalmology is far better today than it has ever been. Beginning with the Diabetic Retinopathy Study, researchers have become more and more sophisticated in the use of appropriate control groups, masking of observers, analysis of data, and the like. The literature is beginning to show a shift from purely descriptive epidemiology toward more quantitation with an increasing role for the biostatistician. The impetus for this important trend has been the National Eye Institute and all due credit should be given the Director and Staff for their help and continued encouragement in this work. Proper studies require months of planning and sometimes years for the accumulation of data. In the long run, however, we can have confidence in the results, and our patients benefit by receiving the best possible care.

J. TERRY ERNEST

1. Lids, Lacrimal Apparatus, and Orbit

Treatment of Ocular Socket Problems

ALLEN M. PUTTERMAN, M.D.

Eye and Ear Infirmary
University of Illinois, Chicago

Ocular socket problems result from loss of the eye. These problems may include a small orbit and cul-de-sac in congenital anophthalmos and microophthalmos, partial and total extrusion of orbital implants, displacement of implants, enophthalmic anophthalmos, partial and total socket contractures, upper eyelid ptosis, and upper eyelid crease-fold asymmetry. In this synopsis I will discuss some of the recent advances in the treatment of these socket abnormalities.

Congenital Anophthalmos

The child born without an eye commonly has a markedly small orbit and palpebral fissure and an extremely shrunken cul-de-sac. The initial treatment of congenital anophthalmos is not surgical, but lies in the hands of a skilled ocularist who effects a gradual expansion of the socket with progressively larger implants. Usually, when the child is 2 to 3 years of age, the palpebral fissure will no longer allow the passage of a larger conformer. At this point, a lateral canthotomy is performed, and the temporal upper and lower lid skin is sutured to conjunctiva. This technique produces a larger horizontal palpebral fissure length and allows the ocularist to expand the socket further with larger conformers.

Once the socket is expanded to its maximal size, lid surgery is performed as needed. This can consist of transmarginal rotation entropion procedures to treat cicatricial entropions, frontalis slings to treat ptosis, and, at times, oral mucous membrane grafts.[1]

Microophthalmos

The problems outlined for congenital anophthalmos also occur with microophthalmos but are less severe. The expansion of the orbit with gradually enlarging conformers also is used to treat microophthal-

11

mos, but does not have to commence until the child is 2 to 3 years of age.

Extruding or Displaced Implants

Extrusion of an ocular implant occasionally occurs. The etiology of this complication includes an oversized implant (20 mm or larger), infection, and suturing of the extraocular muscles over the implant.

If conjunctiva and Tenon's capsule separate over the implant to 8 mm or less in diameter, the extrusion can at times be corrected with a scleral patch.[2]

If the implant has caused a dehiscence greater than 8 mm or if extrusion recurs following a scleral graft, I prefer to remove the ocular implant and replace it with a dermal fat graft.[3] I also recommend doing the same for migrated ocular implants that prevent fitting of an esthetically acceptable artificial eye.

Various other techniques to treat the socket after extrusion or removal of a migrated implant have been performed using secondary implants. These implants are commonly covered with sclera.[4] I have had limited experience with this use, but good results have been obtained in the few I have implanted.

Enophthalmic Anophthalmos

Enophthalmos is another problem that occurs in patients with enucleated sockets. It not only causes the artificial eye to sink inward but also results in a deep supratarsal sulcus, a wide distance between the upper eyelid margin and lid fold, and a narrowed palpebral fissure height.

Initially, enophthalmic anophthalmos should be treated with an adjustment of the artificial eye. The ocularist can frequently enlarge or modify the prosthesis to produce an esthetically acceptable result.

If unacceptable enophthalmos persists after the artificial eye is modified, surgery must be considered. If there is an implant located centrally within the ocular socket, I prefer reducing the enophthalmos with subperiosteal glass beads.[5] I realize that this technique has decreased in popularity during the past few years, but favorable results in my patients continue to make this procedure my first choice of treatment.

If the enophthalmos results from the absence of an ocular implant, I prefer to treat this with a dermal fat graft.[3]

Partial Socket Contracture

Contracture of the ocular socket can result from a chronic socket infection, an extruding implant, radiation, or trauma. However, an old, unpolished artificial eye may also cause contracture. The poorly cared-for artificial eye liberates caustic chemicals that produce brown areas on the prosthetic surface, and that causes chronic conjunctivitis in the ocular socket.

There are various techniques to reconstruct the partially contracted ocular socket. If the contracture is minimal and the patient has enophthalmos secondary to an extruded implant, a dermal fat graft is recommended.[3] If the contracture is more severe, a partial-thickness oral mucous membrane graft is performed to add lining to the ocular cul-de-sac; a stent is used to maintain the space during healing. Probably the main difference in techniques lies in the size and shape of the stent used and whether or not it is secured to the orbital rims or lids. My preference is a modification of the technique that Scott and I described for total socket contractures.[6] A partial thickness oral mucous membrane graft is secured to the remaining conjunctiva. The midperiphery of a C-shaped custom-made conformer is secured to the superior and inferior orbital rims. This forces the posterior periphery deeply into the orbit and creates a spacious cul-de-sac that can easily retain an artificial eye.

Total Socket Contracture

The same etiologies that produce partial socket contracture can also lead to total socket contracture. Patients with total contracture cannot wear an artificial eye and must frequently resort to using a black patch.

One popular technique to reconstruct the severely contracted ocular socket is that described by Vistnes and Iverson.[7] After removing scar tissue and undermining the remaining conjunctiva, a space is formed with blunt and sharp dissection. Holes are drilled through the lateral orbital wall to accept Kirschner wires, and an oral mucous membrane graft is sutured to the remaining conjunctiva. The socket is then injected with vulcanizing Silastic at room temperature. I have not used this technique. Others have reported failures due to contracture of this space and extrusion of the Silastic.[8]

It is my preference to treat total socket contractures by the technique previously reported by Scott and me.[7]

The technique is similar to that described for partial socket contracture except for the size and placement of the graft. A full-thickness mucous membrane graft is wrapped around the custom-made C-shaped conformer and is sutured to itself.

Ptosis

Ptosis of the upper lid frequently occurs in patients with ocular socket problems. The ocularist can usually correct this deformity by modifying the artificial eye. In some cases, however, a residual ptosis persists, and correction with an oversized prosthesis retracts the lower lid.

I have found the most successful method to treat anophthalmic ptosis is with the Muller's muscle-conjunctival resection procedure.[9] Elevation of the upper lid to a normal level with instillation of 10% phenylephrine drops to the upper fornix can determine candidates for this procedure. Seven to 9 mm of conjunctiva and Muller's muscle are clamped and resected above the superior tarsal border, and the remaining conjunctiva and Muller's muscle are sutured to the superior tarsal border.

An alternative method to treat anophthalmic ptosis is with a levator aponeurosis advancement in a ptosis procedure.[10] My results have been better and more consistent with the Muller's resection compared with the levator aponeurosis procedure.

Lid Crease Reconstruction

Many patients with artificial eyes have a deep supratarsal sulcus secondary to enophthalmos. If the enophthalmos is minimal and the lid fold is redundant on the opposite normal upper lid, a satisfactory result can be obtained by operating on the normal upper lid. Skin and orbital fat are excised and the lid crease is reconstructed at a higher level.[11] This achieves symmetry of the upper eyelids and creates the illusion that the enophthalmos is resolved.

Summary

Multiple problems occur in patients with artificial eyes. With the advancement of oculoplastic surgical techniques, nearly all patients who have lost an eye can wear an esthetically acceptable prosthesis rather than having to use a black patch.

References

1. Putterman, A.M.: *Basic Oculoplastic Surgery*. In Peyman, G.A., Sanders, D.R., and Goldberg, M.F. (eds.): *Principles and Practice of Ophthalmology*. Vol. 3. Philadelphia, W.B. Saunders Co., 1980, p. 2270.
2. Zolli, C., and Shannon, G.M.: Experience with donor sclera for extruding orbital implants. *Ophthalmic Surg.* 8:63, 1977.
3. Smith, B., and Petrelli, R.: Dermis fat graft as a movable implant within the muscle cone. *Am. J. Ophthalmol.* 85:62, 1978.
4. Frueh, B.R., and Felker, G.V.: Baseball implant. *Arch. Ophthalmol.* 94:429, 1976.
5. Smith, B., Obear, M., and Leone, C.R.: The correction of enophthalmos associated with anophthalmos by glass bead implantation. *Am. J. Ophthalmol.* 64:1080, 1967.
6. Putterman, A.M., and Scott, R.: Deep ocular socket reconstruction. *Arch. Ophthalmol.* 95:1221, 1977.

7. Vistnes, L.M., and Iverson, R.E.: Surgical treatment of the contracted socket. *Plast. Reconstr. Surg.* 53:563, 1974.
8. Callahan, M.A., and Callahan, A.: *Ophthalmic Plastic and Orbital Surgery.* Birmingham, Aesculapius, 1979, p. 140.
9. Putterman, A.M., and Urist, M.J.: Muller's muscle-conjunctival resection: Technique for treatment of blepharoptosis. *Arch. Ophthalmol.* 93:619, 1975.
10. Jones, L.T., Quickert, M.H., and Wobig, J.L.: The cure of ptosis by aponeurotic repair. *Arch. Ophthalmol.* 93:629, 1975.
11. Putterman, A.M.: *Late Management of Blowout Fractures of the Orbital Floor.* In Aston, S., Hornblass, A., Meltzer, M., and Rees, T. (eds.): Third International Symposium of Plastic and Reconstruction Surgery of the Eye and Adnexa. Baltimore, Williams & Wilkins, 1982, p. 91.

1-1 **Chalazions: Frequency of Spontaneous Resolution.** A chalazion is a chronic inflammatory granuloma caused chiefly by the retention of tarsal gland secretion. David G. Cottrell, Robin C. Bosanquet, and Ivan M. Fawcett (Newcastle upon Tyne, England) reviewed the course of 87 chalazions to determine whether the lesions can resolve without surgery. Twelve patients had 2 lesions and 3 each had 3. Overall, 25% of the chalazions resolved and 57.5% were incised and curetted. Fifteen lesions in 11 patients could not be followed up. The mean ages of the various groups were similar. The mean duration of the chalazion was 6½ months in those treated surgically and 5½ months in those in whom the lesions resolved. The usual conservative measures were topical antibiotic application and hot bathing. The results are summarized in the table.

At least 25% of the chalazions in these patients resolved in a mean of about 6 months with minimal conservative treatment. More elaborate conservative management, including administration of intralesional steroids, reportedly has been successful in more than 50%, and in up to 90% in some instances. The duration of the lesion did not indicate its likelihood of resolving. Thus, treatment can be based on the degree of discomfort and on the patient's attitude toward surgery. Many patients probably would prefer waiting for at least 6 months before undergoing surgery, and in this group a trial of antibiotics and

DURATION OF 72 CHALAZIONS

	Chalazions	
Duration (months)	Resolved (n = 22)	Incised and curetted (n = 50)
<2	4	5
2-4	5	12
4-6	6	14
6-8	2	7
≥8	5	12

(Courtesy of Cottrell, D.G., et al.: Br. Med. J. 287:1595, Nov. 26, 1983.)

(1–1) Br. Med. J. 287:1595, Nov. 26, 1983.

hot bathing is reasonable. However, any atypical lesion should be operated on to rule out malignancy.

▶ [The authors conclude that, for a routine chalazion, waiting 6 months before surgery is reasonable because 25% spontaneously resolve. However, corticosteroid injection is painless and essentially free from complications and it seems to make sense to try it without waiting. Indeed, the newer lesions might be expected to have less capsulation and thus be more likely to respond to corticosteroid injection.] ◀

▶ ↓ In the following 3 articles, noninvasive imaging of the orbit is discussed. The first article is a fine review of computed tomography (CT). We are all now fairly accustomed to having the detailed images to help us with our diagnosis and treatment of orbital disease. Nonetheless, it is important to point out that the x-ray studies with CT result in relatively high doses of radiation to the eye. In the second and third articles, the authors discuss nuclear magnetic resonance imaging (now known as magnetic resonance imaging or MRI) of the orbit. The orbital fat images white with MRI instead of black as with CT, but the detail seems comparable and there is no radiation of any kind. Moreover, the next generation of instruments will give us the MR spectrum and thus information about tissue (especially tumor) metabolism and contribute to histologic diagnosis. In preparation for the new technology, radiology departments are already considering changing their names to "Departments of Medical Imaging" as they jump from the potentially dangerous short x-ray end of the electromagnetic spectrum to the more benign long radio wavelengths. ◀

1–2 **Computed Tomography of the Orbit: Current Status With High-Resolution Computed Tomography.** The high fat content of the orbit makes it an ideal structure for computed tomography (CT) evaluation. G. Wilms, J. Smits, and A. L. Baert (Leuven, Belgium) used a Somatom SD unit to complete an axial series with frontal slices. Contiguous 2-mm slices are made from the floor to the roof of the orbit and from the papilla to the orbital apex. The scan time is 10 seconds. If a lesion is detected, contrast medium is infused. Coronal sections are obtained while the patient is in the supine "hanging head" position. Lens doses have not exceeded 10 rad in the authors' experience.

Ocular neoplasms appear as high-density masses with clear enhancement by the contrast medium. There may be only eccentric thickening of the scleral rim. Low-grade calcification within tumors is well demonstrated by CT. Tumor involvement of the optic nerve is seen as thickening of the entire nerve, a solitary fusiform enlargement, or a separate mass near the orbital apex. Calcification in an optic nerve tumor suggests meningioma. Enlarged ocular muscles are observed in Graves' disease (Fig 1–1). Bilateral changes often are demonstrated when only unilateral disease is suspected clinically. Pseudotumor may be seen on CT as a soft tissue mass, diffuse enlargement of a muscle, or diffuse infiltration of the orbital fat. Orbital infection may appear as diffuse "cellulitis" or an abscess. An underlying predisposing factor (e.g., sinusitis, orbital fracture) may be demonstrated at the same time. Vascular masses such as hemangiomas and dermoid cysts are demonstrated by CT, and primary or secondary

(1–2) Neuroradiology 24:183–192, February 1983.

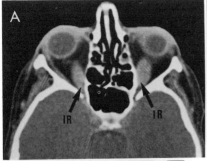
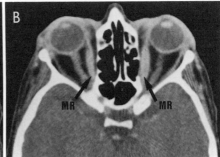
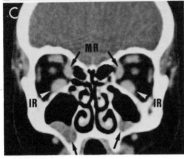

Fig 1–1.—Endocrine ophthalmology. **A** and **B** show axial slices at 2 levels. **C**, coronal slice. There is a marked increase in volume of the inferior *(IR)* and medial *(MR)* rectus muscles on both sides. Mucosal thickening is seen at the bottom of both maxillary sinuses *(arrows)*. (Courtesy of Wilms, G., et al.: Neuroradiology 24:183–192, February 1983; Berlin-Heidelberg-New York; Springer.)

orbital lymphoma can be visualized. The extent of lacrimal gland lesions can be delineated, and various extraorbital lesions are clearly demonstrated.

An excellent level of anatomical detail is obtained with high-resolution CT of the orbit. However, although the method is accurate in detecting orbital disease, it is not as specific as ultrasonography. The use of CT decreases the need for invasive diagnostic procedures. Exact localization of a mass by CT facilitates recovery of biopsy material; furthermore, the need for lateral orbitotomy has declined substantially.

1–3 **Nuclear Magnetic Resonance Imaging of the Orbit.** Ivan Moseley, Michael Brant-Zawadski, and Catherine Mills (Univ. of California, San Francisco) briefly review the principles of nuclear magnetic resonance (NMR) imaging and report its application in the imaging and tissue characterization of the normal human orbit.

The NMR images of the eye demonstrate the lens, aqueous, vitreous, and sclera/cornea. The lens is clearly shown in many images, but the ciliary body is poorly seen, although some images appear to show a structure with NMR properties similar to those of the lens but extending further towards the periphery of the globe. Aqueous and vitreous have essentially the same NMR characteris-

(1–3) Br. J. Ophthalmol. 67:333–342, June 1983.

tics, exhibiting extreme changes in relative intensity with variations in imaging parameters; when the interval between radio frequency (RF) pulses is 1.5 seconds, the intensity of the signal is similar to that of the brain (Fig 1–2). The sclera and conjunctiva also show considerable changes in relative intensity with changes in imaging measurements. With a short echo delay, it is difficult to distinguish the sclera from the vitreous, although there is a suggestion that it gives a stronger signal (Fig 1–2). In addition, derived relaxation time images show that, like the vitreous, the sclera has a long "spin-lattice" time constant (T_1), but, unlike vitreous, has a short "spin-spin" time constant (T_2). The optic nerve can be visualized on both sagittal and axial images (Fig 1–2). All 4 extraocular rectus muscles are clearly identifiable; sagittal sections also allow the levator palpebrae superioris to be distinguished. Both intraconal and extraconal orbital fat appeared as high-intensity images with all imaging techniques used. The superior ophthalmic vein is clearly visualized in images of the upper orbit, the lacrimal gland appears as a rather diffuse zone of mottled reduction in signal intensity from the orbital fat anterosuperiorly in the lateral part of the orbit, straddling the orbital septum, and the soft tissue planes around

Fig 1–2.—Spin-echo images with repetition interval of 1.5 s. Greater contrast is seen between sclera *(long arrow)* and vitreous, and between tendon of lateral rectus *(arrow)* and orbital fat in lower image. (Courtesy of Moseley, I., et al.: Br. J. Ophthalmol. 67:333–342, June 1983.)

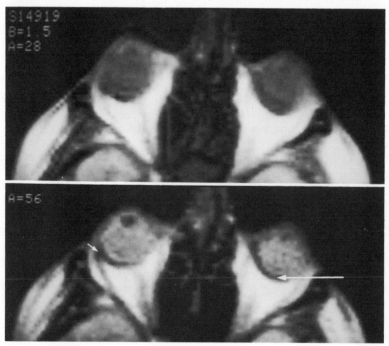

the anterior orbit are well delineated. The bony walls of the orbit essentially give no NMR signal.

The spatial and contrast resolution of NMR imaging of the normal orbit is at least as good as that of early, coarse, but clinically valuable, x-ray CT images. Current preliminary studies indicate that intraocular disease should be clearly visible on NMR images and the possible detection of changes in relaxation time in tissues that appear radiologically normal has considerable significance.

1–4 **NMR Imaging in the Evaluation of Orbital Tumors.** The high image quality obtained with nuclear magnetic resonance (NMR) imaging as well as the absence of ionizing radiation and other hazards make this an attractive method for evaluating orbital disorders. R. C. Hawkes, G. N. Holland, W. S. Moore, S. Rizk, B. S. Worthington, and D. M. Kean (Univ. of Nottingham, England) used a Picker resistive NMR unit to evaluate data on 24 patients with unilateral proptosis and 4 with intraocular melanomas. Nine of the former patients had dysthyroid proptosis, 3 had intraconal tumors, 6 had extraconal tumors, 5 had tumors that invaded the orbit, and 1 had a periorbital lesion. Scans were obtained in a steady-state free-precession sequence. Sections were 1 cm thick and took 2 minutes to produce. The normal appearances are shown in Fig 1–3.

In cases of proptosis, NMR can demonstrate both intracranial and the more usual sinus or nasopharyngeal origin. The method is useful when proptosis is due to encroachment on the orbit by an intrinsic abnormality of the boundary bone. In cases of dysthyroid disease, NMR demonstrates thickened rectus muscles; the coronal view is most helpful. The intraconal or extraconal origin

Fig 1–3.—Axial transverse nuclear magnetic resonance scans of normal subject. **A,** looking right. **B,** looking left. Alteration in position of optic nerves and change in thickness of medial recti are well shown. (Courtesy of Hawkes, R.C., et al.: AJNR 4:254–256, May–June 1983.)

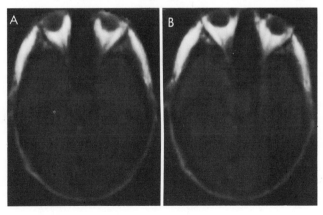

(1–4) AJNR 4:254–256, May–June 1983.

of a mass can be distinguished by NMR imaging, and the shape and sharpness of the boundaries appreciated. Tumors can be clearly identified as arising from the optic nerve. Computed tomography (CT) is helpful in evaluating expansile processes within the orbit. Metastatic disease should be considered in elderly patients who have proptosis. Nuclear magnetic resonance can be helpful in assessing intraocular processes when a vitreous opaque area makes fundus examination impossible or when a retinal detachment is present.

Nuclear magnetic resonance imaging can be as useful as CT in evaluating orbital disease when thinner sections, high-resolution scanning, and spin sequences based on individual parameters are developed. Multiplanar facility and the avoidance of ionizing radiation may make NMR imaging the preferred primary study.

▶ ↓ In the following 2 articles, improved methods for performing the surgical correction of ptosis are described. The most important point, however, is the degree of disease the techniques will correct. In the case of the Fasanella-Servat operation, simple as it may be, the ptosis must be equal to or less than 3 mm and there should be more than 10 mm of levator function. In the case of a levator aponeurosis operation, the ptosis should not exceed 5.5 mm and there should be at least 8 mm of levator function. Following these rules, the authors' results are very good. ◀

1–5   **Fasanella-Servat Operation: Modified Simple Technique With Quantitative Approach.** The Fasanella-Servat procedure is the simplest available operation for ptosis, and is useful in cases of mild ptosis with good levator function. S. M. Betharia, A. K. Grover, and B. R. Kalra (New Delhi) describe a simple, quantitative technique

Fig 1–4 (left).—Cotton sutures are passed close to folded superior margin of tarsal plate.
Fig 1–5 (center).—Other sutures are passed close to lid margin, so as to emerge near superior fornix.
Fig 1–6 (right).—Incision is marked on tarsal plate.
(Courtesy of Betharia, S.M., et al.: Br. J. Ophthalmol. 67:58–60, January 1983.)

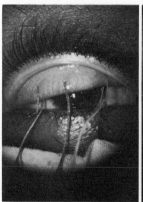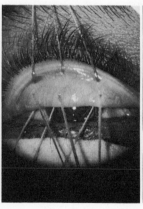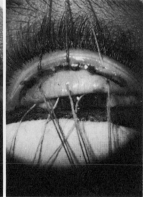

(1–5) Br. J. Ophthalmol. 67:58–60, January 1983.

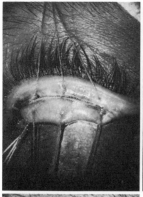
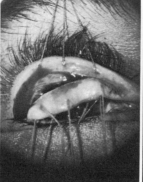
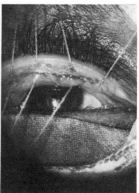

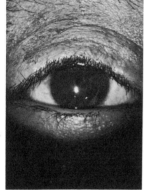

Fig 1–7 (above left).—Initial incision is made in form of groove.

Fig 1–8 (above center).—Excision of tarsal plate is completed.

Fig 1–9 (above right).—Continuous suture is applied with small knots at both ends, cut flush to surface, and buried under wound edges.

Fig 1–10 (left).—Final position of lid margin is assessed. (Courtesy of Betharia, S.M., et al.: Br. J. Ophthalmol. 67:58–60, January 1983.)

that precludes the need for a hemostat or special clamp. It was used in 14 cases of mild ptosis with good levator action and a good lid fold. Ptosis did not exceed 3 mm in these cases, and the levator action exceeded 10 mm.

TECHNIQUE.—With the patient under general anesthesia, cotton sutures are passed close to the folded superior margin of the tarsal plate, as shown in Figure 1–4, and other sutures are passed close to the lid margin, so as to emerge near the superior fornix (Fig 1–5). The incision is planned so that the amount of tarsal plate excision is double the amount of ptosis in the central third of the tarsal plate (Fig 1–6). After completion of the tarsal plate excision (Figs 1–7 and 1–8), suturing is performed with 5–0 plain catgut material. A continuous suture is applied with small knots at both ends, cut flush to the surface (Fig 1–9), and buried under the wound edges. After complete hemostasis has been insured, the final position of the lid margin is assessed (Fig 1–10), and antibiotic ointment is applied. Antibiotics, antiinflammatory drugs, and local hot fomentation are continued for a week postoperatively. If there are signs of corneal irritation by the suture, a soft contact lens is fitted.

This procedure was used in 9 cases of congenital ptosis, 2 of residual ptosis, 2 of complicated ptosis, and 1 of traumatic ptosis. Good esthetic results were obtained except in 1 case of complicated ptosis, in which there was mild central peaking. Complications included corneal abrasion in 3 cases and entropion in 1 case. The tarsal plate is cut in a controlled manner with this technique. Hemostats and clamps are not necessary. The esthetic results have been good in nearly all cases.

1–6 **Levator Aponeurosis Surgery for Correction of Acquired Ptosis: Analysis of 113 Procedures.** Several surgeons obtained success with a levator aponeurosis tuck in patients with acquired and congenital ptosis in whom the aponeurosis had no dehiscence or disinsertion. J. Justin Older (Univ. of South Florida, Tampa) reviewed the results of levator aponeurosis surgery in 113 upper lids of patients with acquired ptosis. The goal was to expose the levator aponeurosis and repair a defect or advance the aponeurosis onto the tarsus. Surgery was done under local anesthesia with 2% lidocaine and epinephrine. A normal-appearing aponeurosis can be tucked or advanced onto the tarsus. The goal was overcorrection by 1 mm. Up to three 6–0 Prolene sutures were used to secure the aponeurosis to the tarsus, with additional sutures placed to form the lid crease.

All but 5 procedures produced a lid height within 1 mm of the desired result, for a success rate of 95%. Most ptoses were involutional in origin, but postcataract ptosis and that of unknown origin also were managed successfully. The range of lid lift achieved is shown in the table. The 5 failures were caused by operative bleeding and friable aponeuroses.

Patients with ptosis and levator function of 5 mm or more often respond to leavator muscle or aponeurosis tightening. Otherwise, a tarsofrontalis suspension or a maximal levator resection usually is indicated. Aponeurosis surgery can be expected to repair up to 5.5 mm of ptosis in patients having 8 mm or more of levator function. The amount of tightening is adjusted at operation, and the correction is assessed in the conscious patient. A

RANGE OF EYELID LIFT FOR ACQUIRED PTOSIS	
Number of Procedures	Amount of Lift (mm)
18	1–1.5
40	2–2.5
26	3–3.5
16	4–4.5
13	5–5.5

(Courtesy of Older, J.J.: Ophthalmology (Rochester) 90:1056–1059, September 1983.)

(1–6) Ophthalmology (Rochester) 90:1056–1059, September 1983.

blepharoplasty can be done at the same time if indicated. Only 1 of the patients in this study required a repeat procedure for postoperative lid drop.

1–7 **Lower Eyelid Blepharoplasty by the Anterior Approach: Prevention of Complications.** Richard K. Dortzbach (Univ. of Wisconsin, Madison) describes an anterior approach to lower eyelid blepharoplasty that can produce good functional and esthetic results with a low rate of complications. Local anesthesia is preferred in most cases, using a mixture of 1% lidocaine with epinephrine and hyaluronidase. An infraciliary incision is used. A skin flap is used if only loose skin has to be excised, and a skin-muscle flap if removal of excess orbicularis muscle and fat is necessary. The incision preferably should not extend beyond the lateral orbital rim or more than 10 mm beyond the lateral canthal angle. The lateral canthal incision is concealed in a "crow's foot" line. The capsule surrounding the fat is opened to allow excess fat to prolapse forward on applying pressure to the orbital tissues, and all bleeding vessels are cauterized before the remaining fat is replaced. The lower lid then is shortened if horizontal lid laxity is present, and excess skin and orbicularis muscle are removed. All bleeding must be stopped before closing the wound. Removal of a narrow strip of orbicularis muscle beneath the skin edges may aid wound closure. Iced compresses are applied to the lids for 48 hours after operation, and the head is elevated to 30 to 45 degrees.

If only excess skin is present, a skin flap is made and the amount of redundant skin judged with a skin-muscle flap. If only fat excision is necessary, as in some younger patients, no skin or muscle is resected. It is not necessary to extend the infraciliary incision into the lateral canthal region in these cases. The skin-muscle flap is undermined inferiorly only so far as is necessary to remove the requisite amount of fat. Where accessory bags overlie the malar area, local excision is performed, making the incisions within the facial wrinkle lines, either alone or in conjunction with a lower lid blepharoplasty with an infraciliary incision.

▶ [In cosmetic lower eyelid surgery, the author makes the important point that the excision of fat may result in bleeding. The bleeding could be so severe that there would be resultant visual loss. To prevent this complication, the author recommends careful cauterization of all bleeding vessels in the fat. Postoperative ice compresses and elevation of the head are also recommended along with frequent measurement of the visual acuity.

1–8 **McCord Procedure for Ectropion Repair.** Because horizontal laxity usually occurs at the lateral canthal tendon, resection of the normal tarsus places more stress on diseased tissue. Therefore, Ralph E. Wesley and John W. Collins used the McCord technique of ectropion repair in which incision is performed at the lateral canthus away

(1–7) Ophthalmology (Rochester) 90:223–229, March 1983.
(1–8) Arch. Otolaryngol. 109:319–322, May 1983.

from the central margin. Eighty-five eyelid procedures were performed in 77 patients who were followed up for 6 to 34 months.

METHOD.—After the lateral canthus is anesthetized, a no. 15 surgical blade is used to perform a lateral canthotomy, splitting the upper and lower lids, carrying the incision down to the lateral orbital rim and extending it 1 cm posteriorly into the skin (Fig 1–11, top right). Any remnants of the lower lateral tendon (Fig 1–11, bottom left) are cut until the lower lid swings down freely. With the lid held taut, the blade may be used to excise 2 to 3 mm; the new cut edge of the tarsus can be seen as a white structure (Fig 1–12, top left). A permanent suture of 4–0 coated polyester suture with a small half-curved needle (4–0 Polydek with an ME-II needle) is placed through the tarsus as a vertical mattress stitch. The other end of the double-armed suture is passed through the periosteum inside the orbital rim, up slightly from the desired position of the lateral canthus to achieve the proper upward and inward orbital curvature. The suture is passed from up and in to down and out so that the knot is buried inferiorly (Fig 1–12, top right). For facial symmetry, comparison should be made with the other lateral canthus with allowance made for some postsurgical sag. Before the knot is cut, forceps may be used to cinch it down deeper into the tissue or to move the mattress suture slightly to make sure it is well buried (Fig 1–12, bottom left). The skin is closed with 7–0 silk interrupted sutures (Fig 1–12, bottom right); the initial skin closure should be placed directly over the buried knot to prevent late erosion or granuloma formation.

Fig 1–11.—McCord procedure for ectropion repair. **Upper left,** sagging ectropion of lower lid is caused by horizontal laxity of lateral canthal tendon. *Dashed line* indicates incision. **Upper right,** lateral canthotomy is carried down to the orbital rim periosteum. Malleable retractors are used to protect the eye. **Lower left,** scissors are used to cut remaining attachments of lower lateral canthus tendon from orbital rim. **Lower right,** lid is stretched tight to determine amount of lateral lid to be resected. (Courtesy of Wesley, R.E., and Collins, J.W.: Arch. Otolaryngol. 109:319–322, May 1983; copyright 1983, American Medical Association.)

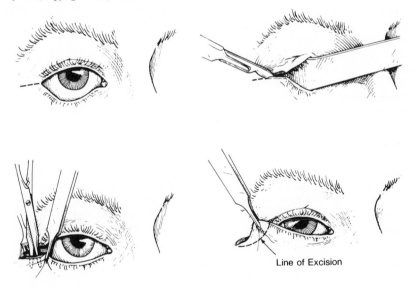

Line of Excision

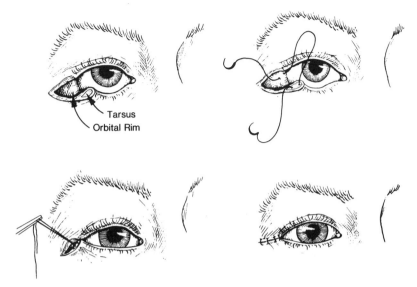

Fig 1–12.—Upper left, cut edge of tarsus to be reattached to orbital periosteum. **Upper right,** vertical mattress suture is made through tarsus to reattach lower lid slightly inside orbital rim. **Lower left,** permanent sutures are tied to reattach lid to the orbital rim. **Lower right,** skin is closed with 7–0 silk at the lateral canthus. (Courtesy of Wesley, R.E., and Collins, J.W.: Arch. Otolaryngol. 109:319–322, May 1983; copyright 1983, American Medical Association.)

In this series, 6 patients had revision of the lid position, 4 had formation of a lateral canthal granuloma, and 1 had a late infection from the permanent stitch.

This procedure involves simple reattachment of the tarsus to the lateral orbital rim. With resection of only a few millimeters of the lower lid, much horizontal tightening is obtained. The technique is especially useful in patients with an artificial eye who require stronger lower lid support. Lower lid tightening is also used as part of lower lid blepharoplasty for dermatochalasis.

Problems in the performance of this procedure usually stem from placing the permanent stitch too low or outside the orbital rim. The lateral lower lid should have an upward and inward contour to the orbital rim. This procedure is contraindicated in ectropion caused by medial canthal tendon laxity because it will pull the punctum over toward the midsection of the lid.

▶ [Eyelid resection in the lateral canthus is markedly improved by attaching the tendon to the periosteum inside the orbital rim with a permanent suture.] ◀

1–9 **Management of Acquired Dacryocystitis** is outlined by J. J. Hurwitz and K. J. A. Rodgers (Univ. of Toronto). Acute dacryocystitis can be a painful and serious condition. Young infants usually have

(1–9)   Can. J. Ophthalmol. 18:213–216, August 1983.

secondary infection in a congenitally obstructed lacrimal tract and are relieved by conservative means, but later cases are due to fibrosis within the lacrimal drainage paths, often due to trauma or infection. Patients are seen with swelling of the lacrimal sac and often have severe pain in the region. Thermography shows hemifacial hyperthermia over an extensive area. Orbital edema may produce orbital displacement or proptosis. A pyocele usually is very tender. A nontender swollen sac, or mucocele, may also enlarge. *Staphylococcus aureus* often is the infecting organism, although *Hemophilus influenzae* is common in children. Passage to the conjunctival sac can be obstructed if the fibrous membrane obstructs the common internal punctum or if lateral swelling of the sac causes the common canaliculus to become kinked.

Pyocele with orbital cellulitis is a life-threatening condition managed by intravenous antibiotics such as cloxacillin and aspiration if necessary to obtain material for culture. Application of hot compresses may be helpful. The sac should be incised if perforation seems imminent. Pyocele alone is managed by oral antibiotic therapy. A mucocele is treated by dacryocystorhinostomy if the patient has tearing or other symptoms or finds the lesion unsightly. When dacryocystitis resolves and the pain subsides, the sac often is still obstructed and dacryocystography should be performed. Dacryocystorhinostomy usually is indicated, although simple probing may be tried if the sac is of normal caliber. The functional integrity of the system can be assessed by lacrimal scintiscanning. If a stone is present, removal and sac drainage will be necessary.

Dacryocystorhinostomy, when indicated, should not be done until at least 4 weeks after the resolution of dacryocystitis. Postoperative antibiotic therapy is recommended. Both a fistula to the skin secondary to the dacryocystitis and a granuloma next to the sac usually resolve spontaneously after dacryocystorhinostomy.

1–10 **Direct Complete Intubation of Lacrimal Ducts in Dacryocystorhinostomy.** K. W. Ruprecht (Univ. of Erlangen, Nürnberg, W. Germany) presents a new variant of the direct complete method of intubation of the lacrimal drainage system. The newly created lacrimal sac and nasal cavity anastomosis is intubated with a U-shaped combined with a Y-shaped silicon tube. The procedure is performed under the microscope showing the common duct orifice. A U-shaped bicanalicular silicon tube is inserted, end to side, into the Y-shaped tubing which is pulled through the lacrimal sac and nasal cavity anastomosis, thus producing a complete intubation of the lacrimal drainage system. The technique has proved successful in 30 operations and is the preferred operation for revisions and so-called improvisations. Four patients had complicated preoperative conditions,

(1–10)   Klin. Monatsbl. Augenheilkd. 182:196–199, March 1983.

whereas 26 patients had an infrasaccular postinflammatory lacrimal duct stenosis.

A mucosal suture is applied over the complete intubation. If this is not possible the anterior broader mucosal wing of the lacrimal sac is sutured to the subcutis of the same side. Through closure of the skin in layers with single-knot sutures the mucosa is indirectly pulled medially toward the opposite side. The canalicular tube system is in itself knotted at the nasal vent of the Y-shaped silicon tubing. This knot is pulled tight with a silk suture and fastened to the thicker intubation; this prevents a looplike pullout of U-shaped cannula during rubbing of the eye in the area of the puncta lacrimalia (Fig 1–13). The Y-shaped tube is removed after 3 months and the U-shaped tube after 6 months.

At the follow-up examinations performed between 4 weeks and 15 months later (average in men, 5.7 months; in women, 6.7 months), a total of 26 cases were found to have unobstructed passage from both the upper and lower puncta. Complete intubation of the lacrimal system permits safe orthograde and retrograde irrigation, promotes the reepithelialization of the new mucosa, and prevents scarring and

Fig 1–13.—Schematic representation of direct complete intubated lacrimal system with bicanalicular U-shaped and Y-shaped silicon tube intubation of lacrimal sac and nasal cavity anastomosis. (Courtesy of Ruprecht, K.W.: Klin. Monatsbl. Augenheilkd. 182:196–199, March 1983.)

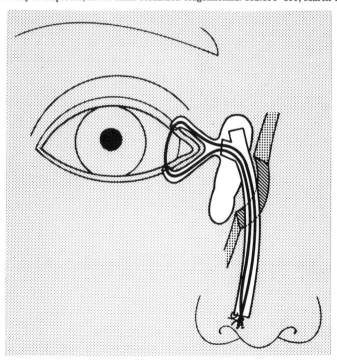

shrinkage in the area of the common duct orifice and the newly formed lacrimal sac and nasal cavity anastomosis.

▶ [Recommended primarily for revisions of failed dacryocystorhinostomies, Ruprecht describes intubation of all the passageways. For these complicated cases, the sac tube must remain in place for 3 months and the canalicular tubes for 6 months.] ◀

▶ ↓ When all else fails, the lacrimal system is bypassed with Lester Jones' tube. The author of the following article suggests placing it under the periosteum and into the lacrimal canal without bone trepanation. The author reports that expulsion or obstruction, or both, are less likely to occur. ◀

1–11 **Treatment of the Lacrimal Duct by Intubation of the Nasolacrimal Canal: Overall Assessment With Seven-Year Follow-Up.** J. C. Talmant (Nantes, France) describes his experience with a procedure derived from L. T. Jones' permanent intubation technique, in which 2 essential modifications are made. A flexible silicone tube can be adapted to each individual case, and the tube can be inserted in a vertical position in the lacrimal canal by a subperiosteal approach. These modifications simplify the operation, bone trepanation is not required, and the drain is stabilized by its declivity and greater length. These 2 modifications have practically eliminated a number of complications encountered in the use of other techniques, such as relatively frequent expulsion of the tube, secondary obstruction, the formation of granulous tissue in the medial canthus, burying of the collar, and notching of the lower rim of the eyelid. An analysis of 21 cases with a 7-year follow-up shows only 4 cases involving expulsion of the drain; in one of these the drain was easily replaced less than 24 hours postoperatively.

Results in this series clearly show that in the presence of a normal medial canthus, drain tolerance is good and drainage effective. In situations such as facial palsy, complex traumatic sequelae, or repairs after tumor, restoration of the anatomical condition is an imperative first step for effective functioning of the drain, the collar of which must be located on a level with the lacrimal stream without rising above the rim of the lower lid. In the 3 failures in this series, 2 were linked to malpositioning of the drain above the lid, which was thus inoperative and bothersome; the complexity of these cases and the particular psychologic context did not allow reintervention. In the third case, which involved a 3-year-old child, a second implantation was performed at a much later date. In the first patients the tube was replaced every 6 months, and subsequently every year. This precaution is now believed to be excessive in light of results of the 7-year follow-up, although results did show that without the tube the drainage becomes immediately ineffective in most cases. Moreover, minimal cooperation is required on the part of the patients, who must ensure hygienic care and regular surveillance, as well as certain precautions when blowing the nose and sneezing, to avoid expulsion of

(1–11) Ann. Chir. Plast. 27:387–393, 1982.

the drain. Among all currently available techniques for treatment of the lacrimal duct, none offers the same advantages of quality and simplicity as does intubation by the nasolacrimal route.

▶ ↓ The debate about early versus late surgery for orbital fractures continues. In the following 2 articles the authors recommend that fractures larger than half the area of the floor should be repaired within 2 weeks even if there is no enophthalmos since it may occur months later and would then be difficult to alleviate. These authors would operate on trapped muscles after 2 weeks if there was no improvement, whereas the authors of the second article recommend immediate surgery in this situation. ◀

1–12 **Surgery on Orbital Floor Fractures: Influence of Time of Repair and Fracture Size.** Michael J. Hawes and Richard K. Dortzbach (Univ. of Wisconsin, Madison) reviewed the results of operations for orbital floor fracture in relation to the time of repair and the extent of injury in 51 patients seen between 1969 and 1979. Most patients had pure blowout fractures of the orbital floor, and all were followed up for at least 6 weeks after repair. Indications for operation included more than 2 mm of enophthalmos or the potential for its development and the presence of diplopia within 30 degrees of the primary position. An intraorbital approach was used in 49 operations and a combined infraorbital and Caldwell-Luc approach in 2. Eight patients were operated on more than 2 months after injury. Seventeen had large fractures.

All but 1 of the 8 patients operated on late had enophthalmos. Three of the 7 were satisfactorily corrected to 2 mm or less of enophthalmos. Three early patients had significant enophthalmos after repair, as did 4 of the late patients. Only patients with large fractures had this finding. All but 3 of 26 early patients with extraocular muscle dysfunction had satisfactory correction, compared with 2 of 5 late patients. This feature was also associated with larger fractures. Two early and 2 late patients had infraorbital nerve dysfunction postoperatively. No patient had reduced vision in relation to operative repair of the fracture.

It is difficult to correct significant enophthalmos that develops some time after orbital floor fracture. Hypocycloid tomography or computed tomography is useful in assessing the extent of injury in blowout fractures of the orbit. Early operation is advantageous in some cases.

1–13 **"Trap-Door" Fracture of Orbital Floor** is discussed by R. Gola, A. Nerini, and Y. Jallut (Marseille, France). Similar to "blowout fractures," the isolated fracture of the orbital floor called "trap-door fracture" is seen primarily in children and adolescents, although it may occur in adults. It is likely that in most cases the trauma simultaneously acts on the globe as well as the suborbital rim (Fig 1–14); elements of the orbital floor, rather than collapsing under the shock, snap back into place, trapping some structures herniated by the intraorbital pressure. In the characteristic fissure-like anteroposterior

(1–12) Ophthalmology (Rochester) 90:1066–1070, September 1983.
(1–13) Ann. Chir. Plast. 27:322–330, 1982.

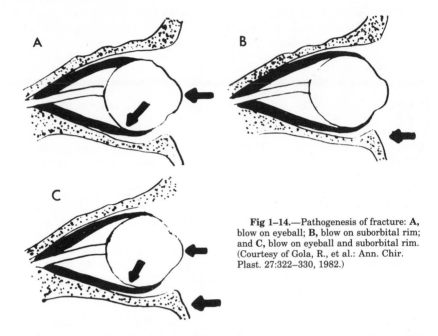

Fig 1–14.—Pathogenesis of fracture: **A,** blow on eyeball; **B,** blow on suborbital rim; and **C,** blow on eyeball and suborbital rim. (Courtesy of Gola, R., et al.: Ann. Chir. Plast. 27:322–330, 1982.)

breach, the inferior oblique muscle and the surrounding anatomical elements are firmly imprisoned over a variably extensive area.

In severe cases the considerable pressure that marks this type of fracture soon leads to permanent lesions, often aggravated by ill-advised and laborious efforts to free the muscle. Dyplopia dominates the clinical picture, and pain upon mobilization of the globe in the absence or paucity of radiologic signs should suggest the diagnosis. Immediate surgical treatment is indicated, since such a situation constitutes an ophthalmologic emergency. Although minor trapping may be managed by a simple liberative intervention, the more serious and extensive cases, frequently reaching the orbital apex, must only be treated after partial removal of the orbital floor to avoid aggravation of the lesions.

1–14   **Reconstruction of the Temporal Canthus** is described by F. J. Steinkogler (Univ. of Vienna). After excision of a tumor infiltrating the temporal canthus and adjacent lid tissue, reconstruction must respect the important role the temporal canthus has in smooth functioning of the eyelids. Suturing the residual tarsal stumps together will lead to a shortened palpebral fissure. Conjunctiva is mobilized from both the upper and lower fornices after excision of the tumor, and the lateral tarsal margins are fixed to the periosteum with 4–0 chromic catgut loops near the origin of the lateral palpebral ligament

(1–14)   Br. J. Ophthalmol. 67:267–269, April 1983.

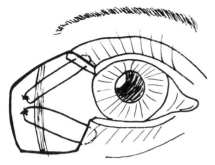

Fig 1–15.—Chromic catgut loops anchoring tarsal plates to periosteum. (Courtesy of Steinkogler, F.J.: Br. J. Ophthalmol. 67:267–269, April 1983.)

to support the tarsal plates (Fig 1–15). A skin flap is then prepared by making 2 lateral incisions extending temporally, both superiorly and inferiorly, from the edges of the defect. The flap is divided into upper and lower segments; the upper one is advanced medially and sutured to the residual upper lid skin, and the lower one is advanced and rotated medially to complete the lower lid. The canthus is anchored to the periosteum. The skin and conjunctiva are co-opted with 8–0 Vicryl to form the lid margin. Skin sutures are made with 6–0 Prolene.

Extensive defects involving the temporal canthus are readily repaired with this approach. The growth of connective tissue in response to the chromic catgut loops allows the reestablishment of tarsal plate function. Complicated tarsal flaps are not necessary, and shortening of the palpebral fissure is avoided. The lid margin remains stable indefinitely.

▶ [Steinkogler reports that the chromic catgut loops anchoring the tarsal plates to the temporal orbital rim stimulate connective tissue which acts as a tarsal substitute. If true, this would solve the problem of palpebral fissure shortening usually resulting from this type of surgical repair.] ◀

1–15 **Ocular and Orbital Complications Following Radiation Therapy of Paranasal Sinus Malignancies and Review of Literature.** Nasser Nakissa, Philip Rubin, Roberta Strohl, and Henry Keys (Univ. of Rochester, N.Y.) reviewed the ocular complications occurring in 30 patients with malignancies of the paranasal sinuses who received supervoltage radiation therapy between 1963 and 1978. A ^{60}Co technique with 1 or 2 lateral fields was used in most instances. Twenty patients were treated for maxillary antral cancer and 9 for ethmoid carcinoma. Two patients were treated palliatively for distant metastasis. Five patients with antral cancer were treated curatively. Most patients had involvement of several adjacent anatomical sites, usually the orbit. Ophthalmic signs and symptoms were the most common clinical abnormalities.

Complications are listed in the table. The acute reactions of the

(1–15) Cancer 51:980–986, Mar. 15, 1983.

COMPLICATIONS

Complication	No. of patients	Dose (rad)
Eyelid and eyelashes		
Lid skin erythema	15/30	3400–6600
Marked edema of eyelid	10/30	5400–7500
Lid margin epilation	6/30	6000
Ectropion	2/30	5400–6000
Entropion	1/30	7500
Fixed lower lid	1/30	5400
Lacrimal gland and duct		
Epiphora due to nasolacrimal duct obstruction	4/30	6572–7500
Lacrimal duct infection	1/30	7500
Xerophthalmia	1/30	6000
Conjunctiva, sclera, globe and lense		
Conjunctivitis	20/30	5500–7500
Keratitis	5/30	3400–7500
Corneal thinning	5/30	4000–6600
Cataract	4/30	

(Courtesy of Nakissa, N., et al.: Cancer 51:980–986, Mar. 15, 1983.)

conjunctiva and sclera were fairly mild and transient. Only 1 of the 4 radiation-induced cataracts had to be extracted. All patients given more than 4,500 to 5,000 rad to the posterior chamber had retinal changes, but most did not have significant visual loss. Eight patients had functional vision after receiving more than 5,000 rad to the retina, but 4 had significantly reduced vision after receiving doses of 6,500 to 7,500 rad. One patient each had macular scarring and vitreous hemorrhage. One patient had ocular muscle involvement related to both the disease process and radiation therapy.

The retina, like other central nervous system tissues, is relatively resistant to radiation damage, but the retinal vessels are not. Careful shielding of the homolateral eye can insure the adequate treatment of known and probable disease in patients with paranasal sinus malignancies. Special shields are used when shielding of the entire eye or part of the eye seems necessary. Posterior ocular complications are rarely significant unless a dose of 5,000 rad is exceeded, and anterior ocular complications are minimal if good technique and high-energy radiation are used.

▶ [When the dose of supervoltage radiation exceeds 5,000 rad, the eye will be affected, but in cases of paranasal sinus malignancies there may be little choice. This article is a fine review of the ocular complications of radiation therapy, although it makes one think that it would be valuable to have an ophthalmologist on the team from the outset to help with shielding and to treat complications as soon as they appear.

1–16 **Contraindications for Further Oculoplastic Surgery.** Alston Callahan (Birmingham, Ala.) points out that some patients have such advanced damage to orbital structures from trauma, cancer surgery, or irradiation that restoration of full function or a near-normal appearance is not possible. These patients may present themselves to many surgeons requesting further surgery. Minor procedures such as tarsorrhaphy or removal of irradiated socket fragments may be indicated, but major surgery is contraindicated. Patients who fit this category include those with a seeing eye fixated in extensive scar tissue; those with grossly contracted sockets with inadequate lid tissue mucosal remnants, or both; and those with destruction or complete loss of function of the levator, combined with a seeing eye that cannot be removed either because of fixation in scar tissue or because of paralysis of the extraocular muscles.

It is futile to attempt to correct a fixated, seeing eye that is embedded in extensive scar tissue since recurrence of scarring and fixation can be anticipated. Patients with this and related conditions commonly visit one surgeon after another in a quest for the return of normal function and cosmesis. Frequently, prosthetic measures are all that can be offered.

▶ [There are some patients that should be told from the outset that no further surgery would be beneficial. Callahan has made this important point for many years but it bears repeating.] ◀

1–17 **Early Treatment of Orbital Anomalies Through Craniofacial Surgery.** Craniofacial surgery, first described by Tessier in 1967, allows for radical treatment of orbital malformations that in years past were repaired by bone integrations only after development was complete. The new techniques permit very early intervention, thereby preventing the anomalies from worsening during the somatic growth of the child. Ernesto P. Caronni (Milan) describes and classifies large malformations of the orbit, describes the techniques used to repair these malformations, and briefly reports 5 illustrative cases.

The orbital malformations can be divided into 3 major classes: (1) those of the roof and the supralateral angle, bound to the sphenoidal area; (2) those of the orbital floor, belonging to the zygomatic-maxillary area; and (3) those of the medial wall, and, therefore, of the ethmoidal area. The first group includes oxycephalia, acrocephalia, trigonocephalia, and scaphocephalia. These primarily involve anterior reduction of the anterior cranial fossa area. Early treatment at about the second year of age must be performed in these cases so that the initial repair will stabilize with cerebral development. In these cases, an ample frontal flap is performed and a fronto-orbital hinge bar is isolated according to Tessier's technique. Modeling of the bar is determined by the particular type of malformation that caused the reduction of the orbital roof surface.

(1–16)   Ann. Plast. Surg. 10:194–199, March 1983.
(1–17)   Ibid., 9:24–31, July 1982.

The second group of malformations includes the Treacher Collins-Franceschetti syndrome and the orbital state of Crouzon and Apert syndromes. In these cases, insufficiency of maxillary development gives rise to inadequacy of the orbital floor and subsequent exophthalmus. Early treatment is limited to patients who also have insufficient development of the anterior cranial fossa. The usual fronto-orbital bar advancement is performed, with maxillary repair by Tessier types II and III osteotomy reserved until the child is 6 or 7 years old. The third group of malformations consists of hypertelorism. Because strabismus can correct itself spontaneously, early treatment is recommended. Olfactory function can be preserved, leaving the perpendicular ethmoidal lamina and nerve endings intact. Although a modest degree of hypertelorism will remain, this can be compensated for by the functional correction.

The good results obtained in the 5 cases presented in this study should encourage repair of the malformations as early as possible. Accurate selection of patients for operative repair is important and should include consultation among neurosurgeons, ophthalmologists, radiologists, and anesthesiologists.

▶ [Early referral to a team seems appropriate for these sad cases. The family needs to be supported and emphasis should be placed on functional results.] ◀

2. Motility

Botulinum Toxin

EUGENE R. FOLK, M.D.
MARILYN T. MILLER, M.D.
LAWRENCE I. CHAPMAN, M.D.

Eye and Ear Infirmary
University of Illinois, Chicago

The use of botulinum toxin in the treatment of disorders of ocular motility has created a great deal of interest in the past several years. Pioneer work in this area was performed by Alan Scott of the Smith Kettlewell Institute. The concept of a toxin that was capable of causing a transient paresis of one of the extraocular muscles has been attractive for a long time. After investigating a number of substances, Scott discovered that the botulinum toxin was ideal for this purpose. The toxin binds closely to the muscle with very little spread into the ocular tissues. The toxin seems to block the release of acetylcholine at the nerve junction. It also seems to provide an effective depletion of calcium, thereby blocking the response of the muscle.

The toxin is injected directly into the muscle using a fine-needle electrode connected to an audio-amplifier. The patient is asked to look in the field of action opposite to that of the muscle being injected. For example, in injecting a medial rectus muscle the patient is asked to look in the abducted position. Ideal placement of the needle is in the junction of the posterior and middle two thirds of the muscle. At this point, the patient is asked to look in the field of action of the muscle and, if the needlle has been properly placed, the increased firing is heard in the audio-amplifier. The muscle is then injected and a decrease in the amplitude sound from the audio-amplifier indicates that the injection has been in the proper location.

Despite the fact that there is audio evidence of a neuromuscular effect, the patient still has a normal range of movement for about 2 or 3 days. At that time a gradually increasing paresis of the affected muscle takes place. This paresis generally lasts for about 3 or 4 months with a slow recovery. This temporary paresis produces a prolonged effect because of the reaction of the antagonist muscle. A spasm of the antagonist similar to that in any paretic squint occurs with the development of a partial contracture producing a lasting effect. Several injections may be necessary to produce the more lasting effect depending on the severity of the initial deviation.

A number of investigators throughout the country have currently been using botulinum injections for some time. There is certainly no question that it is possible to produce a paresis of an extraocular muscle by injecting the toxin, and in concomitant strabismus the hope for a change by contracture of the antagonist does occur. It is possible to produce a fairly permanent straightening of the eyes with the injection of the toxin.

The amounts of toxin used are very small and many times less the dosage which is associated with systemic botulinum toxicity. There have been no reported complications from the toxin itself. The major complication has been a spread of the toxic effect to other extraocular muscles, most notably the upper lid. The levator seems to be unusually sensitive to the toxin and small amounts in that area do produce a ptosis. It is almost impossible, for example, to inject the superior rectus muscle without producing a ptosis. This ptosis can occur even with injections of the horizontal rectus muscles. There are one or two reported cases of penetrating the sclera during the course of attempted injection without any untoward effect. Occasionally, a subconjunctival hemorrhage occurs at the site of injection. The injection is made with the patient under topical anesthesia and is remarkably free of pain. The more experience that the practitioner has with the injection, the fewer the side effects and the less need for repeated injections.

What can be said about the role of botulinum toxin in the treatment of motility problems at this time? It would seem that it is certainly possible to correct concomitant deviations; however, frequently more than one injection is necessary. In the older patient who is a poor candidate for general anesthesia, it would seem that the botulinum injection is the preferred treatment at this time. For the person who is frightened of anesthesia, injection with the toxin offers another option for the treatment of the esthetic deviation. In the older person, however, who is capable of handling a general anesthetic, it would seem that the adjustable suture technique probably presents a more accurate way of correcting the deviation. In addition, there is a definite period following injection when the muscle that has been injected is paralyzed. It is possible that an adult will have troublesome diplopia in that field of action until recovery takes place.

The role of botulinum in children is even more complicated. The only anesthetic that can be used for botulinum injections is ketamine. A general anesthetic tends to eliminate the innervation of the extraocular muscles and, therefore, the audio-amplifier cannot be used to identify the proper insertion of the electrode into the muscle. With ketamine, however, innervation to the muscle is not disturbed and one can judge the placement of the needle for proper injection. However, in children it may take several injections to correct a motility problem. This may mean several injections using ketamine, which use must be balanced against the success rate of treatment of children with horizontal deviations. Certainly I think that our goal of therapy has to be to correct deviations using the fewest number of anesthetics, whether using ketamine or the more frequently used anesthetic agents. Injecting infants (younger than 1 year) in the office by mummifying them has been advocated by some ophthalmologists. This approach eliminates the anesthetic problem, but one wonders about the problem of injecting muscles in a child who may be less than cooperative.

There are some special situations, however, when the use of botulinum toxin seems to be the preferred procedure. In essential blepharospasm, botulinum is the best thing that has come along in many years and its use in this group of patients is truly exciting. It is also helpful in the treatment of patients with hemifacial spasm in which the effects are almost as dramatic. In a theoretic point of view, injections into the medial rectus muscle in patients with acute lateral rectus palsy might potentially prevent a contracture developing in the medial rectus muscle. In the early stages of thyroid disease, a botulinum injection may be helpful in preventing the muscle from becoming fibrotic. Certainly botulinum injections are not effective in the presence of cicatricial disease with limitations of the forced duction test. In the early stages of thyroid disease, however, this may not be true. Botulinum may be helpful in patients who have third-nerve palsies in which an injection into the lateral rectus muscle may enable the patient to have a binocular zone in the straight ahead position. It is certainly an attractive way of attempting to see how the patient reacts to such a narrow binocular zone.

We realize that we are dealing with an exciting tool that certainly has a place in the armamentarium of the physician treating disorders of ocular motility. The exact role of botulinum is not known at this time. Several other possible uses have been indicated and further work is certainly necessary.

2–1 **Medical Management of Accommodative Esotropia** is outlined by Roger L. Hiatt (Univ. of Tennessee, Memphis). Accommodative esotropia can be produced by the convergence associated with accommodation applied to clear the blurred image produced by hypermetropia or by a high accommodative convergence-to-accommodation (AC-A) ratio. Both causes may be present. Patients with a high AC-A ratio have symptoms at near, whereas those with a hypermetropic origin have symptoms at both distance and near. Average age at onset is 2½ years regardless of the cause. Tropicamide, cyclopentolate,

(2–1) J. Pediatr. Ophthalmol. Strabismus 20:199–201, Sept.–Oct., 1983.

homatropine, and atropine are all used as cycloplegic agents in diagnosing and measuring accommodative esotropia.

Atropine can be used as a "medical patch" in these cases and in the "penalization" process. Miotics can be useful as a supplement to glasses when a small amount of residual deviation remains or as a supplement to bifocals in patients with a high AC-A ratio. Miotics can reduce near deviation in patients with a high accommodative convergence ratio if a high AC-A ratio persists. Miotics may be effective postoperatively in patients with uncorrected esotropia and some hyperopia. They are also used when late accommodative esotropia is superimposed on surgically corrected congenital esotropia. Miotics can be used to eliminate the need for glasses intermittently, as for swimming, and to supplement contact lens wear. Most experience has been with Floropryl isoflurophate and phospholine iodide. The formation of cysts on the pupillary border can be countered with dilute phenylephrine solution. Prolonged apnea can occur in miotic-treated patients if succinylcholine-type drugs are given during general anesthesia.

Miotics can be temporarily useful in overcorrected esotropia that does not resolve over time or with patching. In patients with myasthenia gravis and diplopia, miotics may provide intermittent relief from the diplopia.

▶ [This article is a short, concise outline of drugs used for diagnosis and therapy in accommodative esotropia. Hiatt helps us remember to keep miotics as well as glasses available for our young patients and avoid the tendency to use one or the other exclusively.

▶ ↓ In the following 2 articles, the authors discuss their experience in long-term follow-up of esotropia. In the first article, Freeley and others point out that many patients who have recurrent esotropia do so because they have an accommodative component. To make matters worse, the author of the second article points out that adults may not outgrow their hypermetropia and may thus continue to have accommodative esotropia problems. These authors emphasize the importance of long-term follow-up with careful attention paid to refraction in patients with childhood esotropia. ◀

2-2 **Recurrent Esotropia Following Early Successful Surgical Correction of Congenital Esotropia.** Douglas A. Freeley, Leonard B. Nelson, and Joseph H. Calhoun reviewed the occurrence of esotropia in 83 patients with congenital esotropia diagnosed before age 6 months who were operated on between 1976 and 1980. All had alignment to within 10 prism diopters before age 18 months, and were followed up for at least 6 months. Twenty-three patients (28%) had subsequent esotropia (table). The initial deviation in these cases averaged 45 diopters, and the initial refractive error averaged + 1.50. Esotropia developed an average of 14 months after successful alignment of the eyes. The average deviation of the subsequent esotropia was 24.5 diopters. The average refraction at last follow-up had increased by 1.1 diopters. Satisfactory alignment was achieved with

(2–2) J. Pediatr. Ophthalmol. Strabismus 20:68–71, Mar.–Apr. 1983.

RECURRENT ESOTROPIA*

Patient#	Age at presentation (months)	Initial deviation (diopters)	Refractive error spherical equivalent	Age at surgical alignment (months)	Subsequent esotropia (diopters)	Time from surgical correction to subsequent esotropia (months)	Change in refraction	Response to glasses	Comment
1	6	45	+1.50	16	25	6	+1.75	+	
2	8	30	+.50	16	30	2	+1.50	Not given	Surgery
3	9	45	+1.50	12	35	16	no new refraction	N/A	Surgery
4	4	40	No record	7	40	39	+4.50	+	
5	5	40	+3.50	6	25	12	0	+	
6	3	70	+.75	6	20	36	+2.25	+	
7	5	50	+1.00	5	20	35	+1.50	+	Surgery
8	8	45	Plano	10	30	9	+1.25	−	Surgery XT
9	12	45	+.50	19	35	18	+1.75	−	Surgery
10	10	50	+1.00	10	20	7	+.50	−	
11	11	35	+.50	12	20	12	+2.50	+	
12	6	50	+3.00	8	35	6	+.50	+	
13	8	35	+3.00	9	20	5	0	+	
14	6	40	+2.25	7	25	11	+.25	+	
15	3	40	+1.00	4	18	12	0	+	
16	9	60	+5.00	9	14	6	+1.25	+	
17	6	60	+3.25	7	25	6	+.25	−	
18	6	30	+2.50	6	35	12	No new refraction	Not given	Surgery ET
19	12	45	+.50	16	30	19	+1.75	+	
20	12	65	Plano	17	20	8	+1.00	Not given	Surgery XT
21	12	30	+2.00	16	12	24	+2.75	+	
22	9	60	−1.00	11	20	7	+1.50	Not given	Surgery
23	11	35	+.25	13	12	8		+	
Average	7.8	45	+1.50	10.5	24.5	14	+1.10		
Range	3-12	30-70	−1.00-+5.00	4-17	12-40	2-39	0-+2.75		

*XT, exotropia; ET, esotropia.
(Courtesy of Freeley, D.A., et al.: J. Pediatr. Ophthalmol. Strabismus 20:68–71, Mar.–Apr. 1983.)

glasses in 14 cases, indicating that the esotropia was accommodative in nature. Five patients were operated on with no attempt at spectacle correction.

The true incidence of subsequent esotropia in this series probably exceeds 28%. An accommodative cause must be considered in any patient with subsequent esotropia following early successful surgical correction of congenital esotropia. An attempt at spectacle correction should be made in any hyperopia exceeding 1.5 diopters before repeat surgery is considered. It is essential to have a current cycloplegic refraction on which to base the prescription. The cycloplegic refraction at age 1 year may not represent the true refractive state at the time a patient returns with recurrent esotropia. Most children with recurrent esotropia following successful surgical treatment early in life can be cured by antiaccommodative therapy.

2–3 **Accommodative Esotropia Long-Range Follow-Up.** Kenneth C. Swan (Oregon Health Sciences Univ., Portland) reviewed the course of 39 adults treated for accommodative esotropia in early childhood. All acquired an esodeviation when uncorrected high hypermetropia caused excessive accommodative convergence and were classed as having typical, or refractive, accommodative esotropia. The median age at the first manifestations was 26 months. Nearly 50% of the patients had a family history of esotropia. There were 4 pairs and 1 trio of siblings in the series. Most children had constant esotropia when first examined at a median age of 3½ years. The deviation without glasses, with distant fixation, was generally in the range of 20 to 30 prism diopters. The peak median hypermetropia of 5.7 diopters was reached by age 6 years. Twenty-four patients had amblyopia in the deviating eye. Fifteen had anomalous retinal correspondence, with unilateral amblyopia in 10.

The first step in treatment was full correction of the hypermetropia. Bifocals were seldom necessary. Residual esotropia in patients with fusional ability and a deviation of less than 10 prism diopters was managed with base-out prisms. Surgery was done for full correction of larger amounts of residual deviation. With noticeable deviation and poor fusional potential, the goal of surgery was to reduce the deviation to an esthetically acceptable level of esotropia, avoiding full correction. Twenty patients had surgery intended primarily to correct residual esodeviation before age 15 years. In 6 patients exotropia de-

FUNCTIONAL STATUS OF 39 ADULTS WITH TYPICAL
ACCOMMODATIVE ESOTROPIA IN CHILDHOOD

Normal binocular single vision	10
Peripheral fusion—minimal amblyopia and some fusional vergences	6
Gross peripheral fusion—residual amblyopia (20/50–20/200)	8
Abnormal retinal correspondence—suppression	15

(Courtesy of Swan, K.C.: Ophthalmology (Rochester) 90:1141–1145, October 1983.)

(2–3)   Ophthalmology (Rochester) 90:1141–1145, October 1983.

veloped after correction of hypermetropia, and all eventually required surgery. Only 2 patients had less than 3 diopters of hypermetropia in adulthood. Thirteen patients lacking the stabilizing effect of fusion required initial or additional surgery in adulthood. The functional status of the patients is summarized in the table. All but 3 of the 24 amblyopic patients had measurable improvement in visual acuity. Two of the 3 patients who reached presbyopic age have new problems.

Many patients with typical accommodative esotropia do not outgrow their hypermetropia, and their problems are more serious if stable binocular single vision does not develop. Both instruction in relaxing accommodation during such activities as swimming and contact lens wear have been important to many patients.

2–4 **Results of Treatment for Esotropia in Early Childhood.** D. Wieser and H. Hahn (Univ. of Basel, Switzerland) report the findings of a study involving 121 patients with early esotropia who were operated on between the ages of 2 and 4 years. The patients were examined to assess results of surgery and treatment for amblyopia and binocular vision. The recession-resection procedure resulted in alignment, i.e., an angle of less than 5 degrees, in 71% of 77 accurately evaluated patients. Sixteen patients were operated on twice, and 1 patient 3 times. An alignment of ±5 degrees was maintained in 22 patients.

It is important to achieve alignment early, but it makes little difference whether the operation is performed in the second, third, or fourth year of life. The three-muscle surgery showed a greater variability of results and greater secondary divergence than the monolateral combined surgery. Amblyopia treatment by occlusion produced the usual results. The esthetic improvement achieved did not cause the parents to neglect continued treatment.

The binocular result was determined by classifying the patients according to the degree of partial healing. Microtropia with harmonious anomalous retinal correspondence (ARC) was as frequent as residual angle without binocular vision (second and third degree, respectively). These results correspond to those in a group of patients followed up in 1970, who had undergone late orthoptic therapy and surgery.

The authors decided to perform surgery earlier and determine factors responsible for the quality of partial healing. These factors were (1) time of surgery and age (surgery in the fourth year had better results); (2) alignment (there was a definite relationship between the size of the angle and the quality of partial healing); and (3) age when alignment was established (accomplishing alignment early apparently benefits the development of functional partial healing).

The time for surgery can be adjusted to the individual without pressure of time. Surgery in the first year seems unrealistic. Results of

(2–4) Klin. Monatsbl. Augenheilkd. 182:376–378, May 1983.

therapy in 85 patients who acquired esotropia in the first year and had surgery between the second and third year showed that 44 patients had partial second degree healing and 41 had third degree. The age of the patient at the time of surgery seems less important than achieving the angle situation.

▶ [Few would disagree with the authors' conclusion that alignment is the most important factor in the surgical correction of esotropia. Nonetheless, early surgery is considered by many to be performed at 6 months of age and not 2 years. The series would have been of more interest if there had been a group operated on in the first year of life to help resolve the controversy about how early should early surgery be performed in patients with esotropia.] ◄

2–5 **Consecutive Exotropia Following Surgery.** Surgically overcorrected esotropia is a frequent problem. Eugene R. Folk, Marilyn T. Miller, and Lawrence Chapman (Chicago) reviewed the findings in 250 patients seen in 1970 to 1980 with consecutive exotropia. All had manifest exotropia in the primary position exceeding 10 prism diopters or 5 degrees for distance or near. Most patients were younger than age 1 year at the onset of esotropia, but only 5 were operated on before age 1. All surgical procedures were able to produce consecutive exotropia. Most patients had a single operation before developing exotropia, although 33 had multiple procedures before becoming exotropic. A high degree of hyperopia was present in only 11% of cases, but 38% had amblyopia. The interval from surgery to exotropia is shown in the table. Limited medial rectus function was nearly twice as frequent as in patients with normal function and was most distinct in those having multiple operations.

Consecutive exotropia may not develop for years after surgery for esotropia. It is not infrequent after apparently successful esotropia surgery. Amblyopia therapy must be continued after operation, and the smallest hyperopic correction consistent with good vision and straight eyes should be provided. If undercorrection is associated with limitation of the medial rectus, it is best to defer further surgery or plan for a more moderate procedure than is usually done. Exodevia-

---

TIME BETWEEN OPERATION AND APPEARANCE OF EXOTROPIA

Exotropia noted	Number of patients
Overcorrection noted at first postoperative visit	40 (16%)
Overcorrection < 1 year	55 (22%)
Overcorrection 1–4 years	51 (20%)
Overcorrection 5–8 years	31 (12%)
Overcorrection > 8 years	37 (15%)
Unknown	36 (15%)

(Courtesy of Folk, E.R., et al.: Br. J. Ophthalmol. 67:546–548, August 1983.)

(2–5) Br. J. Ophthalmol. 67:546–548, August 1983.

tion in the up and down positions also is a warning sign. It is better to avoid any esotropia surgery than to run a risk of medial rectus limitation unless this is the only way of correcting the deviation. Large resections of the lateral rectus can cause limited medial rectus function. Recessions of the medial rectus exceeding 5 mm should be carefully evaluated.

▶ [It is evident from this article and others that the results of strabismus treatment should be evaluated not only over the short term but also years later for a true assessment of the results.] ◀

2–6 **Intermittent Exotropia: Surgical Results in Different Age Groups.** James M. Richard and Marshall M. Parks reviewed the results of surgery as the sole initial treatment for intermittent exotropia in 111 patients who underwent bilateral rectus muscle recession. Forty-one patients (group 1) were younger than age 3 years at the time of initial surgery, 42 (group 2) were aged 3 to 6 years, and 28 (group 3) were aged 6 to 17 years. All patients had relative emmetropia and no oblique muscle dysfunction or vertical deviation. No orthoptic treatment was given before or after surgery. All patients had at least 15 prism diopters of exodeviation at distance, and the tropic phase of the exodeviation was increasing in frequency and duration.

Based on 10 prism diopters or less of intermittent exotropia while fixating an accommodative target at 20 ft with proper refractive correction, satisfactory results were obtained after initial operation in

TABLE 1.—SURGICAL RESULTS AFTER INITIAL BILATERAL
LATERAL RECTUS MUSCLE RECESSION

	Group I (<3 yrs) [n = 41]	Group II (>3 yrs <6 yrs) [n = 42]	Group III (>6 yrs <16 yrs) [n = 28]
Satisfactory result (10 prism diopters or less of horizontal deviation from ortho)	61% (25/41)	45% (19/42)	64% (18/28)
Unsatisfactory result	39% (16/41)	55% (23/42)	36% (10/28)
Undercorrected	27% (11/41)	50% (21/42)	36% (10/28)
Mean prism diopters residual X(T)*	19	17	18
Overcorrected	12% (5/41)	5% (2/42)	0% (0/28)
Mean prism diopters consecutive E(T)†	13	15	—

*X(T) = intermittent exotropia.
†E(T) = intermittent esotropia.
(Courtesy of Richard, J.M., and Parks, M.M.: Ophthalmology (Rochester) 90:1172–1177, October 1983.)

TABLE 2.—SURGICAL RESULTS AFTER ADDITIONAL SURGERY IN
PATIENTS HAVING AT LEAST TWO YEARS' FOLLOW-UP

	Group I (<3 yrs) [n = 41]	Group II (>3 yrs <6 yrs) [n = 42]	Group III (>6 yrs <16 yrs) [n = 28]
Satisfactory result	89% (8/9)	86% (6/7)	100% (2/2)
Unsatisfactory result	11% (1/9)	14% (1/7)	0% (0/2)
Mean age at time of 2nd operative procedure	4 yrs, 8 mos	6 yrs, 7 mos	7 yrs, 9 mos
Mean length of follow-up (f/u)	3 yrs, 1 mos	2 yrs, 10 mos	3 yrs, 2 mos
Shortest f/u	2 yrs	2 yrs	2 yrs
Longest f/u	4 yrs, 9 mos	5 yrs, 1 mo	4 yrs, 4 mos

(Courtesy of Richard, J.M., and Parks, M.M.: Ophthalmology (Rochester) 90: 1172–1177, October 1983.)

61% of group 1 patients, 45% of those in group 2, and 64% of those in group 3. Half or more of unsatisfactory results in all groups were caused by undercorrection. The results are summarized in Table 1, and the results obtained in patients followed up for at least 2 years after additional surgery are given in Table 2. Final acuity was equal in the 2 eyes in all patients but 1.

Initially satisfactory results can be expected in 56% of the patients with intermittent exotropia who undergo bilateral rectus muscle recession as initial treatment. Most failures are the result of undercorrection and require additional surgery, but satisfactory results ensue eventually in more than 80% of patients. Nearly all overcorrected patients require additional surgery. In all, 95% of patients can have a satisfactory outcome. Delaying initial surgery does not improve the likelihood of obtaining a good result.

▶ [The surgical results in different age groups are all the same. The authors of this careful study thus conclude that, as soon as the patient is seen and the diagnosis made, surgery should be performed. The only question is whether or not there might be a few patients in whom orthoptics would eliminate the need for an operation at any time and if their families might prefer not to take any surgical risk.] ◀

▶ ↓ Even though we are operating on normal tendons attached to normal muscles and the sensory factors are difficult to evaluate but no doubt extraordinarily important, precise measurement of what we are doing seems appropriate. Nonetheless, the following 2 articles raise a number of questions about the quantification of superior oblique muscle surgery. In the first article, the surgeons made measured recession which correlated with decreases in the A-pattern but not with the overactions. In fact, in the second article, the surgeons did not find any difference in the elimination of the A-pattern whether they recessed the superior oblique or just performed a tenotomy. We shall have to wait for further studies to know if it is helpful to measure or not. Perhaps the problem, suggested by Romano and Roholt, is that we don't measure with enough precision. ◀

2–7 **Measured Graduated Recession of Superior Oblique Muscle.**
Paul Romano and Philip Roholt (Univ. of Florida, Gainesville) performed bilateral superior oblique recession in 6 patients with A-pattern strabismus and overacting superior oblique muscles. The technique was modified so that the entire procedure was done through a
single nasal fornix incision. The amount of recession was graduated
and measured both directly from the point of the original incision
anteriorly and indirectly from the nasal corner of the superior rectus
insertion based on anatomical measurements. All patients were followed up for at least 6 months after the operation.

The amount of superior oblique recession, measured directly,
ranged from 10 to 14 mm, and the amount of change in the A-pattern
varied from 27 to 36 prism diopters. The total amount of recession
correlated linearly with the total change in the A-pattern. There were
2 prism diopters of effect for each millimeter of surgery performed
after the first 8 mm. The amount of recession did not correlate with
the reduction in superior oblique overaction, but fair correlation was
observed when the change in overaction was compared with the
amount of overaction present preoperatively. The greater the amount
of overaction present initially, the greater was the change in muscle
action observed regardless of the amount of surgery performed. The
amount of recession measured indirectly did not correlate with the
amount of effect on the A-pattern.

Superior oblique recession can be done through a single superior
nasal fornix incision. The amount of reduction in the A-pattern cor-
relates with the amount of surgery performed when this is measured
directly from the original anterior point of the superior oblique insertion. Superior oblique overaction currently is measured directly in
terms of the degree of misalignment of the corneal light reflexes in
the field of action of the oblique muscles.

2–8 **Superior Oblique Recession Versus Tenotomy: Comparison
of Surgical Results.** The surgical results of superior oblique tendon
recession were compared with those of tenotomy in a retrospective
study undertaken by Edward G. Buckley and John T. Flynn (Univ. of
Miami) using the records of 20 patients from the Bascon Palmer Eye
Institute and data from 2 other published reports. The 20 patients
were aged 2 to 24 years, and 65% were males. After a complete eye
examination was performed, ocular motility measurements were
made using the prism alternate cover test at 20 ft. Cyclotropia was
measured using a double Maddox rod. An "A" pattern determination
was made using measurements from the standard 30-degree upgaze,
the primary, and the 30-degree downgaze positions. For comparison,
measurements taken on the visit 3 days before surgery and those
made 6 months after surgery were used.

(2–7) J. Pediatr. Ophthalmol. Strabismus 20:134–140, July–Aug. 1983.
(2–8) Ibid., pp. 112–117, May–June 1983.

UNILATERAL SUPERIOR OBLIQUE SURGERY—AVERAGE HYPERDEVIATION MEASUREMENTS
(PRISM DIOPTERS)

	Tenotomy (n=5)		Recession (n=4)	
	Average	Range	Average	Range
Primary Position				
Pre-Op	10.6	(6 - 20)	10.75	(0 - 18)
Post-Op	4.4	(0 - 25)	6.0	(3 - 10)
Correction	11.0		6.25	
Downgaze				
Pre-Op	16.8	(6 - 30)	17.25	(10 - 25)
Post-Op	6.4	(0 - 25)	7.5	(0 - 14)
Correction	10.6		9.7	
Greatest Deviation				
Pre-Op	23.2	(15 - 30)	20.25	(15 - 25)
Post-Op	10.2	(0 - 25)	12.0	(10 - 16)
Correction	10.6		9.0	

(Courtesy of Buckley, E.G., and Flynn, J.T.: J. Pediatr. Ophthalmol. Strabismus 20:112–117, May–June 1983.)

Superior oblique tenotomies were performed by the method of Parks and Helveston; the superior oblique recession was done by the method of Caldeira with minor modifications. A summary of the findings is given in the table. Tenotomy produced a much larger effect on hyperdeviation in the primary position than did recession (11 prism diopters vs. 6.25 prism diopters). Both procedures left persistent hyperdeviation in the field of action of the superior oblique tendon that was about half of the preoperative amount. Significant palsy of the superior oblique tendon or marked overaction of the antagonist inferior oblique tendon did not occur with either technique.

Tenotomy and superior oblique tendon recession were equally effective in eliminating "A" pattern strabismus regardless of the initial size of the pattern. Unilateral superior oblique recessions were less erratic than tenotomies but tended to result in slight undercorrection. The type and number of complications were similar for each procedure. A clear advantage of bilateral superior oblique recession over tenotomy could not be demonstrated. Unilateral recession needs further investigation; it may prove useful when combined with the adjustable suture technique.

2–9 **Forced Duction Test in Clinical Practice.** T. H. Oei (Univ. of Amsterdam), W. I. M. Verhagen, and G. P. M. Horsten (Catholic Univ. of Nijmegen, Netherlands) present data on 4 patients with mechanical obstruction of eye movements in whom the forced duction test was helpful diagnostically.

(2–9) Ophthalmologica 186:87–90, 1983.

For this test local anesthesia is administered and the patient is asked to look in the direction of the gaze limitation. The physician holds the eyelids apart and grasps the conjunctiva with a small-tooth forceps as close to the limbus as possible opposite the site of the gaze limitation. Attempts to rotate the globe are made with the forceps further into the gaze position in which the patient has been trying to look. Full and easy rotation of the globe in that direction indicates the agonist muscle is paretic. If the globe can be moved no further than the voluntary gaze will allow and a tightness is felt with the traction forceps, restriction and stiffness of the muscle itself opposite the gaze limitation is indicated. The restriction may also be caused by a reserve "leash" due to scar or muscle tightness on the same side as the gaze limitation.

The 4 patients described had eye movement obstruction due to orbital fracture, ethmoid fracture, or endocrine exophthalmus. All 4 had normal electromyograms. However, in all cases the patient's history in combination with results of the forced duction test provided a strong indication of the cause of the eye movement disorder.

The literature contains data on 1 patient who had a fracture of the floor of the orbit with incarceration of an ocular muscle in whom the incarceration was released by the forced duction test. This simple test, which can be performed in the physician's office in adults and children, should be used whenever eye movement is limited in any direction of gaze.

▶ [Oei and associates clearly describe the method and report that its judicious use has all but eliminated the need for the more invasive electromyography. It seems appropriate to add that the forced duction test may also be valuable at the time of surgery.] ◀

2–10 **Brown's Syndrome: Fusion Status and Amblyopia.** Brown, in 1950, described a syndrome involving a lack of elevation in adduction, with restriction to passive elevation of the affected eye, and postulated that it was caused by a congenital paralysis of the inferior oblique muscle. W. N. Clarke and L. P. Noel (Univ. of Ottawa) reviewed 28 cases of Brown's superior oblique tendon sheath syndrome. Three patients had involvement of both eyes. The average follow-up was 27 months. Thirteen children were thought to have "typical" Brown's syndrome. Five had an anomalous head position but full stereopsis. Superior oblique tenotomy was effective in only 1 of 3 children in this group. Two children had full fusion and stereopsis in forced primary gaze but had large-angle intermittent exotropia and smaller-angle intermittent hypotropia (Fig 2–1). Surgery corrected the intermittent exotropia in 1 case. Eight children had an anomalous head position despite a complete lack of fusion and stereopsis. Seven were amblyopic. Surgery was done in 4 cases. Superior oblique tenotomy led to significant improvement of elevation in adduction in the involved eye.

(2–10) Can. J. Ophthalmol. 18:118–123, April 1983.

Many children with Brown's syndrome retain some ability to elevate the involved eye in adduction. Amblyopia is not commonly described as a significant complication of the syndrome, but it was present in most of the authors' patients who failed to show fusion in their assumed head position or in any field of gaze. The only indication for surgery in Brown's syndrome is a severely abnormal head position. Most of the 8 operated-on patients in the present series had superior oblique tenotomy alone or combined with horizontal rectus surgery

Fig 2–1.—A, full fusion in forced primary gaze. **B,** large-angle intermittent exotropia in forced primary gaze in same patient. **C,** Brown's syndrome of left eye in same patient. (Courtesy of Clarke, W.N. and Noel, L.P.: Can. J. Ophthalmol. 18:118–123, April 1983.)

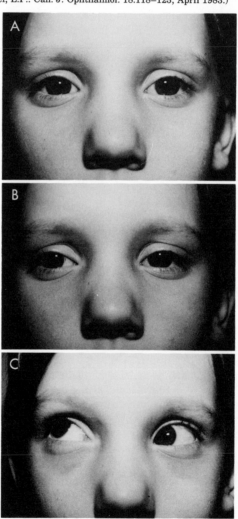

for associated horizontal strabismus. Early surgery may be indicated in severe cases of Brown's syndrome to prevent amblyopia and irreversible changes in the neck musculature and the cervical spine.

▶ [The lack of elevation when the eye is turned in is due to shortening and tightening of the paralyzed inferior oblique muscle's check ligament, the anterior sheath of the superior oblique. The authors' message is that these patients have a high frequency of amblyopia and problems with their neck musculature and cervical spine because of the head tilt. They should consequently be treated early and aggressively with patching and surgery.] ◀

2–11   **Surgical Treatment of Eye Muscle Palsies** is outlined by Henry S. Metz (Univ. of Rochester, N.Y.). Patients with ocular muscle palsy should be observed for 3 to 6 months before any definitive treatment is chosen. Further treatment is indicated if palsy is present without signs of change for 4 to 6 months and symptoms continue. The goals of surgical treatment are to eliminate symptomatic diplopia, produce

Fig 2–2.—Adjustable Harada-Ito procedure. Anterior fibers of the superior oblique tendon have been transposed anteriorly and laterally using an adjustable suture technique *(see inserts)*. (Courtesy of Metz, H.S.: NY State J. Med. 83:319–323, March 1983.)

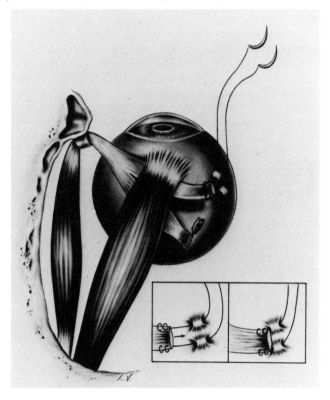

good alignment in the primary position, and provide some improvement in ocular rotation about the midline.

Surgery often is necessary for severe lateral rectus weakness in patients with sixth nerve palsy. Paresis without complete paralysis can be managed by recession of the antagonist muscle and resection of the involved lateral rectus. An adjustable technique may be used in an adolescent or adult to "fine tune" the results after surgery. In complete paralysis, transposition surgery is necessary to achieve some degree of lateral gaze. Any antagonist contracture must be released. Ischemia of the anterior segment can be avoided by performing a Jensen procedure, involving splitting of the superior, lateral, and inferior recti and suturing of the lateral parts of the superior and inferior recti to the upper and lower parts of the split lateral rectus, respectively.

When the third nerve is paretic, it often is possible to achieve good results by lateral rectus recession combined with medial rectus resection. The muscle insertions can be adjusted if a small vertical deviation coexists. The adjustable suture technique is useful. In cases of complete third nerve paralysis, some practitioners have suggested superior oblique transposition to the nasal side of the globe. It is simpler to isolate the superior oblique tendon, cut it medial to the superior rectus, and resect and suture it to the superior nasal quadrant.

Superior oblique palsy with unilateral inferior oblique overaction and a vertical deviation under 15 prism diopters can be managed by inferior oblique recession or myectomy. If the vertical deviation is greater, inferior oblique surgery can be combined with a vertical rectus recession. A modified Harada-Ito procedure for symptomatic cyclotropia resulting from bilateral superior oblique palsy is illustrated in Figure 2–2. The operation provides both increased incycloduction and a controlled effect through use of an adjustable technique.

▶ [This article is a concise review of the various surgical procedures. Prism correction is difficult because the deviations vary with the direction of gaze and the adjustable suture now appears to have vastly improved surgical results.] ◀

▶ ↓ The debate about treating amblyopic eyes by stimulating them with views of a grating is winding down. A great deal of work was done, however, as illustrated by the following 3 articles. Indeed the authors of the first article believe they have evidence that grating stimulation may be better than occlusion in the single case of anisometropic amblyopia. The other studies, however, strongly suggest that the results of treatment are either the same or not as good as the result of classical occlusion. ◀

2–12 **Amblyopia in 4-Year-Old Children Treated With Grating Stimulation and Full-Time Occlusion: Comparative Study.** Gunnar Lennerstrand and Berit Samuelsson compared the effects of grating stimulation procedures (CAM therapy) and full-time occlusion on visual acuity and binocular functions of 38 children aged 4 years with previously untreated amblyopia. The children were placed into

(2–12) Br. J. Ophthalmol. 67:181–190, March 1983.

subgroups according to amblyopia type and fixation pattern, and in each subgroup children randomly received CAM treatment or full-time facial occlusion or occlusion with dimming filters. Grating stimulation treatment was given once or twice a week for 4 to 8 weeks, after which conventional amblyopia therapy was usually started. The children were followed up for at least 6 months.

Grating stimulation was slightly better than occlusion in improving visual acuity of anisometropic amblyopes with central fixation, but both types of therapy were equally effective in strabismic amblyopia with central fixation and in amblyopia with eccentric fixation. Maximal treatment effects were not reached with grating stimulation alone, which was shown at follow-up after continued conventional therapy.

Grating stimulation, or rather short periods of occlusion combined with exercises of concentrated visuomotor activity, is considered valuable at the initiation of treatment, particularly for those with anisometropic amblyopia, but it must be supplemented with occlusion. Full-time occlusion still must be regarded as the prime form of amblyopia therapy.

2–13 **Controlled Study Comparing CAM Treatment With Occlusion Therapy.** The object of this study by K. G. Nyman, Gur Singh, Agneta Rydberg, and Monica Fornander (Stockholm) on 2 groups of 25 amblyopic children, aged 4 to 6½ years, was to compare occlusion treatment with CAM stimulation (looking at a rotating disk with black and white lines) regarding distant visual acuity. Children who showed a difference of at least 2 rows in distant visual acuity between the 2 eyes (as measured by the Snellen E chart) were considered to have amblyopia, provided the weaker eye had an acuity of 0.7 or less. Complete orthoptic assessment was undertaken, and the ocular media and fundus were inspected. Full corrective glasses were provided when indicated. After the glasses were worn for 8 weeks, the patients were examined again and the children who were no longer amblyopic were excluded from the study.

Occlusion therapy consisted of patching over the eye or a semi-

IMPROVEMENT IN VISUAL ACUITY IN CAM AND OCCLUSION GROUPS AFTER TREATMENT

Therapy	Improvement		Number of subjects
	Less than 2 lines	At least 2 lines	
CAM	6	19	25
Occlusion	5	20	25

(Courtesy of Nyman, K.G., et al.: Br. J. Ophthalmol. 67:178–180, March 1983.)

(2–13) Br. J. Ophthalmol. 67:178–180, March 1983.

transparent membrane (Bangerter filter) applied to the front of a spectacle lens. When tropia was present, occlusion of the better eye for 5 days was alternated with occlusion of the amblyopic eye for 2. In the case of heterophoria or orthophoria, a Bangerter filter was worn continuously in front of the better eye. During CAM therapy the vision stimulator marketed by Clement Clark was used. In this therapy the amblyopic eye was shown plates with black and white gratings and the child was asked to identify the correct orientation; the other eye was occluded only during the treatment. The plate with the least contrast that was correctly identified and the 2 of next higher contrast were used in the CAM stimulator. Five to 10 treatments of approximately 7 minutes were given.

The results of treatment in the CAM and occlusion groups (table) indicate that this study did not show a significant difference between the 2 methods of treatment. An improvement of at least 2 lines of the Snellen chart was achieved by both methods in at least 80% of patients. It is not clear whether gratings (CAM) are responsible for visual improvement, as equally good results have been reported with gray disks. However, CAM is a useful alternative when occlusion cannot be used for various reasons.

2-14 **Effect of Minimal Occlusion Therapy on Binocular Visual Functions in Amblyopia.** Sixty amblyopic children aged 5 to 14 years were examined by D. E. Mitchell, E. R. Howell, and C. G. Keith (Melbourne, Australia). After occlusion of the better eye, 33 children were seated in front of a device on which 1 of 6 grating disks was rotated in turn at 1 revolution per minute behind a clear plastic plate on which the child played competitive games with the therapist; the control group of 27 children was treated in the same way, except that the grating disks were replaced by a single stationary gray disk.

The gains in stereoacuity were significant and were usually more obvious than were the small gains in letter visual acuity. Initially, only 21 of 60 children had evidence of stereopsis on either the Titmus or Frisby test, and of these only 7 possessed stereoacuity of 100 seconds or better. On completion of 6 treatment sessions, stereopsis was demonstrated in another 15 children, and 19 others with stereopsis had improved stereoacuity. Thus, after treatment, 36 of 60 children appeared to have stereopsis. The initial and final stereoacuities measured by the Titmus Plates for the 36 patients are shown in Figure 2–3.

The improvement in stereoacuity achieved by children treated with rotating gratings was not significantly different from that in the control group. It does not appear that any of the visual gains were enhanced or promoted by active visual stimulation of the amblyopic eye with rotating gratings during the brief periods of occlusion of the unaffected eye. It is of considerable interest that treatment directed to-

(2–14) Invest. Ophthalmol. Vis. Sci. 24:778–781, June 1983.

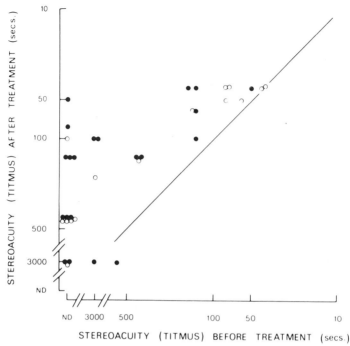

Fig 2–3.—Initial and final stereoacuity scores on the Titmus test after 6 treatment sessions. Score of 3,000 seconds represents the calculated retinal disparity of the "fly" plate. Children who did not have stereopsis before treatment are designated by the letters *ND.* Those who did not have stereopsis after treatment are omitted from the graph. Improvement in stereoacuity is shown by the amount of vertical displacement upward from the line at 45 degrees. Children who viewed rotating gratings during treatment are represented by *filled symbols,* whereas the controls are represented by *open circles.* (Courtesy of Mitchell, D.E., et al.: Invest. Ophthalmol. Vis. Sci. 24:778–781, June 1983.)

ward the amblyopic eye can produce significant improvement in binocular visual functions.

If a sensitive test is desired for the purpose of screening for subtle binocular disorders, a high-dot density random-dot test (e.g., TNO or random-Dot-E) is appropriate because of the exacting requirements. However, for quantifying the stereoacuity of patients with abnormal binocular vision or with oculomotor problems, a test with large fusion cues is more suitable.

2–15 **Eye Movements of Preschool Children** are discussed by Richard N. Aslin, Kenneth J. Ciuffreda, James L. Dannemiller, Martin S. Banks, Benjamin R. Stephens, E. Eugenie Hartmann, Eileen Kowler, and Albert J. Martins. Aslin (Indiana Univ.) and Ciuffreda (State Univ. of New York), in response to the report by Kowler (Rutgers Univ.) and Martins (Univ. of Maryland) that the eye movements of

(2–15) Science 222:74–76, Oct. 7, 1983.

preschool children are considerably less accurate than adult eye movements under identical viewing conditions, disagree with the views that normal children are significantly deficient in oculomotor control and have only a limited ability to use eye movements to acquire visual information. Only 2 children were tested, and their results were compared with those of just 1 adult. Young children are notoriously poor at maintaining attention during tasks, even for brief periods. Dannemiller, Banks, Stephens, and Hartmann (Univ. of Texas, Austin) suggest that it is not reasonable to claim that the shape of the contrast sensitivity function in young infants results from oculomotor immaturity alone. Changes in shape with age, particularly in the peak shift, are more probably related to postnatal changes in retinal anatomy and to progressive narrowing in the spatial tuning of pattern mechanisms.

Kowler and Martins believe that there is insufficient reason to alter their chief conclusions, i.e., that children's eye movements differ from those of adults and that the differences are relevant to an understanding of visual development. The children tested were attentive and cooperative, and performed in a helpful manner in many tasks. The observations of higher smooth eye speeds during fixation of a stationary target in children and of longer lags when the target changed direction during smooth pursuit could not be attributed to failure to cooperate. The children tested continue to be free of any visual or oculomotor abnormality. A contribution of neural maturation to the development of visual performance has not been ruled out. Quantitative determinations of the effects of eye movements on visual processing require simultaneous measurements of both visual performance and retinal image position and velocity. Studies in preschool children can be as useful as those in infants because visual acuity is not fully developed until age 5 or later.

▶ [This article is actually a series of 3 papers with 2 groups attacking the conclusions of the third. The controversy arose because Kowler and Martins suggested that eye movements of children differ from eye movements of adults and that they are not fully developed until about age 5 years. The debate, not yet resolved, is whether the higher eye speeds affect a child's visual performance. The definitive answers await further studies.] ◀

3. Vision, Refraction, and Contact Lenses

The Reliability of Retinal Visual Acuity Measurements Behind Cataracts

DAVID L. GUYTON, M.D.

The Wilmer Ophthalmological Institute
Johns Hopkins University School of Medicine

Many methods have been used to assess the functional integrity of the retina behind cataracts: direct viewing by ophthalmoscopy, ultrasonography, the pupillary light reflex, electrophysiologic tests, entoptic imagery, color perception, and direct measurement of the retinal visual acuity. Direct acuity measures are performed by projecting a test target or pattern through a relatively clear area, or "window," in the eye's optics. An ordinary pinhole aperture can sometimes isolate such an area, but the accompanying decrease in light entering the eye often compromises the retinal acuity obtained. New instruments, the interference fringe instruments and the Potential Acuity Meter, compensate for this light loss by projecting narrow beams of bright light directly through accessible windows.

The interference fringe instruments[1] use narrow beams of laser light (Rodenstock Retinometer, Randwal Acuiometer), or white light (Haag-Streit Lotmar Visometer), to form round patches of interference fringes on the patient's retina 1.5 to 8 degrees in diameter. These red and black, or white and black gratings are made finer and finer until the patient can no longer identify the correct orientation, thereby measuring a form of "grating" visual acuity expressed in decimal or Snellen notation.

The Mentor Guyton-Minkowski Potential Acuity Meter,[1, 2] in which the author has proprietary interest, uses a narrow beam of white light to project an ordinary Snellen visual acuity chart through the cataract onto the retina. Snellen acuity is determined in the customary manner.

Although the interference fringe instruments and the Potential Acuity Meter yield actual numbers for expected visual acuity after cataract surgery, the predictions are not always reliable. The visual acuity prediction can be falsely poor (a "false negative" prediction) or falsely good (a "false positive" prediction). Anticipating these erroneous results is possible, though, if one understands the mechanisms by which they arise.

Falsely poor visual acuities are usually due to blocked light beams. Mild or moderate cataracts, those yielding best correctable visual acuity of 20/200 or better, usually allow accurate measurement,[2] but advanced or mature cataracts often do not have adequate windows for light beam penetration. If good vision *is* measured through a dense cataract, all is well, but if poor vision is obtained, the light beam may have been blocked. With the Potential Acuity Meter, and to some extent with the interference fringe instruments, penetration of the light beam can be monitored by the examiner with the slit-lamp microscope as the beam traverses the crystalline lens. If the beam traverses the lens cleanly and disappears into the vitreous, the resulting acuity measurement should be reliable, whether indicating good retinal vision or poor retinal vision. If, however, the lens is blocked by lens opacity, the lens will light up with scattered light, and a poor visual acuity reading may be obtained even in the presence of a 20/20 retina. Thus the examiner should learn to judge, by slit-lamp observation, when the beam penetrates and when it does not. If the beam penetrates well, the retinal acuity obtained is highly reliable.

Falsely *good* acuities may be obtained in 3 situations: with macular scotomas, with macular edema, and with irregular refraction. Because failure to achieve the predicted visual acuity after cataract surgery is a major disappointment to both patient and surgeon, it is particularly important to understand the mechanisms for these "false positive" predictions.

Only with the interference fringe instruments are false positives obtained with macular scotomas (amblyopia, field cuts through fixation, dry forms of macular degeneration, etc.). These appear due to the large stimulus size produced by these instruments, with the patches of interference fringes subtending a visual angle of as much as 5 to 8 degrees. As we and others have recently discovered, visual acuity measurements with large cards filled with uniform illiterate Es (the "Full Field" E test[3]), as well as measurements with cards covered with square-wave black-and-white gratings, are often 2 to 3 times better in the presence of macular scotomas than are measurements with random illiterate Es arranged in lines ("linear Es"). The large homogenous stimuli obviate the need for fixation. This allows measurement of the best resolution possible of any remaining retinal area, even though the patient has not learned, or cannot learn, to fixate with that area. Our old assumption that patients spontaneously fixate with the best remaining area of retina appears to be wrong in many cases. Whatever the case, the large stimulus size appears to be the reason that the interference fringe instruments often yield falsely good retinal acuity in cases of amblyopia, field defects, ocular histoplasmosis, and dry forms of macular degeneration.

Macular edema can result in falsely good retinal acuity with both the interference fringe instruments and the Potential Acuity Meter. This appears to be due to intraretinal light scattering. With full-pupil viewing, many rays of light converge toward each retinal image point. The edematous inner layers of retina scatter these light rays, blurring each image point at the photoreceptor layer. The image as a whole appears "washed out" to the patient. If, on the other hand, the light entering the eye is restricted to a small light beam, as with the interference fringe instruments and the Potential Acuity Meter, the light traveling to each retinal image point is scattered much less, resulting in a clearer overall image at the photoreceptor layer. If the photoreceptor layer is still healthy, good retinal acuity will thus be obtained, whereas good acuity cannot be obtained with full-pupil viewing. Although such a false positive reading by the interference fringe instruments or the Potential Acuity Meter may indeed be a valid measure of the potential visual acuity of the photoreceptor layer, this acuity cannot be realized unless the macular edema resolves. Diabetic macular edema and postoperative cystoid macular edema are commonly recognized, but macular edema can also accompany intraocular inflammation, subretinal fluid, wet forms of macular degeneration, and newly reattached retina. The presence, or possible presence, of any one of these forms of macular edema should invoke informed caution in the interpretation of retinal acuity measurements.

Finally, irregular corneal refraction or a residual posterior capsule after extracapsular cataract surgery can result in an apparent false positive retinal acuity. This occurs not only with the interference fringe instruments and the Potential Acuity Meter, but with ordinary pinhole testing as well. Each of these tests can bypass irregular refraction or residual opacity by the pinhole effect, resulting in a better visual acuity than can be measured otherwise. Unless the presence of irregular refraction or residual opacity is suspected, thee potential acuity device will be blamed for falsely predicting a good retinal acuity. The retinal acuity is indeed good; the problem is still in the optics of the eye.

Occasionally my colleagues with an interference fringe instrument or a Potential Acuity Meter tell me that a particular patient obtained much poorer vision after surgery than predicted. I ask them, "Why?" They appear dumbfounded, as if I am supposed to assume there is something wrong with the instrument. I then ask them, "Did you repeat the potential acuity test after surgery?" They say, "No, I never thought of that." I continue, "How clear and regular is the retinoscopic reflex?" They say, "I don't know; my assistant refracted the patient." The point is that false positive predictions do not just happen; there are definite reasons for them.

Once the above mechanisms for false positive readings are understood, residual problems with postoperative vision can be sorted out with certainty. Also, false positive readings can often be anticipated preoperatively, tempering overenthusiastic predictions and increasing the reliability of the preoperative evaluation. The new instruments are good, but they can be so much better when combined with a little knowledge of how they work.

References
1. Guyton, D.L.: Instruments for measuring retinal visual acuity behind cataracts—1982. *Ophthalmology* 89(8S):34–39, 1982.
2. Minkowski, J.S., and Guyton, D.L.: Potential acuity meter using a minute aerial pinhole aperture. *Ophthalmology* 90:1360–1368, 1983.
3. Robins, D., Harris, M., Walsh, P., et al.: Full field acuity testing in nystagmus and amblyopia. Submitted for publication.

3–1 **Risks and Difficulties of Treatment of Aphakia in Infancy.**
D. S. I. Taylor (London) reviewed data on 105 bilateral infantile aphakic patients fitted with contact lenses between 1976 and 1982, with particular reference to 43 randomly selected patients for whom records were complete.

Ten eyes of the 43 children had severe acute episodes of infection, and 5 of these eyes showed residual visual effects. Apical ulceration occurred in 3 eyes. Circumferential pannus of 0.5 mm or less was recorded in 18 patients, and 3 patients showed pannus of 1 mm or more. Incorrect optical correction, sometimes due to an inadequate gap in the capsule, also occurred. In addition to these risks to the eye and vision, some families had economic, social, and emotional difficulties. Geographic location was sometimes a problem. Some parents had problems with occlusion, drop therapy, lens insertion and removal, and appreciation of the risks of treatment.

Difficulties for the ophthalmologist included the need for close cooperation between the surgeon and the contact lens team. Lenses were costly and had an average lifespan of 9 weeks, making it desirable to change to spectacles once the child is 3 or 4 years old, a time when the refractive error is less, the child is more cooperative, and the risk of amblyopia development within a few days of optical defocussing of the eye is much less. Surgical problems included whether to perform lensectomy or lens aspiration. Follow-up examinations were difficult from the time the child starts resisting at about 6 months until about 3 or 4 years, when he or she is more cooperative.

Despite all these risks and difficulties, there is increasing evidence that the visual prognosis is greatly improved and that reduction of the visual handicap from amblyopia in aphakic infants by the use of contact lenses is justifiable on both social and economic grounds. Thus, infants are fitted with continuous-wear soft lenses. When the parents are able to insert and remove the lenses, daily-wear soft or

(3–1) Trans. Ophthalmol. Soc. U.K. 102:403–406, 1982.

high gas-transfer hard lenses are used until the child is able to wear spectacles or high gas-transfer hard lenses. All patients are treated symmetrically.

▶ [The difficult and expensive treatment of aphakic children with contact lenses continues to improve. This is a good thing since use of infant intraocular lenses raises questions about long-term eye tolerance as well as growth of the eye.

3–2 **Visual Acuity, Spectacle Blur, and Slit-Lamp Biomicroscopy on Asymptomatic Contact Lens-Wearing Recruits.** Contact lens use is becoming increasingly popular among young persons. A. J. P. Rouwen, A. J. L. G. Pinckers, A. A. I. v't Pad Bosch, H. Punt, W. H. Doesburg, and W. A. J. G. Lemmens reviewed refraction data on 644 Dutch Army and Air Force recruits who wore contact lenses or spectacles. The 476 contact lens wearers and 168 spectacle wearers were similar in age and training unit. Contact lens wearers were not refracted until after 3 days without lens wear. Nearly 60% of them wore hard contact lenses.

Acuity frequently was reduced in contact lens wearers, especially those using soft lenses, because the lenses were not or were no longer powerful enough. There was less spectacle blur with gas-permeable hard lenses than with nonpermeable lenses and practically none with soft lenses. Conventional hard lenses in myopic individuals tended to be stronger than prescribed glasses after 3 days without lens wear. The contact lens power and trial lens power were closest with gas-permeable hard lenses. The average cylinder power in refraction after 3 days without soft lens wear was only half that with conventional hard lenses. Residual astigmatism was found in 7% of the soft lens wearers. Staining of the corneal epithelium was less frequent with gas-permeable lenses. Corneal neovascularization, anterior stromal opacification, and papillary changes were found in a relatively large number of soft lens wearers.

The optical properties of rigid contact lenses are superior to those of soft lenses, but mechanical irritation of the eye is a problem with rigid lenses. Gas-permeable hard lenses are an improvement. Corneal pathologic change is observed in a significant number of asymptomatic soft lens wearers. Contact lens wearers, especially those using soft lenses, should have slit-lamp biomicroscopic evaluation every 6 months.

▶ [Rouwen and colleagues found a surprisingly large amount of pathologic change in asymptomatic soft lens wearers. They concluded that gas-permeable rigid lenses are the best optically as well as in terms of corneal pathologic change.] ◀

3–3 **Philosophy of Permanent Wearing of Soft Hydrophilic Lenses, 1981–1982,** is discussed by F. Kreis-Gosselin (Paris). The ametropic individual, acutely aware of the value of good vision, desires permanent correction. Thanks to the recent development of soft hydrophilic lenses (SHL), permanent correction has become possible. Therapeutic success with SHL has been shown in a certain number

(3–2) Graefes Arch. Clin. Exp. Ophthalmol. 221:73–77, October 1983.
(3–3) J. Fr. Ophthalmol. 6:75–85, 1983.

of corneal conditions. Permanent wearing is achieved when the lens is left in place for 1, 3, and 6 months at a time, in contrast to discontinuous daily wearing when the lens is removed each night. Such permanent use would seem particularly desirable for elderly subjects and for infants after cataract surgery—that is, whenever manipulation is problematic.

For successful permanent use of a contact lens certain physiologic conditions must be considered, particularly oxygenation, supply of metabolites to the cornea, and the elimination of cellular and metabolic waste products. These functions are mainly accomplished by the lacrimal film and are hampered by placement of a lens on the eye. Material that is permeable to oxygen and contains a high percentage of water must be used, and the lenses must be kept as thin as possible. The lens must be mobile to enable renewal of the lacrimal film and elimination of waste products. In view of the persisting technical difficulties, the permanent wearing of contact lenses should be restricted to those cases in which it is indispensable, in consideration of the classical contraindications to the use of contact lenses in the first place. Permanent use increases the potential risks, which occur mainly as a result of hypoxia, such as the constriction syndrome, conjunctival and corneal complications, and vascular neoformation.

The use of permanent lenses should only be recommended when distinct benefits justify the risks, such as in cases of elderly, young, or physically handicapped patients.

▶ [Extended contact lens wear appears to mean 24 hours or more and permanent contact lens wear is usually meant to be about a month. The clearest criteria are for monocular aphakia in which an intraocular lens is contraindicated and the patient is physically handicapped and cannot handle the daily care of a contact lens. It is obvious by the large numbers prescribed that more liberal criteria are being applied. Cosmesis and convenience appear to be important considerations. One would hope the continuous-wear contact lens would be tried before radial keratotomy is considered. Following are 5 articles on extended-wear contact lenses.] ◀

▶ ↓ In the following 2 articles, the authors discuss extended-wear contact lenses for aphakic patients. In the first article the patients were carefully selected, while the patients described in the second article were selected randomly. In both series, the success rate was extraordinarily high, although the patients using contact lenses need more follow-up care with corneal lens inspections and lens cleaning. ◀

3–4 **Extended-Wear Soft Contact Lenses for Aphakic Correction.** Neil F. Martin, Gregory P. Kracher, Walter J. Stark, and A. Edward Maumenee (Baltimore) report the results obtained in 320 aphakic eyes of 135 male and 126 female patients, aged 7 months to 92 years (mean, 65 years), who received a perfilcon A lens (Permalens) and were followed up for 4 to 48 months (mean, 23 months). In addition, 24 eyes were fitted with a lidofilcon B lens (Sauflon PW) and 25 with a silicone lens (Silsoft).

Of the 320 eyes fitted with a perfilcon A lens, 33 were dropped from the study because of a lens-related problem such as poor lens fit or

(3–4) Arch. Ophthalmol. 101:39–41, January 1983.

EYES SUCCESSFULLY FITTED WITH EXTENDED-WEAR APHAKIC CONTACT LENSES

Type of Lens	No. of Eyes Fitted	Success Rate, %
Perfilcon A lens (Permalens)	320	89
Lidofilcon B lens (Sauflon PW)	24	91
Silicone lens (Silsoft)	25	92
Total	369	89

(Courtesy of Martin, N.F., et al.: Arch. Ophthalmol. 101:30–41, January 1983; copyright 1983, American Medical Association.)

poor visual acuity. Seventeen patients (21 eyes) discontinued use for other reasons, and 266 continued wearing the lens for at least 4 months. With the use of spectacles in addition to the contact lenses, the visual acuity was 20/40 or better in 89% of the patients. Failure to achieve this level of acuity was due to previous posterior segment abnormalities.

Complications included "tight-fit" syndrome (32 cases), conjunctivitis with (15) or without (38) sterile corneal infiltrate, and corneal vascularization (3). There were no infectious corneal ulcers, no scarring, and no permanent vision loss. Lens replacements, which averaged about 1.4 lenses per eye per year, were required for poor fit or poor visual acuity (50%), lens loss (23%), lens deposits (14%), lens damage (8%), and red eye (8%).

The lenses were removed at 1- to 3-week intervals in 24% of patients, at 1- to 3-month intervals in 46%, and at 4- to 6-month intervals in 30%. Success rates were similar with the 3 types of lenses (table); many of the patients fitted with lidofilcon B or silicone lenses had not been able to use the perfilcon A lens successfully. Overall, 94% of the patients were successfully fitted with one of the 3 types of lenses.

The perfilcon A lens is usually tried first, using the flattest lens consistent with the production of stable vision. The lidofilcon B lens has the largest optical zone of the 3, making it useful after sector iridectomy. The extremely high oxygen transmissibility of the silicone lens makes it useful if the cornea is compromised from Fuchs' dystrophy or if penetrating keratoplasty has been performed. A lens need not be removed for routine cleaning and sterilization if it fits well and is free of noteworthy deposits. Patients reporting discomfort or a red eye should be examined at once.

3–5 **Intraocular Lenses Versus Extended-Wear Contact Lenses in Aphakic Rehabilitation: A Controlled Clinical Study.** Peter Bernth-Petersen and Torben Sørensen (Univ. of Aarhus, Denmark) compared intraocular lens implantation with extended-wear contact lens use in 61 patients aged 70 years and older who had bilateral cataracts and were admitted for first-eye cataract extraction. None

(3–5) Acta Ophthalmol. (Copenh.) 61:382–391, June 1983.

had a history of other ocular disorders. Thirty-one patients were selected at random to undergo implantation of a four-loop iris-clip intraocular lens, while 30 others used the Scanlens 75, a high water-content extended-wear lens with a spherical power of + 15.0 diopters (D). An attempt at early postoperative contact lens fitting was made.

Lens implantation proved impractical in 5 cases, and these patients were rehabilitated with aphakic spectacles. One patient required removal of a dislocated lens implant. One patient chose to have aphakic spectacles rather than an extended-wear lens; another had rupture of the anterior hyaloid membrane and corneal contact and underwent a vitrectomy. Three other patients stopped wearing the lens, 2 because of hypermobility and 1 because of recurring corneal edema. Final acuities were similar in the 2 groups. The inflammatory response to surgery tended to last longer in the lens implant group. Iritis developed in 5 implant patients. Final visual functioning was similar in the 2 groups. All of the contact lens wearers and all but 2 of the lens implant patients were satisfied with the outcome. These 2 patients had cystoid macular edema and reduced visual acuity.

The extended-wear contact lens probably is safer than the iris-clip intraocular lens if strict aftercare instructions are observed. Further surgery seldom is necessary in patients who are rehabilitated with contact lenses. The cataract extraction procedure is simpler when contact lenses are to be fitted. The lens implant is more convenient for the patient and is comfortable. It probably is less expensive than rehabilitation with contact lenses during the patient's lifetime. Contact lenses may be used in alert, cooperative patients who have ready access to ophthalmic care and are sufficiently mobile to seek such care.

▶ ↓ In the following 2 articles the authors have used extended-wear contact lenses for myopic patients with a success rate of approximately 50% to 80%. These patients were obviously carefully selected and highly motivated, but the success rate is still extraordinary. ◀

3–6 **Extended-Wear Contact Lenses for Myopes: Follow-up Study of 400 Cases.** Laurent Lamer (Univ. of Montreal) retrospectively re-

TABLE 1.—ADVERSE REACTIONS DURING 4 YR, 9 MO
IN 400 PATIENTS USING EXTENDED-WEAR
CONTACT LENSES FOR MYOPIA

Neovascularization	1	0.2%
Edema	2	0.5%
Giant papillary conjuctivitis	6	1.5%
Cleaning solution	11	2.7%
Corneal staining	70	17.5%
Red eye	110	27.5%

(Courtesy of Lamer, L.: Ann. Intern. Med. 98:13–20, January 1983.)

(3–6) Ophthalmology (Rochester) 90:156–161, February 1983.

TABLE 2.—OUTCOME FOR PATIENTS INITIALLY FITTED
IN 1979 OR EARLIER

Still wearing (under our care)	81%
Lost to follow-up	5%
Dropped out for variety of reasons	14%

(Courtesy of Lamer, L.: Ann. Intern. Med. 98:13–20, January 1983.)

views the results obtained in 294 women and 106 men, aged 12 to 63 years (average, 28.4 years), who were fitted with and wore perfilcon A (Permalens) extended-wear contact lenses for up to 4 years, 9 months.

The patients had degrees of ametropia ranging from −1.00 to −11.50 diopters (D). Some had astigmatism of +0.50 to +2.50 or greater (equivalent to more than 20% of the spherical values). The patients were motivated, demonstrated good personal hygiene, and had no anterior segment disease incompatible with the wearing of soft contact lenses. Recent patients were given lenses with a radius of curvature 0.3 mm flatter than the flattest K reading, or the flattest radius they felt comfortable with during the first week of wear.

Almost all patients wore the lenses continuously for a mean duration of 2 weeks, and a significant number wore them for as long as 4 weeks. Optimal or best-corrected visual acuity was obtained in 94.7% of the patients. The 400 patients used a total of 1,990 lenses during the study period, of which 25.7% broke and 14.8% were lost, showing that the lens is fragile and requires careful handling. Most complications (Table 1) were due to tight fitting in the early years of the study, which was recommended by the manufacturer. Of the 98 patients initially fitted at least 3 years ago, 81% are still wearing perfilcon A lenses (Table 2).

The main disadvantages of the perfilcon A lens are its fragility (with breaks, losses, and deposits occurring in more than 40%), short lifespan (average 13.73 months), limits of correction (no toric or presbyopic lens), limits of range (−1.00 to −19.50 D), and a single available diameter of 13.5 mm, which may not fit a large cornea. However, the high rate of success among well-selected patients far outweighs the risks of radial keratotomy as it is known today. Informed patients usually opt for this method of optical correction and remain with it despite the necessary frequent replacement of the lenses.

3-7 **Myopic Extended-Wear With the Hydrocurve II Soft Contact Lens.** Perry S. Binder (San Diego) reviewed the results obtained with a Hydrocurve II (bufilcon A) 55% contact lens, fitted in 1,099 myopic patients by 42 investigators for extended wear. A total of 533 patients

COMPLICATIONS IN PARTICIPATING PATIENTS WITH HYDROCURVE
EXTENDED-WEAR LENSES*

Complication	Time (Months)					
	1	2–6	7–12	13–24	25–36	37–48
Edema	3%	0.7%	0.7%	0.4%	0.1%	0.8%
Vascularization	0.4	2.7	3.5	4.5 †	2.6 †	7.0†
Red eye	0.8	1.0	0.4	0.9	1.1	3.4
Epithelial stain	11.9	12.8	12.3	9.7	7.6	4.0

*Findings represent percentage of slit-lamp examinations confirming compli-
cation during postfitting period. Complications were significant at FDA grades of
>1.
†More than half of these complications were reported by two investigators.
(Courtesy of Binder, P.S.: Ophthalmology (Rochester) 90:623–626, June 1983.)

(48%) have continued to wear the lenses for 3½ years. Patients were chiefly interested in extended-wear lenses for esthetic reasons. A majority had previously used hard or soft contact lenses successfully.

More than 90% of active patients had no change in contact lens acuity, as compared with spectacle acuity, during lens wear. Only 0.4% of patients lost more than one line of acuity, and the reductions in acuity were transient. No patient experienced a permanent change in acuity. Acuity of 20/20 or better was achieved by 84% of patients, and acuity of 20/30 or better by 98%. An increase in minus power of 0.25 to 1.00 diopters was necessary to achieve best-corrected vision in most patients. An average of 1.3 lenses per eye per year were replaced; this is comparable to daily-wear lenses. The most common reason for withdrawal from the study was lack of interest. Only 6% of patients were excluded because they could not be fitted. Complications are shown in the table. Complications developed in 12.4% of the patients who withdrew from the study and in 6.4% of all those entering the study. In one patient a confirmed case of microbial keratitis developed.

The Hydrocurve II 55% soft contact lens is a safe, effective modality for the correction of myopia. The major patient motivation seems to arise from the desire to eliminate both glasses and the need for daily contact lens cleaning. Complications have been infrequent, and permanent visual complications have not occurred. The extended-wear lens should be offered to a patient who is considering such convenient alternatives to daily-wear contact lenses and spectacles as orthokeratology and radial keratotomy. Highly satisfactory results can be obtained with appropriate patient selection, fitting, and follow-up.

3–8 **Corneal Swelling Response to Contact Lenses Worn Under Extended-Wear Conditions.** Most conventional hydrogel lenses sufficiently restrict corneal oxygen supply to cause corneal swelling. How-

(3–8) Invest. Ophthalmol. Vis. Sci. 24:218–226, February 1983.

ever, the wearing of these lenses on a daily basis (lens removed overnight) is considered acceptable so long as the extent of corneal swelling is no greater than the degree of physiologic swelling of the cornea that occurs during overnight sleep (about 4%). Recently, both high water-content and extremely thin hydrogel lenses have come under consideration as extended-wear lenses. Brien A. Holden, George W. Mertz, and John J. McNally (Univ. of New South Wales, Sydney) measured corneal thickness changes in 10 subjects during a 36-hour period of no contact lens wear and during 7 days of continuous wear using 1 of 3 types of hydrogel contact lenses of different back-vertex powers.

Measured on awakening, the diurnal variation in central corneal edema ranged from 1.4% to 5.1% (mean, 3.0% ± 1.2%). After sleep with lenses, the mean overnight central corneal swelling ranged from 9.7% to 15.1% for the various lenses (mean, 12.0% ± 1.9%). Higher minus-power Soflens 04 lenses caused significantly greater corneal swelling than did lower-power lenses ($P < 0.01$). The degree of corneal swelling was 10.3% ± 0.6% with the −1.25 diopter (D) lenses, 13.1% ± 0.9% with the −6.00 D lenses, and 15.1% ± 0.8% with the −9.00 D lenses. These lens power–related differences were not observed with the Hydrocurve II or Permalens lenses. No decrease in overnight corneal edema was detected during the 7 days of extended wear for any of the lenses. The mean daytime edema level with lenses ranged from 1.6% to 5.8% for the various lenses (mean, 4.0% ± 1.3%). Subjects wearing the Soflens 04 lenses, but not those wearing the Hydrocurve II or Permalens lenses, showed a gradual increase in mean daytime corneal swelling ($P < 0.01$). Obvious signs of stromal edema persisted with high minus-power low and medium water-content lenses throughout the study. Comparison of the extent of edema at eye opening with that noted 12 hours later showed that deswelling of the cornea was reasonably consistent for all lenses (mean, 8.2% ± 1.1%). Thus the level of daytime corneal edema was primarily influenced by the degree of overnight swelling.

As the results of long-term studies of the edema cycle associated with continuous contact lens wear are not yet available, it is suggested that 8% is the desirable maximal level of overnight swelling with extended-wear contact lenses, since this level allows the cornea to regain normal thickness during the day.

▶ [The bad news is that the corneas swell with full-time contact lens wear, most likely due to some deficiency in oxygen. We do not know what the long-term effect of minimal corneal edema might be, but the extended-wear contact lens patients should be carefully followed up, probably indefinitely.

3–9 **Managing Geriatric Vision Disorders: Where to Get Help.** As the population continues to age, patients with geriatric visual problems will be seen more frequently by the primary care physician, according to Frank J. Weinstock (Canton, Ohio). Recent advances (e.g.,

(3–9) Geriatrics 38:96–102, May 1983.

intraocular lens implantation or laser therapy) will benefit some of these visually impaired patients; advice concerning optical aids, sources of information, and resources that might help the visually handicapped to better cope with their situation is valuable. All patients with visual problems should receive a complete eye examination. Many vision problems can be alleviated with corrective lenses; others require medical or surgical intervention. Of equal importance is psychological support and reassurance, because most eye conditions in the elderly do not progress to the point of complete loss of sight and light perception. The legal definition of blindness requires medical verification that visual acuity is 20/200 or less, and that the visual field is restricted to less than 20 degrees. All legally blind patients are entitled to an extra income tax deduction.

A number of organizations supply products or services for visually impaired patients. Also, frequently there are local agencies that provide transportation for the visually impaired. Many public libraries carry large-print publications, and some have recorded books available on audiotape together with the necessary equipment to play them. Various local nonprofit agencies offer services to the visually handicapped, and it is recommended that the physician have a list of these organizations available. The American Academy of Ophthalmology provides information, training, and referrals for physicians treating visually handicapped patients; furthermore, the Society of Geriatric Ophthalmology is currently preparing guidelines for the geriatric ophthalmology examination.

▶ [As ophthalmologists we may sometimes forget the need to care for the entire patient and the older, visually handicapped have serious problems and specialized rehabilitation needs. Knowledge of one's community resources can make it easier for our patients with poor vision.] ◀

▶ ↓ In the following 2 articles the authors point out that there are artifacts in measuring strabismus with ophthalmic prisms. The prisms must be held properly, not superimposed on each other, and patient spectacle corrections must be compensated for. ◀

3–10 **Ophthalmic Prisms: Measurement Errors and How to Minimize Them.** John T. Thompson and David L. Guyton (Johns Hopkins Univ.) believe that the variable results obtained in strabismus surgery may be due in part to errors in measuring strabismic deviations with ophthalmic prisms. The prismatic deviation of a given prism depends on its angular position as it is held before the patient's eye. Errors can occur if a prism is used in a position for which it is not calibrated. Another source of error arises from adding or stacking 2 prisms together in the same direction to measure large strabismic deviations.

Prisms commonly are used (1) in the Prentice position, with the posterior face perpendicular to the line of sight of the deviating eye; (2) in the position of minimal deviation, in which the visual axis inside the prism is perpendicular to the line bisecting the apex angle of

---

(3–10) Ophthalmology (Rochester) 90:204–210, March 1983.

the prism; and (3) in the frontal plane position, with the posterior face of the prism held in the frontal plane of the patient. Deviation in the position of minimal deviation is very close to that in the frontal plane position; that in the Prentice position is much greater, however, and small changes from this position produce relatively large changes in deviation. The difference in deviation increases with large prisms. The frontal plane position would appear to be the most practical position, since the position of minimal deviation can be difficult to judge in clinical practice.

The deviation produced by the sum of 2 plastic prisms will always be greater than that produced by the sum of the calibrated values, since these prisms are calibrated for the position of minimal deviation. The same usually is true for glass prisms. There is no simple means, apart from using a table, to add 2 prisms accurately in the same direction. Substantial errors in prism measurement also occur when adding the effects of 2 large prisms held 1 each before each eye. There is no practical way of estimating accurately large strabismic deviations using prisms.

3–11 **Artifacts Introduced by Spectacle Lenses in the Measurement of Strabismic Deviations** are discussed by Kirk D. Scattergood, Mary H. Brown, and David L. Guyton (Johns Hopkins Univ.). The use of Prentice's rule in calculating the amount of prismatic effect obtained with decentration of a lens is well known. The induced phoria in the reading position with anisometropic spectacle corrections is readily calculated, but spectacles may add to or subtract from the apparent deviation in a strabismic patient because both visual axes of the eyes of such a patient must pass through noncorresponding areas of the respective spectacle lenses (Fig 3–1). A simplified model was used to estimate the measurement error introduced by spectacle lenses. The measured deviation of 25 mm from the center of rotation of the eye is equal to the true deviation altered by an amount proportional to the power of the glasses.

Predictions from this model were compared with what can be expected in clinical situations, using ray tracing analysis with typical front and back curvatures for commonly used spectacle lenses of -20, -10, $+10$, and $+20$ diopters. The arbitrary value of true deviation was 30 prism diopters. Measured surgical correction per millimeter of surgery was greater for patients with myopia and less for those with hyperopia. In exotropia surgery the clinical data corresponded almost exactly with predictions from the model. In esotropia surgery the data corresponded less well, with more effect than was predicted by the model. The slope of the regression line, however, was within 2 SE of the predicted slope, and the clinical results were not significantly greater than expected from analysis.

The peripheral prismatic effects of corrective spectacle lenses intro-

(3–11) Am. J. Ophthalmol. 96:439–448, October 1983.

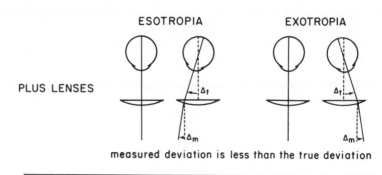

measured deviation is less than the true deviation

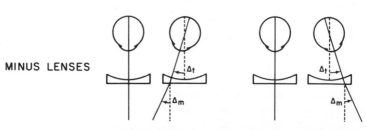

measured deviation is greater than the true deviation

Fig 3–1.—Effect of spectacle lenses on measured deviation (Δ_m) with respect to true deviation (Δ_t) in horizontal strabismus. Plus lenses always reduce deviation, whether it is esodeviation or exodeviation (or hyperdeviation); minus lenses always increase the measured deviation. (Courtesy of Scattergood, K.D., et al.: Am. J. Ophthalmol. 96:439–448, October 1983.)

duce an artifact when strabismic deviations are measured, and the effect starts to be clinically significant with lenses having powers exceeding ±5 diopters. Correcting for the artifacts should enhance the predictability of strabismus surgery in patients with significant ametropia.

3–12 **Interobserver Variation in Refraction and Visual Acuity Measurement Using a Standardized Protocol.** Reproducible measures of visual acuity and refraction are necessary to obtain valid results in clinical and population studies of ocular disorders. Ronald Klein, Barbara E. K. Klein, Scot E. Moss, and David DeMets (Univ. of Wisconsin, Madison) assessed interobserver differences in measurements made according to the Early Treatment of Diabetic Retinopathy Study (ETDRS) protocol by an experienced ophthalmologist, an optometrist, and an ophthalmic technician. The charts used were smaller versions of those described by Ferris et al. (1982). Two of the 3 examiners tested each subject in a prescribed order. No clinically significant interobserver variation was found for either refraction or visual acuity measurements among the 3 observers. The maximal dif-

(3–12) Ophthalmology (Rochester) 90:1357–1359, November 1983.

ference in refractive error was 0.19 diopter, and that in visual acuity was 1.7 letters.

This study failed to show clinically important interobserver variation when experienced examiners of differing professional backgrounds used the standardized ETDRS protocol to measure refraction and visual acuity. It appears that standardized protocols, with a training program, can yield reproducible results, at least for these ocular variables.

▶ [This work stems from the current popularity of clinical studies performed by multiple examiners in different clinics to pool data for better reliability. It has not been possible to study measurements reliably, such as cup-to-disk ratios, macular pigment, nuclear sclerosis, and the like, in multiple clinics with several investigators. Visual acuity, however, appears to be a measurement that can be successfully standardized.] ◀

3–13 **Evaluation of Night Vision Mobility Aids.** Night blindness is a major symptom of retinitis pigmentosa and other disorders that impair peripheral vision, such as advanced glaucoma and diffuse chorioretinitis. Use of a flashlight is often ineffective because of visual field restriction. Diane L. Morrissette, Michael F. Marmor, and Gregory L. Goodrich evaluated 2 night vision aids designed for use by the visually impaired, the ITT Night Vision Aid (NVA), a hand-held monocular device that amplifies light electrically to produce an image on a phosphor screen, and the Wide Angle Mobility Light (WAML), a rechargeable flashlight producing a broad, bright beam. The mobility of 24 patients with various conditions and an average acuity of 20/100 was assessed during walking over a 6-block course of residential sidewalk with poor to fair street lighting. Twelve other patients with retinitis pigmentosa, fields constricted horizontally to less than 20 degrees in diameter, and an average corrected visual acuity of 20/60 were also evaluated. Furthermore, 33 patients using the WAML were interviewed.

Error scores with the NVA did not differ significantly from the unaided nighttime results. Most patients preferred the WAML, but no significant effect of this device at night was observed in the patients with retinitis pigmentosa. The survey of 33 handicapped persons who had used a WAML for 4 to 14 months showed that all but 1 were continuing to use the device, and that a large majority believed that their confidence was greater when walking with the WAML. Twelve users reported walking more often at night than they did before using the aid. Three subjects reported malfunctions.

User acceptance of the WAML as a mobility aid exceeds that of the NVA, which must be hand held in front of the eye and is a monocular, monochromatic device. The WAML, though heavier, permits the subject to use binocular vision within a lighted zone. Patients should be given an opportunity to try all available aids.

▶ [The authors of this article have performed a careful review of use of 2 visual aids,

(3–13) Ophthalmology (Rochester) 90:1226–1230, October 1983.

but they also make the important point that patients must be shown all available aids and helped to select the best for their needs. This requires time, but the reward is great if patients with decreasing vision can be helped to maintain their independence and productivity.] ◄

3–14   **Visual Prognosis of Disciform Degeneration in Myopia.** Disciform degeneration is believed to develop in up to 10% of myopic eyes with an axial length exceeding 26.5 mm, but its visual prognosis is unclear. G. Robert Hampton, Davut Kohen, and Alan C. Bird undertook a retrospective study of the visual outcome after subretinal neovascularization of recent onset in 39 myopic patients. Forty-two eyes with angiographically proved subretinal neovascularization had been symptomatic for 6 months or less, and in all but 4 cases, 3 months or less. All had a diagnosis of Förster-Fuchs spot. No other ocular disease was present. Most of the 27 evaluable patients had refractive errors of -10 to -15 diopters.

The neovascular disease initially was subfoveal in 58% of eyes, juxtafoveal in 23%, and extrafoveal in 19%. Nearly 80% of all complexes were 400 μ or more in diameter. At last follow-up, vision had improved in 1 eye, was unchanged in 11, and had deteriorated in 29. The group had lost an average of 1.6 lines since presentation. Presenting acuity was inversely related to size of the neovascular complex. Larger neovascularizations were likelier to be subfoveal. Patients older than age 30 had a significant reduction in vision at follow-up. Forty-two percent of the eyes were potentially treatable at presentation, and only 35% of these subsequently became untreatable.

Disciform degeneration in myopia appears to have a poor visual prognosis. Final vision is related to the distance of the fovea from the neovascular complex and inversely to the size of the disciform lesion. Most patients have deteriorating or stable vision after presentation. The findings challenge the view that laser treatment is unnecessary in these cases because of a generally good visual outcome, although few treatable patients had significant visual loss during follow-up.

► [It is evident that disciform degeneration in myopia has a poor prognosis and consequently ranks with senile macular degeneration, diabetic retinopathy, and glaucoma as a major cause of blindness. Laser therapy, as in senile macular degeneration, is only effective in the few patients who have active neovascular membranes distant from the fovea.] ◄

(3–14)   Ophthalmology (Rochester) 90:923–926, August 1983.

4. Conjunctiva

Blepharitis

JOEL SUGAR, M.D.

Eye and Ear Infirmary
University of Illinois, Chicago

While our recent annual reviews have covered new topics, these are sometimes difficult to find and not of broad interest in the area of the conjunctiva. For this reason and because the editor of this book suffers from blepharitis, we have decided to review briefly the categories and treatments of blepharitis.

Staphylococcal blepharitis is significantly less common than is seborrheic or mixed seborrheic and staphylococcal blepharitis.[1] Clinically it is associated with the presence of brittle crusts and fibrinous scales as well as collarettes around the lashes. Lid margin telangiectases, poliosis, and broken and absent lashes are seen. Chalazia and hordeolae are frequent. Angular involvement can occur and papillae are infrequently seen in the conjunctiva. Corneal changes include punctate staining, especially at the four o'clock and eight o'clock position where the eyelid crosses the limbus; catarrhal ulcers, and phlyctenules.

Seborrheic blepharitis is characterized by the presence of greasy scales, scurf (oily debris), foam along the lid margin, and lid margin erythema. These patients also have facial seborrhea including scaling of the scalp, brows, forehead, and nasolabial folds. Mixed blepharitis, that is, combined seborrheic and staphylococcal blepharitis, is very common.

Meibomianitis, rather than predominantly involving the anterior lid margin which is seen with staphylococcal and some seborrheic blepharitis, involves the meibomian glands with excess secretions and plugging of the glands. These patients experience more burning, mattering, and ocular redness. Ocular signs include those of seborrheic blepharitis in addition to plugging and stagnation in the meibomian glands, papillary conjunctivitis, superficial punctate keratopathy, and rapid tear film breakup time. Meibomitis may be observed frequently with seborrheic blepharitis, and rosacea is commonly associated. Rosacea is an entity characterized by facial erythema, telangiectases, papular and pustular skin eruptions, and hypertrophy of sebaceous glands without the presence of comedones (blackheads). When advanced hypertrophy involves the skin of the nose, it is called rhinophyma. Eyelid involvement combines seborrheic and meibomianitis changes. Corneal involvement resembles that seen with phlyctenular disease with small, white intraepithelial infiltrates and superficial vascularization. Ulceration and even perforation can occur. Alkaline tear pH has been reported[2] but more recent studies have not confirmed this.[3] Abnormalities in the lipids present in the meibomian glands of patients with meibomianitis and rosacea have been investigated and some changes in the lipids have been found, although these changes have not as yet been well characterized.[4]

Other entities may be associated with blepharitis including atopic keratoconjunctivitis and infectious diseases involving the eyelids such as primary herpes simplex and herpes zoster. The use of systemic retinoids (Acutane) for acne has also been associated with blepharitis, which we discussed in last year's YEAR BOOK.

Treatment can be broken down into both general treatment of blepharitis and specific treatment. General treatment is that which is helpful for all forms of blepharitis. This includes warm compresses usually for 5 to 10 minutes twice daily and lid scrubs. We recommend lid scrubs with a moist cotton-tipped applicator and a small amount of baby shampoo to create a lather along the closed lid margins immediately following application of the warm compresses. This therapy is of benefit, in general, to all forms of blepharitis. Staphylococcal blepharitis, especially ulcerative staphylococcal blepharitis, may respond well to topical antibiotics. Meibomianitis, especially that seen with rosacea, is impressively responsive to systemic tetracycline, which is given initially in a dose of 250 mg by mouth 4 times daily on an empty stomach. Chalazia, which can occur with all the forms of blepharitis that we have discussed, may respond to lid hygiene alone. If they do not, it is our preference to inject a small amount of intralesional corticosteroid which is often exceedingly effective.[5] It is unusual for surgical excision to be necessary.

While we have reviewed only basic information on blepharitis, we believe that this review may be beneficial because of the frequency with which blepharitis is encountered in ophthalmic practice.

References
1. McCulley, J.P., Dougherty, J.M., and Deneau, D.G.: Chronic blepharitis: classification and mechanisms. In Proceedings, Immunology of the Eye: Workshop III. Suran, A., Gery, I., and Nussenblatt, R.B. (Eds.) *Immunol. Abstr.* (Spec. Suppl.), 1981.
2. Abelson, M.B., Sadun, A.A., Udell I.J., et al.: Alkaline tear pH in ocular rosacea. *Am. J. Ophthalmol.* 90:866–869, 1980.
3. Browning, D.J.: Tear pH in ocular rosacea. *Invest. Ophthalmol. Vis. Sci.* 25(Suppl.):41, 1984.
4. Dougherty, J.M., and McCulley, J.P.: Comparative analysis of the free

fatty acid component of meibomian secretions from normals and patients with chronic blepharitis. *Invest. Ophthalmol. Vis. Sci.* 25(Suppl.):191, 1984.

5. Pizzarello, L.D., et al.: Intralesional corticosteroid therapy of chalazia. *Am. J. Ophthalmol.* 85:818–821, 1978.

4-1 **Dry Eye and Tear Deficiency** are discussed by David W. Lamberts. The tear film is composed of a lipid layer, an aqueous layer, and a mucous layer. A tear deficiency exists when 1 or more of these 3 components is present in insufficient quantity to maintain the health of the epithelium. Lipid deficiency is rare. Aqueous-deficiency diseases are common and form part of the triad (together with xerostomia and rheumatoid arthritis) that constitutes Sjögren's syndrome. Mucin-deficient dry eyes are less common than the aqueous-deficient types. The final common pathway of all dry-eye diseases, regardless of origin, is desiccation and necrosis of the corneal and conjunctival epithelium, with the cornea ultimately responding with vessel ingrowth and scarring.

Clinical findings that are common in dry-eye diseases include tear film floaters, which are desquamated epithelial cells from the cornea and conjunctival surface. Filaments, which are epithelial-covered mucin strands attached to the corneal epithelium, make blinking uncomfortable. Corneal mucous plaques are flat, transparent, or opaque deposits on the surface of the cornea. Papillary conjunctivitis is also common in dry-eye diseases.

Dry-eye syndromes are common and may initially be unilateral. Rose-Bengal staining is the best single test for diagnosing these syndromes. It stains dry, dying epithelial cells, filaments, and mucus strands, and, in dry-eye states, triangles of stain can be seen within the interpalpebral fissure, with the bases directed toward the limbus. Schirmer's test tends to give variable results and is most useful if repeated measurements give consistently low results.

All dry-eye diseases are treated similarly, using tear replacement, preservation, or stimulation. Many artificial teardrop preparations are available that are basically similar in function. A new type of artificial tear preparation that some patients have found useful consists of a small pellet of hydroxypropyl methylcellulose (Lacrisert) that is inserted in the inferior cul-de-sac and dissolves over several hours, releasing the artificial tear polymer.

Methods used to preserve tears include punctal occlusion (usually via electrocautery), punctum plugs (not readily available in the United States), plastic wraps and swimmer's goggles (useful in homebound, moribund, and comatose patients), and soft contact lenses (most useful for patients whose eyes are mucin-deficient but still wet enough to provide a milieu for the lens, and for patients with exposure keratitis and filaments).

(4–1) Int. Ophthalmol. Clin. 23:123–130, Spring 1983.

Orally administered bromhexine hydrochloride shows promise as a lacrogenic agent. Other medications given for systemic effect that may stimulate the lacrimal gland into greater production include eledoisin, psysalaemin, and pilocarpine.

▶ [This is a brief but fine review of the dry eye which is a common and difficult therapeutic problem. In this, and the following article, the slow-dissolving hydroxypropyl methylcellulose pellet is described. Only 50% of a group of difficult practolol-therapy patients with dry eyes (oculomucocutaneous syndrome) continued to use the pellet, although there were essentially no complications from the insert. Patients did struggle to keep the pellet in the cul-de-sac, but the dry-eye problem is so serious that treatment with an insert appears to be beneficial for some patients and a trial seems reasonable for selected patients.] ◀

4–2 **Slow-Release Artificial Tear Inserts in Treatment of Dry Eyes Resulting From Oculomucocutaneous Syndrome.** Patients with dry eyes resulting from the oculomucocutaneous (OMC) syndrome present a therapeutic challenge. In most cases, frequent instillation of preservative-free tear substitutes is the only therapy. P. Wright and R. Vogel (London) evaluated the therapeutic efficacy of a slow-release artificial tear insert in 11 patients (mean age, 64.5 years) with the OMC syndrome. The insert consists of a 5-mg rod of hydroxypropyl cellulose, approximately 1 × 3 mm in size, that is inserted into the inferior fornix where it imbibes water from the conjunctiva. Within a few minutes after insertion, the rod swells to form a small soft mass (Fig 4–1), which dissolves to coat the conjunctiva and cornea with a hydrophilic film that stabilizes the tear film and hydrates and lubricates the cornea.

All but 1 of the patients were using tear substitutes more often

Fig 4–1.—Slow-release artificial tear insert in lower fornix is seen as an ovoid which initially is a rod that swells to form the small soft mass. (Courtesy of Wright, P., and Vogel, R.: Br. J. Ophthalmol. 67:393–397, June 1983.)

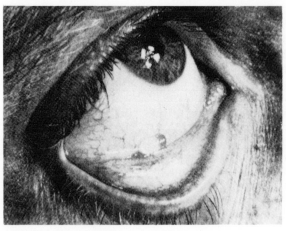

than once every 30 minutes at the time of the prestudy examination. Observations and symptoms were scored on a 0 to 3 scale: 0 = absent, 1 = very slight, 2 = moderate, 3 = very troublesome. Patients with an absence of or with slight symptoms had a total score of 16 at the time of the prestudy examination. After 5 weeks of use of the slow-release artificial tear inserts, the total score in this group of patients had increased to 29. Conversely, 5 weeks of insert use in patients with moderate or very troublesome symptoms resulted in a decrease in the total score from 29 to 16. Scoring for precorneal tear film and marginal strip and for rose-Bengal staining showed a similar pattern.

All patients in the study had some degree of fornix shortening and all but 1 experienced some difficulty from ejection of the inserts. However, all found some means to overcome this problem and no patient left the study solely because they were unable to retain the insert. Only 5 patients completed the study protocol. All 6 who withdrew from the study before its completion reported that they experienced more instant relief from eyedrops than from the inserts. Two of these 6 patients also were unable to tolerate the inserts. There were no adverse local or systemic reactions to the inserts. The slit-lamp appearance of the inferior fornix remained unchanged and the visual acuity was unaltered on the average during the study.

The level of acceptance of this new treatment system in this extremely difficult to treat group of patients is encouraging. The use of this system or similar inserts would be worth considering in the management of patients with troublesome dry-eye symptoms.

▶ ↓ In the following 2 articles, the same authors discuss the epidemiology, clinical findings, and treatment of patients in an outbreak of acute hemorrhagic conjunctivitis. Topical corticosteroids were not helpful and isolation and good hygiene were apparently not only important but the only defense against rapid spread of the disease. ◀

4–3 **Acute Hemorrhagic Conjunctivitis: Investigation of a Large-Scale Community Outbreak in Dade County, Florida** is reported by Peter A. Patriarca, Ida M. Onorato, Virgil E. F. Sklar, Lawrence B. Schonberger, Rose M. Kaminski, Milford H. Hatch, David M. Morens, and Richard K. Forster. Acute hemorrhagic conjunctivitis (AHC) was not recognized in the western hemisphere until Southeast Asian refugees entered the United States in 1980. An explosive outbreak occurred in the Miami region in September 1981. The diagnostic criteria included an onset within 48 hours of known exposure, foreign-body sensation, watery discharge, swelling of the eyelids, bilateral involvement, follicular involvement, and subconjunctival hemorrhage. A total of 2,689 cases were reported by 44 outpatient clinic surveillance sites in a 4-month period. The outbreak was due to enterovirus type 70. There was 1 case of Bell's palsy, but no radiculomyelitis was reported, and there were no marked ocular sequelae attributable to AHC.

(4–3) JAMA 249:1283–1289, Mar. 11, 1983.

The risk of AHC was increased in younger persons, members of larger households, and the poor. The infection was most likely to be introduced into households by schoolchildren, and reported cases declined sharply after exclusion of all affected children from school. Acute hemorrhagic conjunctivitis spread readily among family members, but simple hygienic measures were associated with lower attack rates.

This is the first known outbreak of AHC in a major metropolitan area in the United States. Spread of infection was facilitated in the home and schools also were important sites of transmission. Acute hemorrhagic conjunctivitis is a highly contagious illness that warrants attention by public health officials and clinicians in this country. Whether it will become endemic is uncertain, but experience in developing countries suggests that this may occur. Control measures are best directed at residents of densely populated, poor neighborhoods, where simple hygienic measures may reduce transmission of the infection.

4–4 **Clinical Findings and Results of Treatment in an Outbreak of Acute Hemorrhagic Conjunctivitis in Southern Florida.** Among the Southeast Asian refugees who arrived in the United States in 1980 were some who showed symptoms of hemorrhagic conjunctivitis. The first epidemic of this readily transmitted infection occurred in Miami in September 1981 and involved about 800 confirmed and 2,500 suspected cases.

INITIAL SYMPTOMS AND SIGNS OF ACUTE HEMORRHAGIC CONJUNCTIVITIS

Findings	No. of Patients
Symptoms	
Discharge	97
Foreign-body sensation	92
Burning	82
Sensation of eyelid swelling	80
Signs	
Follicular reaction	94
Eyelid edema	84
Superior conjunctival hemorrhage	82
Inferior conjunctival hemorrhage	70
Preauricular adenopathy	67
Bilateral involvement	58

(Courtesy of Sklar, V.E.F., et al.: Am. J. Ophthalmol. 95:45–54, January 1983.)

(4–4) Am. J. Ophthalmol. 95:45–54, January 1983.

V. E. F. Sklar, P. A. Patriarca, I. M. Onorato, M. P. Langford, S. W. Clark, W. W. Culbertson, and R. K. Forster report that most patients lived in a poor neighborhood and were between the ages of 10 and 29 years. Nearly 60% of the patients were female. Enterovirus was considered the causative agent in the outbreak. The most common symptoms included a profuse, predominantly watery discharge, foreign-body sensation, burning, swelling of the eyelids, and pain in the upper eyelid. Most patients noted onset of symptoms within 24 hours of known exposure to affected individuals; coryza was frequent but fever, myalgias, and headaches occurred in less than 5% of patients. Initial symptoms and signs of acute hemorrhagic conjunctivitis are summarized in the table.

To determine optimal treatment methods, 100 consecutive patients were placed in groups of 20: group 1 applied cold compresses 4 times each day and was used as a control to determine the natural course of the disease; the other 4 groups were treated with artificial tears, a decongestant (Vasocon A), prednisolone acetate (Pred Forte, 1%), or a combination of decongestant and prednisolone acetate 1%. All medications were applied topically 4 times a day.

Comparison of the data from all 5 groups indicated that the time course of acute hemorrhagic conjunctivitis was not significantly changed by any of the topical therapeutic regimens described. Mean time of resolution varied from 3 to 10 days; the follicular conjunctival reaction was slowest to improve.

To help prevent widespread dissemination of this readily disseminated infection it is recommended that patients remain home for 7 days after onset of symptoms and that they be given instructions describing proper hygienic precautions to avoid contamination of family members.

4–5 **Conjunctival Eosinophils in Allergic Ocular Disease.** It frequently is difficult to diagnose ocular allergy clinically. Mark B. Abelson, Nalini Madiwale, and Judith H. Weston (Boston) reviewed the findings in tarsal conjunctival scrapings from both eyes of 317 patients with ocular allergy. The diagnosis was based on the patient and family histories and on the presence of pruritus, chemosis, and vasodilation of scleral and conjunctival vessels. Scrapings were obtained before and after 1 week of treatment with a combination product of 0.05% naphazoline and 0.5% antazoline, the vasoconstrictor alone, the antihistamine alone, or a phosphate-buffered saline solution placebo. The diagnosis was vernal conjunctivitis in 27 cases, hay fever conjunctivitis in 147, atopic keratoconjunctivitis in 68, and nonspecific allergic conjunctivitis in 75. Eosinophils were present in scrapings from 63% of patients with vernal conjunctivitis, in 45% of those with hay fever conjunctivitis, and in 25% of each of the other groups. Eosinophils were found in biopsy specimens taken from a pa-

(4–5) Arch. Ophthalmol. 101:555–556, April 1983.

tient with vernal keratoconjunctivitis, despite their absence in conjunctival scrapings from the same eye.

Eosinophils are not consistently found in conjunctival scrapings from patients with allergic ocular conditions, especially those with milder states, and their absence should not preclude a diagnosis of allergic ocular disease. The diagnosis should be based on the history, symptoms, and signs of disease. The presence of eosinophils in scrapings of the conjunctiva supports the diagnosis of allergic ocular disease.

▶ ↓ Allergic conjunctivitis is caused by pollens, molds, animal dander, and the like. In the first of the following 3 articles the authors point out that the diagnosis usually cannot be connfirmed by eosinophils in conjunctival scrapings since they are located deep in the tissue. The diagnosis is based on the seasonal nature of the disease with chemosis, vasodilation, and an absence of lid or corneal involvement.

Literally millions of bottles of decongestants are sold each year. In the following 2 articles, several therapeutic products are assessed. Not surprisingly, there is little difference between the popular brands containing both a vasoconstrictor and a decongestant. Cromolyn, however, at least for the milder cases of allergic conjunctivitis associated with ragweed, seems efficacious and has few side effects. ◀

4-6 **Double-Masked Comparison of Ocular Decongestants as Therapy for Allergic Conjunctivitis.** During episodes of allergic conjunctivitis, the conjunctiva and eyelids become edematous and hyperemic, accompanied by itching, watery rhinorrhea, nasal obstruction, and sneezing. B. Q. Lanier, N. Tremblay, Judson P. Smith, and J. M. deFaller (Fort Worth, Texas) conducted a prospective, randomized, double-masked study of 3 commercially available ocular decongestants to compare their relative efficacies in the treatment of allergic conjunctivitis.

The 3 drugs tested were Albalon-A, Vasocon-A, and Naphcon-A. The first 2 preparations contain 0.05% naphazoline HCl and 0.5% antazoline phosphate, whereas Naphcon-A contains 0.025% naphazoline HCl and the antihistamine, pheniramine maleate, 0.3%. Baseline values of the following ocular signs were graded: lid swelling without

MEAN COMPOSITE SCORES FOR OCULAR SIGNS AND SYMPTOMS

a. Ocular signs

Treatment group	Pretherapy	30 Minutes	Day 1
Preparation No. 1	1.2738	0.2976*	0.2222*
Preparation No. 2	1.3500	0.1111	0.0500
Preparation No. 3	1.3889	0.1500	0.1333

b. Ocular symptoms

Treatment group	Pretherapy	30 Minutes	Day 1
Preparation No. 1	0.9643	0.1905*	0.1250
Preparation No. 2	1.0611	0.0611	0.0667
Preparation No. 3	1.1222	0.1056	0.0833

*Statistically significant differences, $P < .05$.
(Courtesy of Lanier, B.Q., et al.: Ann. Allergy 50:174–177, March 1983.)

(4–6) Ann. Allergy 50:174–177, March 1983.

erythema, palpebral conjunctival inflammation, and bulbar conjunctival inflammation. Ocular symptoms of tearing, itching, and discomfort were also graded. Eighty-nine patients were randomly assigned to 1 of the 3 treatment groups. Two drops of the assigned medication were instilled into the affected eyes; after 30 minutes, ocular signs and symptoms were again graded. The patients were then released and instructed to instill 2 drops of the assigned medication into each eye 4 times daily for 1 week. Follow-up examinations were conducted on days 1 and 7 with grading of signs and symptoms as well as evaluation of response to treatment.

Ocular signs and symptoms scores were averaged for both eyes of each patient. After which, a composite score was calculated; the mean composite scores are given in the table for each treatment group. All patients using Vasocon-A and Naphcon-A had excellent to good follow-up impressions after 30 minutes and 1 day. Results in 3 patients using Albalon-A were rated poor after 30 minutes; by day 1, 4 patients had discontinued treatment in this group, and the result in 1 patient was rated poor.

All drugs produced statistically significant ($P < .01$) reduction of lid swelling, palpebral and bulbar conjunctival inflammation, tearing, itching, and discomfort. Albalon-A, however, produced excessive stinging and burning with topical instillation. All 3 preparations contain a vasoconstrictor and an antihistamine, which accounts for their efficacy; the remaining components of the 3 preparations show considerable differences, which may account for the differences in comfort described. The physician should be familiar with the ingredients and strengths of available preparations and prescribe the lowest concentration of any drug to achieve the desired therapeutic effect.

4–7 **Treatment of Ragweed Allergic Conjunctivitis With Cromolyn Sodium 4% Ophthalmic Solution.** Cromolyn sodium is effective in the prophylaxis of asthma, allergic rhinitis, and other histamine-mediated conditions and has been reported to be effective in treating allergic conjunctivitis. Gilbert A. Friday, Albert W. Biglan, David A. Hiles, Stephen M. Murphey, D. Lee Miller, Craig Rothbach, and Stephen Rand (Pittsburgh) conducted a randomized, double-blind, placebo-controlled trial to assess its efficacy in preventing and treating ragweed allergic conjunctivitis in 19 male and 12 female patients aged 8 to 53 years who had required symptomatic medication for this condition for 2 to 30 years, had skin sensitivity to ragweed pollen, and had serum levels of IgE ragweed antibody of 2 to 1,316 ng/ml.

The trial began 1 week before the usual onset of the ragweed pollen season and ended 45 days later. Patients received 4% cromolyn sodium or placebo, 2 drops in each eye 4 times daily, for a total dosage of 25.6 mg of cromolyn sodium per day.

Preseason serum levels of IgE antibody to ragweed were found to

(4–7) Am. J. Ophthalmol. 95:169–174, February 1983.

predict drug response. Of 16 patients with ragweed IgE values of less than 100 ng/ml, the 9 treated with cromolyn had significantly fewer symptoms during the trial than the 7 treated with placebo. Of the 15 patients with ragweed IgE levels of more than 100 ng/ml, the 8 treated with cromolyn improved but the difference between their symptom scores and those of the 7 patients treated with placebo was not significant.

Analysis of the low ragweed IgE subgroups showed significant differences in favor of cromolyn treatment for itchy eyes, ocular irritation, total ocular symptoms, stuffy nose, total nose symptoms, and use of chlorpheniramine. Side effects included mild burning of the eyes when the drops were instilled, reported by 13 patients in each treatment group, and incidental reports of nasal symptoms and red eyes.

Patients with ragweed conjunctivitis, particularly those with low but significant ragweed IgE levels, may benefit from topical treatment with an ophthalmic solution of cromolyn sodium, either alone or in combination with other medications to treat the disease. The greatest benefit of the drug may be in the reduction of corticosteroid use by patients with severe symptoms.

4–8 **IgG-Specific Antibodies to Rye Grass and Ragweed Pollen Antigens in Tear Secretions of Patients With Vernal Conjunctivitis.** Vernal conjunctivitis has been shown to be an atopic ocular disorder with an IgE-mediated pathogenesis. Hypothesizing that other immune mechanisms may play a role in its pathogenesis, Mark Ballow, Peter C. Donshik, Louis Mendelson, Pamela Rapacz, and Kenneth Sparks (Univ. of Connecticut, Farmington) measured specific IgG antibodies to 2 inhalant pollen allergens, rye grass and ragweed antigen E, in the tears of 25 male and 5 female patients, aged 8 to 34 years (mean, 13 years) who had vernal conjunctivitis and in 24 control subjects (8 without atopy, 4 with seasonal rhinitis, and 12 with allergic conjunctivitis). An enzyme-linked immunosorbent assay was used for the studies.

Of the 30 patients with vernal conjunctivitis, 18 (60%) had significant levels of IgG antibodies to rye grass and 20 (67%) had significant levels of IgG antibodies to ragweed antigen E. Control subjects had only low levels of specific IgG antibodies to these 2 pollen antigens in their tears. Total IgG and IgM were also increased in patients with vernal conjunctivitis.

To evaluate whether these immunoglobulins and specific IgG antibodies were produced locally by the conjunctival tissues, transferrin was used as a marker for leakage of plasma proteins into the tears. These studies showed that 20% to 99.9% of the specific IgG antibodies to one or both of the allergens were produced locally, supporting the hypothesis that the external eye can produce a local immune response even in the absence of systemic immunity.

(4–8) Am. J. Ophthalmol. 95:161–168, February 1983.

Specific IgG antibodies to rye grass or ragweed antigen E, or both, were found in the tears of 14 and 17 (82%) patients with vernal conjunctivitis and undetectable pollen-specific IgE antibodies in their tears but in only 9 of 13 (69%) with measurable IgE antibodies. Both IgE- and IgG-mediated immune mechanisms may be important in the pathogenesis of vernal conjunctivitis.

▶ [IgG antibodies to rye grass and ragweed antigen may be produced in the conjunctiva of patients with vernal conjunctivitis. If true, this immune mechanism may be an important part of the disease process and may suggest new therapeutic and prophylactic approaches.] ◀

▶ ↓ In the following article, the authors suggest another approach to vernal conjunctivitis. They believe that the prostaglandins may be involved and they thus treated patients with aspirin to inhibit its synthesis. The authors' results are impressive and it seems reasonable to try aspirin, especially if there is a chance to decrease or eliminate the use of corticosteroids. ◀

4–9 **Aspirin Therapy in Vernal Conjunctivitis.** Prostaglandin D_2 is a secondary mast cell mediator that causes redness, chemosis, mucous discharge, and eosinophil chemotaxis in the eye and may play an important role in allergic ocular disease. Histamine is a key mediator of allergic inflammation, but antihistamine therapy provides only symptomatic relief. The pathophysiology of both mastocytosis and vernal conjunctivitis involves mast cell abnormalities, and aspirin therapy is beneficial in patients with mastocytosis. Aspirin acetylates the enzyme cyclo-oxygenase, thereby preventing formation of prostaglandin D_2.

Mark B. Abelson, Salim I. Butrus, and Judith H. Weston (Boston) evaluated the effectiveness of adding aspirin therapy to the treatment regimens of 3 patients, aged 9 to 17 years, with intractable vernal conjunctivitis. Aspirin was given in doses of 325 mg every 2 hours, 81 mg every 3 hours, or 650 mg 3 times a day. Within 2 weeks, 1 week, or 2 days, respectively, there was dramatic improvement in conjunctival and episcleral redness and resolution of keratitis and limbal infiltration.

A trial of orally administered aspirin is recommended as adjunctive therapy for patients with recalcitrant vernal conjunctivitis and for those who require long-term use or high doses of corticosteroids for control.

4–10 **Contact Lens-Induced Giant Papillary Conjunctivitis.** T. Neuhann (Univ. of Mainz, W. Germany) describes the characteristic features of contact lens-induced giant papillary conjunctivitis observed in 64 patients between 1978 and 1980. The main symptoms are increasing lens intolerance with foreign body sensation, mucous discharge, and reduced vision. The typical subtarsal sign is cobblestone formation resembling vernal conjunctivitis. Indentation and edema of the conjunctiva form giant papillae of irregular limits with a diame-

(4–9)   Am. J. Ophthalmol. 95:502–505, April 1983.
(4–10)   Klin. Monatsbl. Augenheilkd. 182:46–50, January 1983.

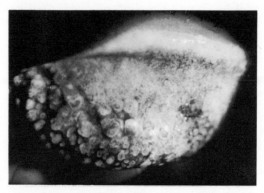

Fig 4–2.—Conjunctiva of upper lid in 27-year-old woman wearing silicon lenses for 18 months. Numerous definite giant papillae are seen covering the greater part; stage III. (Courtesy of Neuhann, T.: Klin. Monatsbl. Augenheilkd. 182:46–50, January 1983.)

ter larger than 1 mm and several blood vessels in the center (Fig 4–2). Discontinuing lens wear is sufficient only in the less pronounced cases (stage I and II).

Although postobservational periods are too short and patient numbers too small for a final assessment, 9 patients wear contact lenses without problems. Two patients experienced difficulties after 4 to 6 months and currently wear contact lenses only occasionally and glasses the rest of the time. One patient (stage IV) needed surgery and wears glasses only. In the fully developed cases (12 patients) additional cryocoagulation of the lesions proved to be effective.

This author's observations coincide closely with those of Spring (1974) and Allansmith et al. (1977); however, 2 differences should be noted. In this study, the complaint-free period prior to conjunctivitis is longer than the one reported by the other authors. The most likely reason is the difference in the method of cleaning and disinfection. At the time of the study in the United States, boiling after cleaning with saline solution was the only accepted procedure for soft lenses. The patients included in this study cleaned and disinfected their lenses with a chemical solution. Saline solution will not remove material from the lens surface and boiling makes the remaining particles adhere firmly to the lens. With chemical cleaning a thorough removal of the deposit is possible, and by storing the lenses in a disinfecting solution additional cleaning is accomplished. Also according to this study, therapy must achieve complete disappearance of the conjunctival lesion to avoid recurrences. The difference in the clinical pattern between this group of patients and that of Allansmith et al. (1977) support the opinion that surface deposits on the contact lenses are pathogenically of prime importance.

▶ [Contact lens deposits are implicated in the lens-induced giant papillary conjunctivitis. If this is so, one wonders if the incidence of the disease is going to increase with increased use of the long-wear contact lenses. It is disappointing to learn that discontinuing lens wear did not cure the more severe cases, but cryotherapy seems a little severe for the disease in question.] ◄

▶ ↓ The following is a concise and reasonably informative review of Reiter's syndrome. It's unfortunate that a disease first described almost 70 years ago should still be an enigma. ◄

4–11 **Reiter's Syndrome** according to Yehudi M. Felman and James A. Nikitas (State Univ. of New York, Brooklyn), is a disease of unknown cause, but it is secondary to either an enteritis or an infection of the genital tract due to sexually transmittted disease. The only organism isolated from patients has been *Chlamydia trachomatis.* Rheumatic disorders are more frequent in the families of affected patients, and up to 90% of patients with Reiter's syndrome have the histocompatibility antigen HLA-B27. Both venereal and dysenteric forms of the syndrome occur, the latter predominating in the United States and Europe. The disorder is seen throughout the world and affects both sexes and all ages.

Urethritis is the initial manifestation of the venereal form of Reiter's syndrome. It is followed in a few days by conjunctivitis in fewer than 50% of cases, and by a polyarticular, asymmetric arthritis. In dysenteric cases these abnormalities occur nearly simultaneously. The conjunctivitis usually is bilateral and mild and resolves within a month. It can recur with persistence or relapse of the syndrome. Corneal ulceration and keratitis occasionally develop. Anterior uveitis can occur late in the course in association with chronic sacroiliitis. About 25% of patients develop lesions on the glans penis and foreskin, and fewer have keratotic lesions on the soles. Buccal mucosal lesions are also seen in 10% of cases. The course is characterized by exacerbations and remissions and by recurrences more severe than the initial attack.

The treatment of Reiter's syndrome is directed at reducing symptoms. The urethritis is treated with tetracycline. Mydriatics and corticosteroid eyedrops are generally used for iritis, and systemic corticosteroid therapy may be necessary if posterior uveitis develops. Most patients require an antiinflammatory agent such as indomethacin for the arthritis. Prednisone is considered in refractory cases. Concomitant sexually transmitted diseases must be treated at the same time.

4–12 **Adult Polio-Like Syndrome Following Enterovirus 70 Conjunctivitis (Natural History of the Disease).** The epidemics of an unusual type of conjunctivitis that occurred in the Indian subcontinent in 1971 and 1981 were caused by Enterovirus type 70 (EV 70), which has neurovirulent properties. B. C. Katiyar, S. Misra, R. B. Singh, A. K. Singh, Saroj Gupta, A. K. Gulati, S. Christopher, and T. Jacob John evaluated data on 79 patients seen at Banaras Hindu Univ. in Varanasi, India, with neurologic complications developing as

(4–11) Cutis 31:152–156, 164, February 1983.
(4–12) Acta Neurol. Scand. 67:263–274, May 1983.

a result of the 1981 epidemic. Most of the 54 males and 25 females were aged 15 to 45 years. The disorder began with an episode of conjunctivitis (Fig 4–3) that was mild except in 9 patients who had severe hemorrhagic conjunctivitis; its mean duration was 5 days. A preparalytic stage lasting for 4 or 5 days with fever, pain, and fasciculations was followed by a paralytic stage of acute onset, with limb or cranial nerve involvement. Paralysis progressed from the upper to the lower extremities, or the reverse, or from one side to the other; it usually was asymmetric and flaccid. The deep reflexes were sluggish or absent. Forty patients had cranial nerve involvement, primarily of the seventh or the fifth nerve. Recovery usually was slow in patients with limb involvement.

Mild leukocytosis and an elevated sedimentation rate were the only frequent laboratory abnormalities. The cerebrospinal fluid (CSF) levels of lymphocytes and protein were increased in the first month of disease. Electrophysiologic studies suggested a proximal lesion at the level of the anterior horn cells or the motor roots. Terminal latencies were prolonged, motor conduction velocities were slightly reduced, and the amplitude of the motor action potentials was decreased; sensory conduction was normal. Electromyography showed active denervation and evidence of reinnervation in some cases. Serum and CSF titers of antibody to EV 70 were elevated in patients with limb or cranial nerve involvement, but serum titers were also high in some controls. Muscle biopsy specimens from patients with limb involvement showed "group atrophy" of muscle fibers and normal or hypertrophied fibers, as well as segmental necrosis and aggregation of muscle cell nuclei and changes of regeneration. Lymphocytic infiltration was found in a few biopsy specimens.

This disorder seems related to damage to the anterior horn cells of the spinal cord or cranial nerve nuclei caused by EV 70. Specific ther-

Fig 4–3.—Natural history of the conjunctivitis that developed after Enterovirus 70 infection. (Courtesy of Katiyar, B.C., et al.: Acta Neurol. Scand. 67:263–274, May 1983.)

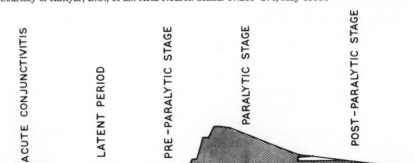

apy is unavailable, suggesting the need to develop a vaccine for immunization.

▶ [For those of us old enough to remember the devastation of polio, this syndrome, heralded by conjunctivitis, is frightening to contemplate. It is important to note that there were cases of the Enterovirus conjunctivitis in Florida during the 1981 global epidemic.] ◀

5. Cornea and Sclera

Refractive Surgery

RONALD E. SMITH, M.D.

University of Southern California,
Los Angeles

Surgical procedures designed to modify the shape of the cornea and correct refractive errors have received increasing attention during the past year.

Techniques for surgically modifying the refractive power of the cornea are not new. More than 20 years ago, Jose Barraquer (Bogota, Colombia) developed the keratophakia and keratomileusis surgical procedures to correct aphakia and high degrees of myopia using cryolathed corneal lenticules. Only within the past few years, however, have these techniques been introduced in the United States, and results are now being published. Radial keratotomy for low degrees of myopia was introduced in Japan in the 1950s (Sato) and in Russia in the 1970s (Fyodorov) and has become the subject of a great deal of controversy concerning its safety, efficacy, and predictability of outcome.

At the outset, I think it is important to emphasize that regardless of the results of long-term clinical trials of these various techniques and their ultimate usefulness, the increased interest in surgically modifying the shape of the cornea by various surgical techniques has resulted in a related technological explosion. Diamond knives, ultrasonic pachymeters, keratoscopes, operating keratometers have all been developed primarily to facilitate refractive surgical procedures. Thus, ophthalmologists, whether they perform these operations or not, will benefit from this new technology. Also, please note that this introductory discussion of a few of the refractive surgery techniques represents my personal views of these procedures and should be interpreted in that light.

Keratophakia and Keratomileusis

These procedures are not only technically complex but require expensive instrumentation. In keratophakia, a lamellar button (lenticule) from a donor cornea is prepared with a microkeratome and lathe-cut on a cryolathe unit to specifications determined by keratometry and other measurements. A lamellar resection of the anterior portion of the patient's cornea is then removed with a microkeratome. After this is done the donor tissue lenticule is thawed or rehydrated and positioned in the host bed; the anterior cap of the host cornea is sutured back in place. The additional stromal thickness created by the lamellar implant adds to the dioptric power, thereby correcting a great deal of hyperopia in the aphakic eye. However, the recovery of good acuity generally takes several months, possibly related to keratocyte repopulation problems or to swelling of the stroma. A major drawback of this procedure is the need for specialized instrumentation and a high degree of skill and technical knowledge on the part of the surgeon. These requirements may eventually be reduced if commercial laboratories can supply preshaped lenticules to the specifications of the operating surgeon. But, assuming these advances, keratophakia will still have to compete with improvements in extended-wear contact lenses and intraocular lenses for aphakic patients. However, older patients who are not candidates for intraocular lenses or who are unable to wear contact lenses represent a small but important population which would probably benefit from keratophakia.

Keratomileusis, on the other hand, requires the use of specialized instrumentation and lathing *at the time* of the procedure. A lamellar button is removed from the patient's own cornea, is frozen, cryolathed to a specified shape, thawed, and resutured in the stromal bed. This procedure, when first introduced in the United States a few years ago, was fraught with numerous technical difficulties and complications. However, during the past 2 years there has been some improvement in the clinical results, and the procedure is now returning to popularity among corneal refractive surgery specialists. Because the patient's *own* cornea is used, return of the best possible vision is usually more rapid than that following keratophakia. However, there are limitations imposed by the patient's preoperative corneal curvature.

Results of both keratophakia and keratomileusis are rather unpredictable, and undercorrection or overcorrection commonly occurs. Improvements in technology and refinement of the surgical technique will undoubtedly make these procedures more reliable in the future.

Alloplastic Lenticules

Attempts have been made by some investigators to use nonhuman corneal lenticules in keratophakia and keratomileusis. For example, to determine their potential usefulness, precut hydrophilic lens materials have been used as lenticules in animal studies. Theoretically, such material would be preferable to the use of living cornea simply because it is more readily available and is lathed and prepared in a more reliable fashion, but the search for the ideal material continues. However, at the present time, use of an ideal material is only a potential solution to a technically difficult problem.

Radial Keratotomy

Unlike the previously mentioned procedures that require cryolathe techniques and sophisticated instrumentation, radial keratotomy is becoming increasingly popular because of its relative simplicity; it can be performed under topical anesthesia on an outpatient basis and requires a minimal amount of instrumentation. Ultrasonic pachymeters that provide more accurate corneal thickness measurements and use of diamond knives have improved the safety of the procedure from a technical standpoint. Most surgeons who perform this procedure use a 3- to 3.5-mm optical zone and 4 or 8 radial corneal incisions. The deeper the incision (90% corneal thickness) the better the result. The exact mechanisms of refractive change is unclear, but the procedure produces a central flattening of the cornea with a relative bulging of the corneal periphery which seems to account for the reduction of myopia.

Unlike keratomileusis, in which the range of correction can be from 15 to 30 diopters, radial keratotomy corrects only low degrees of myopia, i.e., in the 2- to 5-diopter range. Unfortunately, the correction is not predictable and there are great variations in results among patients with the same degree of myopia. While results have been reported by many surgeons, results of the NIH-sponsored Prospective Evaluation of Radial Keratotomy (PERK) Study are not yet available. Functional complications include glare and fluctuating visual acuity, both of which tend to decrease after several months. Undercorrections and overcorrections also occur. In addition, severe complications such as cataract, corneal ulcers, and endophthalmitis have been reported, and one of the potential major complications is long-term damage to the corneal endothelium. This particular change was observed in patients undergoing the early Sato versions of the procedure, which involved incisions not only from the external side, but also from the endothelial side. Eighty percent of patients who had this procedure developed bullous keratopathy after 20 years. It is unlikely that this would be a major complication with current radial keratotomy techniques, but it is possible that certain subpopulations of patients will experience progressive endothelial cell loss over a long period. Unfortunately, it is impossible to predict at this time which patients are at risk. Despite these risks, however, most patients are extremely happy with the outcome, even in the face of overcorrection, undercorrection, or functional problems such as glare and fluctuating vision.

In the long term, it is likely that radial keratotomy in some form will be a part of the armamentarium of some ophthalmologists.

In the final analysis, each ophthalmolgist will have to decide for himself or herself what level of risk is acceptable in a procedure which, in my opinion, addresses an esthetic problem. Remember, the cornea itself is "normal" in these patients with low degrees of myopia.

Epikeratophakia

Epikeratophakia was developed in Herbert Kaufman's laboratory in an effort to overcome some of the technical difficulties associated with operations requiring use of a cryolathe. "Epi" techniques make use of a prelathed donor cornea which is sutured in place over an intact Bowman's membrane (epithelium removed). A small groove is made in the periphery of the patient's cornea and the "epi" button is sutured in place. Preoperative lathing can be done for correction of aphakia or myopia. Since the lenticule is sutured on the surface of the cornea, it seems to have the advantage of correcting a wide range of refractive errors, unlike the anterior lamellar resection in kerato-phakia, for example, which is too small to vault the lenticule, which is pushed posteriorly, resulting in decreased correction. While tech-nically much less difficult than the keratophakia and keratomileusis procedures, this technique still requires significant surgical skill and there is a potential for epithelial complications or sloughing of the epikeratophakia button if technical problems with suturing occur or vascularization of the wound ensues. Although the use of a corneal press (Kaufman) to compress the "epi"-button before transplantation has improved accuracy of the correction, predictability and reliability are problems. Slow return of acuity may well be overcome by modifi-cations in technique but is currently a factor in using this procedure for aphakic infants (congenital cataracts) and other individuals who require rapid return of visual acuity. Research on keratocyte repopu-lation and on methods for preserving such epikeratophakia buttons is now being performed at our Institution (David J. Schanzlin). A great advantage of the epikeratophakia procedure is its reversibility; the button can be removed at any time and the patient's own cornea will reepithelialize without complications.

Of all the procedures under current evaluation and investigation, epikeratophakia may well have the most potential. More laboratory investigation and extensive clinical trials are needed before it will be useful to the general ophthalmologist. However, in my opinion, it has great potential as an attractive alternative to the currently more standardized cryosurgical techniques.

The next decade will undoubtedly provide us with many innovative and exciting changes in refractive surgery of the cornea. It is likely that a better artificial material will be found that can be introduced into the cornea to modify its shape successfully, thus precluding the need for human donor lenticules. It is likely that some modification of radial keratotomy will be found to make it a more predictable, reliable, and safe procedure. It is likely that epikeratophakia, or a variant of it, will evolve into a procedure which will predictably correct high degrees of refractive error.

Throughout this "Decade of the Cornea," it is important for all of us to maintain a critical view of these procedures and to insist on high-quality publications reporting their techniques, safety, and results. Studies which present the "mean" or "average" refractive change should be viewed with some suspicion, as the *range* of corrections is a more accurate and clinically meaningful measure of predictability and reliability. Studies in which the *surgeon* is also the postoperative *data collector* should be rejected since there is a well-established bias inherent in any such study, no matter how well-intentioned. Studies that are reported orally at various meetings without benefit of adequate discussion by a qualified discussant should be considered, at best, scientific anecdotes rather than good science.

But despite all the caveats noted, and while maintaining a critical view of these new procedures, I think it is safe to say that refractive surgical procedures in one form or another are here to stay. We all look forward to modifications and improvements that will bring these procedures to the general ophthalmologist as useful methods to help some patients.

5–1 **Herpes Simplex Keratitis** is discussed by H. E. Kaufman, Y. M. Centifanto-Fitzgerald, and E. D. Varnell (Louisiana State Univ., New Orleans). Most herpetic disease seen clinically is secondary herpes. Although up to 90% of the population may be infected with herpes, only 20% to 30% are clinically affected. Multiple ganglia typically are infected, all by the same strain of herpesvirus. Isolates have been obtained at autopsy from patients without a history of clinical herpes. Studies in rabbits indicate that previous infection with an avirulent strain protects against the development of severe corneal epithelial disease on challenge with a virulent strain. Avirulent virus can infect and multiply in an experimental setting and colonize the ganglia. Previous infection with avirulent virus appears to prevent a virulent strain from colonizing the ganglia. There would appear to be a host response that is chiefly responsible for stromal disease and that is a function of the antigenicity of the infecting viral strain. Most strains of human herpesvirus may be relatively avirulent; usually, therefore, herpesvirus appears to be a well-adjusted parasite that produces disease only if the immune system is markedly disrupted or if infection by a more virulent strain occurs.

Vidarabine and idoxuridine are relatively insoluble drugs that are active against epithelial herpes, but they have no demonstrable effect on stromal disease or iritis. Trifluridine is a soluble, highly potent agent that prevents stromal disease in rabbits when given early enough. Large geographic or ameboid ulcers respond better to triflur-

(5–1) Ophthalmology (Rochester) 90:700–706, June 1983.

idine treatment than to administration of vidarabine or idoxuridine. It may be worthwhile trying this drug in patients with stromal disease before resorting to steroids and other measures. Acyclovir and E-5-(2-bromovinyl)-2'-deoxyuridine are representatives of a new class of drugs having great potential for the treatment of stromal disease and iritis. They are systemically active with very low toxicity, and also are highly effective when used topically. However, the development of virus resistance to these agents in the laboratory is possible; even so, the mutant viruses that may develop could be less virulent than those causing the primary infection.

▶ [This is a fine review and the authors suggest that the new class of drugs which includes acyclovir may be a cause for hope in the treatment of herpes simplex keratitis. Virus converts the drugs to potent antiviral agents, while normal cells do not. Thus the drugs are highly specific and effective. Further research is expected to give us more information about combined effects, viral mutation, and the like.] ◀

5–2 **Topographic Analysis of the Cornea: Ten Caveats in Keratorefractive Surgery.** J. James Rowsey reports that the newer keratorefractive operations require thorough understanding of refractive changes at the cornea-air surface. The corneascope can be used to quantify surgically induced changes in corneal contour. The normal cornea flattens over any incision, whether traumatic or surgical, and decreased plus power results. If the incision is near the limbus, as in cataract operations, inadequate corneal closure produces wound gaping in this area. Incisions around the visual axis produce considerable flattening in the center of the cornea and less in the midperiphery. Radial incisions flatten the adjacent cornea and also the cornea 90 degrees away. The flattening effect is greater as incisions approach the visual axis, and incisions near the visual axis result in maximal flattening of the cornea in the area of the incision. Disparate degrees of flattening are seen along radial incisions, with a midperipheral "knee" present in the cornea.

The cornea flattens directly over any sutured incision. The limbal cornea flattens adjacent to loose sutures and also 180 degrees away, and it steepens 90 degrees away from the incision. Corneal steepening is observed adjacent to tight sutures and 180 degrees away, and flattening is present 90 degrees away from the incision. Against-the-rule astigmatism may be reversed during cataract extraction when tight suturing is performed. The cornea flattens over any wedge resection or corneal tuck, and it steepens anterior to wedge resections or tucks.

Tissue removal, traumatic or surgical, produces corneal flattening over the site of removal. Tight sutures in the area of removal produce considerable corneal flattening in the immediate area, and substantial steepening can occur adjacent to the area of trauma. Addition of full-thickness corneal tissue produces corneal steepening over the site

(5–2) Int. Ophthalmol. Clin. 23:1–32, Winter, 1983.

of the addition and flattens the adjacent cornea. The radius of curvature of the cornea can be effectively reduced in a site of tissue supplementation.

▶ [These are helpful concepts for ophthalmic surgeons wishing to modify the corneal curvature (or not modify it) during cataract surgery or the experimental procedures reported in the following articles.] ◀

5–3 **Update on Keratophakia.** Miles H. Friedlander, Aran Safir, Marguerite B. McDonald, Herbert E. Kaufman, and Nicole Granet (Louisiana State Univ., New Orleans) report the results of keratophakia in 27 consecutively seen patients operated on for the correction of surgical aphakia. Donor corneal tissue, lathed at the time of surgery, was used in the first 5 cases, and stored lenticules were used in the remaining cases. Cataract extraction was combined with keratophakia in most cases. Patients selected had a corrected acuity of 20/40 or better in the fellow eye and were unable or unwilling to wear a contact lens. The fellow eye was either phakic or aphakic with a lens implant. Patients were followed up for 1 to 4 years after keratophakia. The prepared tissue was inserted intrastromally after a superficial keratectomy was performed, with subconjunctival gentamicin used as antibiotic coverage. A tarsorrhaphy no longer is performed.

Seventeen of the 23 evaluable patients had a final acuity of 20/40 or better with spectacle correction a year or more after operation. Four patients had an acuity of 20/50. The average residual overrefraction was 1.9 D. Postoperative astigmatism was increased by a mean of 1.7 D. No graft rejections or infections occurred and no eyes were lost. Two patients had their lenticules removed because of corneal edema secondary to increased intraocular pressure; 1 of these had a history of mild glaucoma. Four patients had nonprogressive depositis of epithelial material at the edge of the lenticule.

Keratophakia may be preferable to secondary intraocular lens implantation in the monocular aphakic patient who has had either an intracapsular or an extracapsular cataract extraction. The procedure is an alternative to bilateral intraocular lens implantation, and it may be preferable in young aphakic patients. Further improvements are needed to improve the predictability of the outcome and to minimize induced astigmatism. Hyperopic epikeratophakia has an advantage over keratophakia in that the visual axis of the cornea is avoided. The complexity of keratophakia and the time needed to achieve best-corrected acuity are disadvantages of this approach.

▶ [Keratophakia is the lathing of a donor cornea into a lenticule and then inserting the lenticule intrastromally in the host cornea. The host's own corneal epithelium is theoretically undisturbed. Visual rehabilitation usually takes 4 to 6 months, but the authors of this article believe it still may be better for the young patient and for the secondary as well as for the bilateral intraocular lens-implant patient.] ◀

▶ ↓ In the following 5 articles the authors discuss radial keratotomy. The procedure

(5–3) Ophthalmology (Rochester) 90:365–368, April 1983.

is controversial, but the National Eye Institute is sponsoring a multicenter clinical trial to attempt an evaluation of the surgery. In the first article the authors are very enthusiastic about the procedure. They report a 6-month follow-up with rare complications and 73% of the 156 eyes in their study achieving 20/40 or better vision. In the second study, however, the enthusiasm was less. A longer follow-up to 19 months resulted in a postoperative visual acuity of 20/40 or better in only 48% of the eyes. In the third study, with a 2-year follow-up, while 50% had an uncorrected visual acuity of 20/40 or better, 34% had 20/200 or worse. Detailed study of these 3 articles is recommended for the ophthalmic surgeon thinking of performing the procedure.

The final 2 articles in this series present in complete detail the rationale and design of the National Eye Institute's clinical trial of radial keratotomy. It is obvious that this clinical trial is important and we should all support the various clinics involved. ◀

5-4 **Visual, Refractive, and Keratometric Results of Radial Keratotomy.** A prospective evaluation of radial keratotomy was conducted using data on 101 consecutive patients (156 eyes) by Peter N. Arrowsmith, Donald R. Sanders, and Ronald G. Marks. Only patients aged 18 years or older were included, and operations were performed on an outpatient basis. Preoperative myopia ranged from a spherical equivalent (SE) of −1.50 to −16.0 diopters (D), with a mean of −5.0 D. The mean change in SE 6 months after surgery was +4.8 D. Preoperative uncorrected distance visual acuity of 20/200 or worse was evident in 96% of patients, and 51% had uncorrected acuity of less than 20/400. Six months after surgery, 73% of eyes had 20/40 or better uncorrected distance acuity, 43% having uncorrected distance acuity of 20/20 or better. A strong relationship was shown between

REFRACTIVE RESULTS 6 MONTHS AFTER SURGERY VERSUS PREOPERATIVE MYOPIA GROUP				
Group (N)	1 (38)	2 (70)	3 (36)	4 (12)
Preoperative Spherical Equivalent, Diopters				
Range	−1.5 to −2.9	−3.0 to −5.9	−6.0 to −9.9	−10.0 to −16.0
Mean	−2.2	−4.3	−7.0	−12.6
Spherical Equivalent Change, D				
Mean	+2.6	+4.7	+6.0	+8.6
SD	1.0	1.6	2.8	2.6
Minimum	+1.3	+0.4	+1.5	+5.3
Maximum	+5.5	+8.4	+15.8	+13.9
Spherical Equivalent Range v % of Eyes				
Myopia > 2.0 D	0	6	36	75
−1.1 D to −2.0 D	5	7	14	0
−0.1 D to −1.0 D	18	19	11	8
0.0 D to +1.0 D	61	36	14	8
+1.1 D to +2.0 D	11	23	14	8
+2.1 D to +4.0 D	5	6	8	0
Hyperopia > 4.0 D	0	4	3	0

(Courtesy of Arrowsmith, P.N., et al.: Arch. Ophthalmol. 101:873–881, June 1983; copyright 1983, American Medical Association.)

the degree of preoperative myopia and the change in SE 6 months after surgery. Eyes were classified into 4 groups based on the degree of preoperative myopia. As the mean preoperative SE increased from groups 1 through 4, there was a corresponding increase in the mean change in SE 6 months after surgery (table). When preoperative myopia was less than 6.0 D, the 6-month uncorrected acuity was 20/20 in 53% and 20/40 or better in 84% of eyes; 63% of eyes were within 1.0 D of emmetropia. Keratometric changes were similar to, but consistently less than changes in SE with a ΔSE/Δ K equal to 1.3 six months after surgery.

Microperforations in 55 (35%) eyes were the result of attempting deep corneal incisions. In 78% of these eyes, there were 3 or fewer microperforations, most usually occurring during redeepening incisions. No complication resulted in reduced best-corrected acuity, and most were transient and well tolerated. Early postoperative complications included epithelial erosion in about 50% of the eyes, usually resolving within 1 to 3 days after operation. Moderate pain was common during the first 24 to 48 hours postoperatively. Tearing, photophobia, and decreased acuity were usually moderate, resolving within 1 to 2 weeks. Intermediate and late complications included glare, overcorrection or undercorrection, induced astigmatism, and occasional recurrent pain. Most patients reported fluctuating vision at some period during the first 6 months after surgery.

Radial keratotomy can be effective for reducing myopia over a range of approximately 10 D. Predictability of outcome appeared best when preoperative myopia was less than 6 D. Improvement in uncorrected visual acuity was usually dramatic, and most patients could eliminate use of corrective lenses. Radial keratotomy appears safe in the short term; further evaluation is necessary to determine its long-term safety and effectiveness.

5–5 **Ongoing Prospective Clinical Study of Radial Keratotomy.** Verinder S. Nirankari, Leeds E. Katzen, James W. Karesh, Richard D. Richards, and Vinod Lakhanpal (Univ. of Maryland, Baltimore) reviewed the results of radial keratotomy in 58 eyes of 33 patients. Six eyes were subjected to 2 operations. All patients were aged 18 years and older and had 1.75 to 12.50 diopters (D) of stable myopia and no more than 2.50 D of astigmatism. The emphasis was placed on selecting patients who required specified uncorrected acuity for occupational reasons. A diamond blade currently is used. Eight incisions have been increasingly used rather than 16 incisions in the past year. A 3-mm central optical zone continues to be used; incisions are made from the central zone to within 1 mm of the limbus. The mean follow-up period is 19 months.

In 50% of the operated-on eyes 8 incisions, and in the other 50% 16 incisions, were made. Most patients had uncorrected acuity of 20/400

(5–5) Ophthalmology (Rochester) 90:637–641, June 1983.

LONG-TERM COMPLICATIONS OF RADIAL KERATOTOMY

Perforations	0/58
Endothelial cell loss	1/58
Corneal scarring	3/58
Deep corneal vascularization	2/33
Epithelial cysts	6/58
Overcorrection	4/58
Induced astigmatism	5/58
Regression of flattening	7/58

(Courtesy of Nirankari, V.S., et al.: Ophthalmology (Rochester) 90:637–641, June 1983.)

or worse preoperatively. About 50% of the operated-on eyes achieved uncorrected acuity of 20/40 or better. The average change in refractive error was 2.70 D of myopic decrease, a highly significant change. The average amount of corneal flattening was 1.51 D. The outcome was not related to the number of radial incisions made nor the depth of the incisions. The best results were obtained in patients with initial refractive errors of 5 D of myopia or less. Complications are listed in the table. No microperforations occurred. One of the 3 patients with central scarring experienced a decrease in best-corrected vision to 20/30. Epithelial cysts and deep corneal vascularization along the incisions have not occurred in the last 25 operated-on eyes.

Radial keratotomy leads to a reduction in refractive myopia and flattening of the cornea, but it is unclear whether the results can be accurately predicted and whether they can be maintained during the long term. Questions also exist regarding the effect of the procedure on corneal function.

5–6 **Three Years' Experience With Radial Keratotomy: The University of California at Los Angeles Study.** Kenneth J. Hoffer, John J. Darin, Thomas H. Pettit, John D. Hofbauer, Richard Elander, and Jeremy E. Levenson (Univ. of California, Los Angeles) reviewed the results of 16-incision keratotomies performed over 2 years as well as those of the more recent 8-incision procedure. Fifty-two eyes receiving 16 incisions were followed up after a mean of 25 months; 63 eyes receiving 8 incisions were followed up for a mean of 9 months.

In the 16-incision group, the mean myopia initially was −5.20 diopters (D) and the mean reduction was 3.85 D. Half of the eyes had an uncorrected acuity of 20/40 or better, and a third had acuity of 20/200 or worse. The best results were obtained in patients with preoperative myopia of 5 D or less. Long-term endothelial cell loss was not significant. Fourteen eyes retained a hyperopic cycloplegic refractive error at follow-up; 4 eyes ranged from +2.50 to +5.75 D. Microper-

(5–6) Ophthalmology (Rochester) 90:627–637, June 1983.

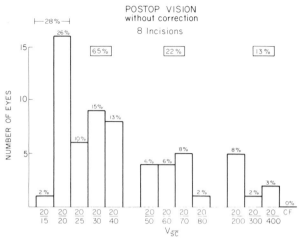

Fig 5–1.—Unaided visual acuity postoperatively in 62 eyes treated by 8-incision keratotomy. (Courtesy of Hoffer, K.J., et al.: Ophthalmology (Rochester) 90:627–637, June 1983.)

foration occurred in 19%, with no adverse effects to date. In the 8-incision group, 47 patients were operated on using primarily diamond blades and optical zones of 3 to 3.5 mm; 15 were treated bilaterally. In 65% of all patients in the 8-incision group, an uncorrected acuity of 20/40 or better was achieved, whereas 13% had vision of 20/200 or worse (Fig 5–1). The results were better than those in the 16-incision group because of patient selection. No microperforations occurred in this series, and glare was a lesser problem than in the 16-incision group. The severity of overcorrection hyperopia was greatly reduced in the 8-incision group. An incisional bacterial corneal ulcer was successfully treated in 1 patient. Three surgeons obtained similar results with radial keratotomy in this series.

Radial keratotomy with 16 incisions should no longer be performed on a routine basis; fewer side effects occur with the present 8-incision procedure, and less distinct overcorrection hyperopia is produced. Comparable rates of good unaided acuity are obtained when patients with less than 5 D of myopia are operated on. The procedure can be considered for patients seeking improvement in unaided vision for specific reasons if they understand that the long-term safety of the operation is not establiished.

5–7 **Design Features of the Prospective Evaluation of Radial Keratotomy (PERK) study** are described by George O. Waring III, Juan J. Arentsen, Linda B. Bourque, Henry Gelender, Richard L. Lindstrom, Steven D. Moffitt, William D. Myers, Stephen A. Obstbaum, J. James Rowsey, Aran Safir, and David Schanzlin. The PERK study is

(5–7) Int. Ophthalmol. Clin. 23:145–165, Fall 1983.

Participants in Prospective Evaluation of Radial Keratotomy (PERK) Study

Study Centers and Groups	Investigators and Monitors	Coordinators and Staff
Bascom Palmer Eye Institute, Miami, FL	Richard K. Forster, M.D. Henry Gelender, M.D. William Culbertson, M.D.	Teresa Obeso Gustave Garmizo, O.D. (Paul Ajamian, O.D.) (Howell Finley, O.D.)
University of California, Los Angeles, CA— Psychometric Center	Linda B. Bourque, Ph.D.	
Emory University, Atlanta, GA	George O. Waring, III, M.D. H. Dwight Cavanagh, M.D., Ph.D. William H. Coles, M.D., M.S. Louis A. Wilson, M.D.	Eugene Steinberg, L.D.O., C.O.T.
Louisiana State University Eye Center, New Orleans, LA	Marguerite McDonald, M.D. Herbert E. Kaufman, M.D. Joseph A. Baldone, M.D. Rise Ochsner, M.D. (Aran Safir, M.D.) (Rudy Franklin, M.D.) (John Linberg, M.D.) (Barry Kassar, M.D.)	Deborah Poloson, L.D.O., O.T. (Mike Ostrick, O.D.)
University of Minnesota, Minneapolis, MN	Donald J. Doughman, M.D. Richard L. Lindstrom, M.D. J. Douglas Cameron, M.D. J. Daniel Nelson, M.D.	Pat Williams, C.O.T.
Mount Sinai School of Medicine of the City University of New York, NY	Stephen A. Obstbaum, M.D. Steven M. Podos, M.D. Penny Asbell, M.D. (Michael J. Newton, M.D.) (George Pardos, M.D.)	Norma Justin, C.O.A.
National Eye Institute, Bethesda, MD	Robert Sperduto, M.D. Ronald G. Geller, Ph.D. Ralph J. Helmsen, Ph.D.	
University of Oklahoma, Oklahoma City, OK	J. James Rowsey, M.D. Hal D. Balyeat, M.D. James Hays, M.D. (Wayne F. March, M.D.)	Jack Whiteside (Douglas Corley) (Beth Kuns) (Becky Hewett, C.O.A.)
University of Southern California, Los Angeles, CA	David J. Schanzlin, M.D. Ronald E. Smith, M.D. James J. Salz, M.D. Douglas L. Steel, M.D. Richard A. Villaseñor, M.D.	Jan Reinig, L.V.N., C.O.T.
William Beaumont Eye Clinic, Royal Oak, MI	William D. Myers, M.D. John Cowden, M.D. Robert C. Arends, M.D. Paul Fecko, M.D. William T. Sallee, M.D. Robert L. Stephenson, M.D.	Vicki Roszka, C.O., C.O.M.T.
Wills Eye Hospital, Philadelphia, PA	Peter R. Laibson, M.D. Juan J. Arentsen, M.D. Michael A. Naidoff, M.D.	Nubia Cantillo, C.O.
Coordinating Center, Emory University, Atlanta, GA		
Clinical	George O. Waring, III, M.D.	Ceretha S. Cartwright, Dr.P.H. Nancy E. Hayes, B.A.
Statistical	Steven D. Moffitt, Ph.D.	Portia J. Griffin, B.S. Michael Lynn, M.S. Angela Morman
Reading Centers		
Photokeratography: University of Oklahoma, Oklahoma City, OK	J. James Rowsey, M.D.	Roy Montux (Michael Isaac, B.Sc.)
Specular Microscopy: Emory University, Atlanta, GA	George O. Waring, III, M.D.	Vickie Shadix
Clinic Monitoring Group	Jay H. Krachmer, M.D. Ceretha S. Cartwright, Dr.P.H. Robert J. Hardy, Ph.D. James P. McCulley, M.D. Steven D. Moffitt, Ph.D. Robert D. Sperduto, M.D. Walter J. Stark, M.D.	
Data and Safety Monitoring Board	Richard A. Thoft, M.D. James V. Aquavella, M.D. Jules L. Baum, M.D. Robert J. Hardy, Ph.D. Jay H. Krachmer, M.D. Steven D. Moffitt, Ph.D. Robert D. Sperduto, M.D. Joel Sugar, M.D. James Ware, Ph.D. George O. Waring, III, M.D.	

(Courtesy of Waring, G.O., III, et al.: Int. Ophthalmol. Clin. 23:145–165, Fall 1983.)

a 5-year multicenter collaborative trial of radial keratotomy for myopia that is designed to include about 500 patients. The organizational structure follows that of several previous multicenter trials. The participating centers are listed in the table.

Patients aged 21 years and older who prefer keratotomy to spectacles or contact lenses and have no residual, recurrent, or active eye disease are eligible for the study. All have a corrected visual acuity of 20/20 or better and no pathologic myopia. The current cycloplegic refraction must be between − 2.00 to − 8.00 diopters (D) with 1.50 D or less of astigmatism. The spherical part of the refraction should not have changed more than 0.5 D in the past year. Central keratometry readings should be stable within ± 0.5 D in 3 measurements made at least 1 week apart in contact lens wearers. The procedure is done with the use of an operating microscope. It is recommended that the second eye not be operated on for a year after operation on the first eye unless asymmetry of vision significantly disrupts function.

A specially designed visual acuity box is used to assess acuity. A manifest and cycloplegic refraction is done at each visit, without knowledge of the previous findings. Central keratometry and photokeratoscopy are performed. It is planned for 100 patients to receive evaluations twice the same day to quantify fluctuations in acuity during the day and detect their source. Glare is quantified with a glare tester, and slit-lamp examination is routinely performed. Corneal thickness is measured ultrasonically. Endothelial specular microscopy is used to assess the central endothelium. Scleral rigidity is calculated from applanation measurements and tonometry. Psychometric evaluation also is performed. The results will be reported throughout the course of the 5-year PERK study.

5–8 **Rationale for and Design of the National Eye Institute Prospective Evaluation of Radial Keratotomy (PERK) Study.** George O. Waring III, Steven D. Moffitt, Henry Gelender, Peter R. Laibson, Richard L. Lindstrom, William D. Myers, Stephen A. Obstbaum, J. James Rowsey, Aran Safir, David J. Schanzlin, and Linda B. Bourque (PERK Study Group) describe the organization of a 5-year, multicenter clinical trial of radial keratotomy for myopia that is under way at 9 clinical centers throughout the United States. About 500 patients aged 21 and older with − 2.00 to − 8.00 diopters (D) of physiologic myopia are being recruited into the study. In all cases, acuity in each eye is correctible to at least 20/20 with spectacles or contact lenses. There are 1.50 D or less of refractive astigmatism in each eye. The spherical part of the refraction in each eye has not changed more than 0.50 D during the past year, or more than 1.00 D during the past 3 years. No randomization of patients is performed. Surgery on the second eye is delayed for a year after surgery on the first eye.

(5–8) Ophthalmology (Rochester) 90:40–58, January 1983.

A new, diamond-bladed micrometer knife is used to make 8 radial incisions in the anterior cornea. The diameter of the central clear zone is determined by the degree of myopia present, and the proper depth of the incisions is estimated by intraoperative ultrasonic pachymetry. If regular astigmatism is induced by the procedure it is corrected optically. If irregular astigmatism is produced and the patient's activities demand it, attempts are made to fit contact lenses. Most cases of undercorrection will be managed by spectacles, and overcorrection is also managed by spectacles.

Investigators other than the surgeon gather all preoperative and postoperative data in the PERK study. Refractions are verified by a second observer. Corneal curvature is measured by keratometry and photokeratoscopy. Glare is quantified using a glare tester. Changes in endothelial-cell size are monitored by specular photomicrography. Formal psychometric testing also is performed to assess subjective responses to the procedure.

▶ ↓ In the following 2 articles the authors discuss corneal transplantation in aphakia and in the special case of pseudophakia. Indeed, the incidence of corneal edema requiring transplantation is rapidly increasing in the pseudophakic population. The posterior chamber lens may have better results, however, and may decrease the incidence of corneal edema to standard aphakic patient levels. The surgery is complicated, usually requiring Healon, and it appears best not to try and remove the intraocular lens. ◄

5–9   **Results of Penetrating Keratoplasty in 123 Eyes With Pseudophakic or Aphakic Corneal Edema.** Corneal edema after cataract surgery is an increasingly frequent indication for penetrating keratoplasty (Fig 5–2). George O. Waring III, Spencer N. Welch, H. Dwight Cavanagh, and Louis A. Wilson (Emory Univ., Atlanta) reviewed experience with penetrating keratoplasty for corneal edema in 35 pseudophakic eyes from which an intraocular lens had been removed and 88 aphakic eyes that never contained an intraocular

Fig 5–2.—Frequency of penetrating keratoplasty for aphakic and pseudophakic corneal edema at 3 institutions. (Courtesy of Waring, G.O., III, et al.: Ophthalmology (Rochester) 90:25–33, January 1983.)

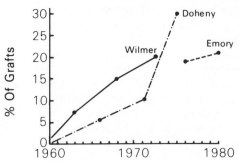

(5–9)   Ophthalmology (Rochester) 90:25–33, January 1983.

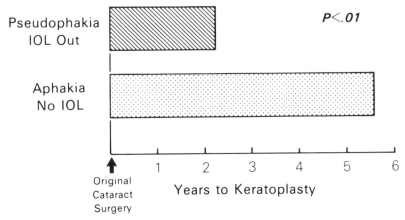

Fig 5–3.—Interval between cataract surgery and penetrating keratoplasty was shorter in pseudophakic eyes from which intraocular lens was removed than in aphakic eyes that had no intraocular lens (IOL). (Courtesy of Waring, G.O., III, et al.: Ophthalmology (Rochester) 90:25–33, January 1983.)

lens. The mean follow-up period was 17 months. The 2 groups were similar in age, sex, and length of follow-up, and the preoperative findings were comparable. Anterior vitrectomy was performed with the use of either a vitrectomy instrument or cellulose sponges and scissors. The eyes in the 2 groups were anatomically similar at the end of keratoplasty surgery.

The interval between initial cataract surgery and penetrating keratoplasty was shorter in the pseudophakic group than in the aphakic group (Fig 5–3). A large majority of the intraocular lenses were iris-supported lenses. Corneal grafts remained clear in 84% of all eyes. The final corrected visual acuity was better overall in the aphakic group without intraocular lenses. Postoperative maculopathy was more frequent in the pseudophakic group. Intraocular pressures were not significantly different in the 2 groups.

Corneal grafts remained clear after penetrating keratoplasty in 91% of previously pseudophakic eyes in this study and in 81% of aphakic eyes. The final visual acuity was better in the aphakic group, and maculopathy was less frequent in this group than in eyes from which intraocular lenses had been removed. The intraocular lens now often is retained if it is in good anatomical position and has not produced chronic ocular inflammation.

5–10 **Pseudophakic Bullous Keratopathy (PBK),** or irreversible corneal edema in an aphakic eye with an intraocular lens, is rapidly becoming the chief indication for penetrating keratoplasty. Daniel M. Taylor, Barry F. Atlas, Kenneth G. Romanchuk, and Alan L. Stern (Univ. of Connecticut, Farmington) performed 81 penetrating kera-

(5–10) Ophthalmology (Rochester) 90:19–24, January 1983.

TABLE 1.—Factors Predisposing to Pseudophakic
Bullous Keratopathy in 42 Eyes

I. Preoperative
   A. Corneal endothelial guttata ... 9 (21%)
   B. Glaucoma (no prior surgery) (one patient had both) ... 5 (12%)
   13 (31%)

II. Operative
   A. Vitreous loss ... 4 (9%)
   B. Endothelial trauma (two patients had both) ... 10 (24%)
   12 (29%)

III. Postoperative
   A. Uveitis/Vitritis ... 29 (69%)
   B. CME ... 13 (31%)
   C. Glaucoma ... 7 (16%)
   D. Trauma (IOL subluxation) ... 8 (19%)
   31 (74%)

CME, cystoid macular edema; IOL, intraocular lens.
(Courtesy of Taylor, D.M., et al.: Ophthalmology (Rochester)
90:19–24, January 1983.)

TABLE 2.—Incidence of Pseudophakic
Bullous Keratopathy

Binkhorst	45/1005	4.5%
Worst	44/1813	2.4%
Hirschman	36/1011	3.6%
Jaffe	5/500	1.0%
Drews	2/300	0.7%
Tennant	4/160	2.5%
Shepard	9/500	1.8%
Duffner	65/623	10.5%
Berkowitz	14/226	6.2%
Baggeson	13/203	6.4%
Williamson	3/200	1.5%
Gentry	3/103	2.9%
Total	240/6644	3.6%

(Courtesy of Taylor, D.M., et al.: Ophthalmology
(Rochester) 90:19–24, January 1983.)

toplasties for PBK on 66 eyes in 1977 to 1981. Forty-two eyes were from an average cataract population and had undergone intracapsular extraction and implantation of an iris-supported intraocular lens. The 32 women and 10 men had an average age of 76 years. The mean interval from cataract surgery to the appearance of PBK was 23 months, and the average follow-up period after keratoplasty was 18 months.

All but 5 of the 42 eyes evaluated ultimately had clear grafts. The intraocular lens was removed from 7 eyes. Ten patients required regrafting, 6 of them because of irreversible rejection. Five of the regrafts were clear when last evaluated. Spectacle acuity was obtained by 31 of the 37 patients with clear grafts. Sixteen of these patients have vision of 20/80 or better, and 10 of these have an acuity of 20/40 or better. The most common causes of acuity worse than 20/100 in patients with a clear graft were senile macular degeneration and chronic cystoid macular edema.

The etiology of PBK often is multifactorial (Table 1). The incidence in various series is given in Table 2. Half the present cases were unavoidable and due to the presence of an intraocular lens. Most patients had clear grafts after penetrating keratoplasty, but the visual results were less satisfactory. The occurrence of PBK should lead to a reduction in the use of iris-supported intraocular lenses. Eyes with guttate or chronic glaucoma and those previously operated on should have a careful assessment of endothelial status by specular microscopy before intraocular lens implantation is considered. The question of whether to remove the lens implant at the time of keratoplasty remains unanswered.

5–11   **Keratoprosthesis: Long-term Review.** J. J. Barnham and M. J. Roper-Hall (Birmingham, England) reviewed the results of 55 keratoprosthesis (KP) insertions in 35 patients, 39 of which were initial KP operations. The mean follow-up period was 2.3 years, and all but 4 patients were followed up for 6 months or longer. A penetrating KP was inserted on 49 occasions, and an intralamellar disk in 6 cases. The penetrating implants included 28 one-piece Cardona-Choyce implants, 15 two-piece implants, and 6 polymethylmethacrylate cylinders supported by tooth or silicone rings. The KPs usually were placed in a lamellar pocket dissected from the limbus with a central trephine opening. Twenty patients had a diagnosis of bullous keratopathy; 16 of these had undergone cataract extraction. Six patients had a history of glaucoma. All but 5 patients had had previous surgery. Nineteen patients had light perception only preoperatively, and 2 others had no light perception. Only 3 patients had vision of 6/60 or better.

DURATION OF IMPROVED VISUAL ACUITY

Single or multiple surgery
(Postop. 2 (5·4%) were worse and 6 (16·2%) were similar)

0 to 6 months	7 (18·9%)
6 months to 1 year	4 (10·8%)
1 to 5 years	6 (16·2%)
5 to 10 years	8 (21·7%)
10 to 15 years	4 (10·8%)

(Courtesy of Barnham, J.J., and Roper-Hall, M.J.: Br. J. Ophthalmol. 67:468–474, July 1983.)

(5–11)   Br. J. Ophthalmol. 67:468–474, July 1983.

After operation, 42% of patients had unaided vision of 6/60 or better, and 27% had acuities of 6/24 or better. With spectacles, 53% of patients had vision of 6/60 or better, and 36% had acuities of 6/24 or better. The duration of improved acuity is shown in the table. More than 50% of the patients had corneal erosion of varying degrees, with or without partial exposure, and about 34% had spontaneous extrusion. About 34% of the patients had retroimplant membranes or deposits, and many had anterior epithelial overgrowth. Cataract developed in the only patient having phakic KP insertion. Only 34% of patients did not require further surgery after first-time penetrating KP insertion. Forty-three percent of all penetrating KP implants remained in place after a mean follow-up period of 2.3 years; 11 of these implants were followed up subsequently and were retained. Four of the 6 intralamellar implants remained in place.

Keratoprosthesis surgery is indicated in patients with corneal blindness that is not amenable to conventional measures. Close, continued follow-up is necessary. Although further surgery often is necessary, some long-term successes can be achieved in patients with otherwise untreatable conditions.

▶ [This heroic procedure clearly has a place in desperate cases, but careful follow-up must be continued indefinitely. The basic problem is the plastic-cornea interface, but newer substances are continually being devised and the problem may one day be resolved.] ◀

5–12 **Topical Versus Subconjunctival Treatment of Bacterial Corneal Ulcers.** Jules Baum and Michael Barza (New England Med. Center, Boston) compared the effectiveness of the topical and subconjunctival approaches in sterilizing corneal ulcers produced in rabbits by injections of *Staphylococcus aureus* and *Pseudomonas aeruginosa*. Drug therapy was begun 24 hours after corneal inoculation. Staphylococcal ulcers were treated with gentamicin or cefazolin, and pseudomonal ulcers were treated with gentamicin. Either drops were placed in both eyes, or one eye received subconjunctival injections of antibiotic. Treatment was continued for 9 or 17 hours. The subconjunctival dose of cefazolin was 100 mg, and that of gentamicin was 40 mg. Cefazolin eyedrops contained 33.3 mg/ml, and gentamicin drops, either 3 or 14 mg/ml.

Corneal antibiotic concentrations were significantly higher 1 hour after subconjunctival injection than when given topically, but, by the 17th hour, corneal concentrations were lower in the subconjunctival group. Both types of treatment markedly reduced bacterial counts in corneal ulcers compared with control eyes, and there were few significant differences in bacterial counts between the 2 routes of therapy. The more concentrated gentamicin eyedrops produced much higher corneal and serum drug levels than did the less concentrated preparation. The concentrated drops were significantly more

(5–12) Ophthalmology (Rochester) 90:162–168, February 1983.

effective in reducing colony counts in pseudomonal ulcers at 9 hours.

Fortified antibiotic eyedrops, instilled every 15 to 30 minutes, should be used alone in cases of mild, early corneal ulceration, if compliance can be assured. Compliance can often be a problem, however, especially in pediatric cases. It may be better to anesthetize a child daily for several days to administer subconjunctival injections than to rely on drops. The risk of general anesthesia is minimal when compared with that of undertreating a bacterial corneal ulcer. Ketamine may be a reasonable alternative to a general anesthetic.

▶ [The efficacy of topical and subconjunctival administration of antibiotics is the same, but hourly compliance versus daily injections must be carefully weighed. Sustained release antibiotic inserts might solve part of the problem, if they can be manufactured.] ◀

5–13 **Demographic and Predisposing Factors in Corneal Ulceration.** David C. Musch, Alan Sugar, and Roger F. Meyer (Univ. of Michigan, Ann Arbor) examined the factors involved in corneal ulceration in a series of 224 patients hospitalized with corneal ulcers seen between 1975 and 1981. The male-female case ratio was 1.2. A striking bimodality was evident in the age distribution, with peaks at ages 20 to 29 and 65 to 74 years. The causes of the ulcers are listed in Table 1. More than half of the bacterial isolates were *Pseudomonas aeruginosa* and *Staphylococcus aureus*. Predisposing ocular factors were identified in most patients (Table 2). Two thirds of the postsurgical ulcers developed after penetrating keratoplasty procedures. Herpes simplex keratitis was a predisposing factor in 18% of the patients and steroid therapy in 11%.

Age at admission was inversely related to both visual acuity at that time and acuity after discharge. In the 78 patients for whom complete information was available, the prognosis for improved vision in those with light perception or less in the ulcerated eye was not good. It was appreciably better for patients with hand motions or greater acuity

TABLE 1.—Causes of Corneal Ulcers

Cause	No. (%)
Bacterial	35 (35)
Postherpetic	17 (17)
Posttrauma	8 (8)
Neurotrophic	5 (5)
Fungal	3 (3)
Neuroparalytic	2 (2)
Miscellaneous	12 (12)
Unknown	18 (18)
Total	**100 (100)**

(Courtesy of Musch, D.C., et al.: Arch. Ophthalmol. 101:1545–1548, October 1983; copyright 1983, American Medical Association.)

(5–13) Arch. Ophthalmol. 101:1545–1548, October 1983.

TABLE 2.—Frequency of Predisposing Ocular
Conditions

Predisposing Ocular Conditions	% of Patients†
Trauma	**49**
Postsurgery	15
Contact lenses	11
Acute abrasion	10
Penetration/laceration	5
Thermal burns	3
Unspecified	5
Corneal states	**42**
Herpetic keratitis	18
Keratitis sicca	8
Bullous keratopathy	7
Keratitis (other)	6
Anesthesia	3
Lacrimal obstruction	**4**
Dacryocystitis	2
Unspecified	2
Entropion	**4**
Spastic	1
Cicatricial	1
Unspecified	2
Exophthalmos	**4**
Conjunctival states*	**8**
Sjögren's syndrome	5
Stevens-Johnson syndrome	2
Xerophthalmia	1
Blepharitis	2
Lagophthalmos	2

*The following factors were sought, but not found: vernal catarrh, trachoma, pemphigoid.
†n = 100.
(Courtesy of Musch, D.C., et al.: Arch. Ophthalmol. 101:1545–1548, October 1983; copyright 1983, American Medical Association.)

at the time of admission, but these patients were younger than the others. The only variable significantly associated with length of hospitalization was the presence of hypopyon at admission.

Both age and visual acuity at admission are significant prognostic factors for final visual acuity in patients with corneal ulceration. Important predisposing factors in the present series included ocular trauma, herpetic keratitis, contact lens wear, steroid use, keratitis sicca, diabetes, rheumatoid arthritis, and bullous keratopathy. The series was biased toward patients with more serious or complicated conditions and toward a midwestern locale.

▶ [It is not surprising but it bears emphasizing that corticosteroid therapy is an important predisposing factor for serious corneal ulceration. Indeed, did any herpetic eyes perforate before administration of corticosteroids? Probably not.] ◀

5–14   **Effects of Swimming Pool Water on Cornea.** To define better

(5–14)   JAMA 249:2507–2508, May 13, 1983.

the nature and extent of corneal changes that occur in swimmers, Jeffrey R. Haag and Richard G. Gieser (Loyola Univ., Maywood, Ill.) performed eye examinations in 37 males and 13 females, average age 21, immediately before and after swimming in a chlorinated pool.

METHOD.—The concentration of free chlorine gas in the pool is kept at about 1.0 to 1.5 ppm, and the pH stays close to 7.5. Electronic sensors constantly monitor pH and chlorine content; manual tests are performed twice daily. Before swimming, the visual acuity of the study population was measured for each eye, and a slit-lamp examination of the cornea was performed that included instillation of fluorescein and use of a cobalt blue filter to evaluate the condition of the corneal epithelium. Participants were asked to look at the ceiling lights every 5 minutes while swimming and to watch for the appearance of rainbows or halos around the lights. If these symptoms appeared, the swimmers were to note the elapsed time since they entered the pool. Another assessment of visual acuity and a slit-lamp examination were done immediately after the swimmers left the pool. No one wore protective goggles or contact lenses.

The average swim time was 34 minutes. Visual acuities remained within the preswim range of 6/6 to 6/30. Halos or rainbows around the lights were seen by 34 (68%) swimmers after 5 to 30 minutes in the pool. These symptoms disappeared within 30 minutes of leaving the water. Fluorescein staining of the cornea was observed in 47 (94%) swimmers; it was primarily consistent with superficial punctate erosions most prominent in the lower third of the cornea. The hypotonicity of the swimming pool water was considered to be the cause of this corneal edema. After the corneal epithelium imbibes water, these cells may slough off, resulting in punctate keratitis that stains with fluorescein. Friction of the water against the cornea and disruption of the tear film may also contribute to corneal epithelial erosion and edema.

▶ [A contact lens study would be interesting since it should eliminate the friction factor, although it might compound the chlorine problem.] ◀

5–15 **Corneal Endothelium—Morphology, Function, and Clinical Importance** are discussed by M. Stur and G. Grabner (Univ. of Vienna). The corneal endothelium consists of a single layer of flat, hexagonal cells covering the posterior surface of the cornea. It has prominent functions in the maintenance of corneal integrity and transparency. These cells produce Descemet's membrane, dehydrate the corneal stroma, have a barrier function against the aqueous humor, and possess active glucose transport mechanisms. In children a regular hexagonal endocell pattern with a density of 2,000 to 4,000 cells per mm is found. With aging, some cells are lost and, to maintain the barrier function, the cells must be replaced by enlargement of neighboring cells. Since this process differs in speed, inference to age cannot be made; however, older patients frequently develop a cornea guttata (Fig 5–4).

(5–15) Wien. Klin. Wochenschr. 95:274–276, Apr. 15, 1983.

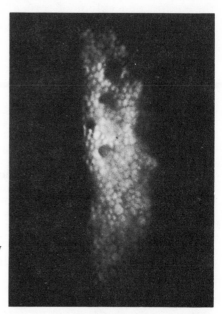

Fig 5–4.—Cornea guttata senilis. (Courtesy of Stur, M., and Grabner, G.: Wien. Klin. Wochenschr. 95:274–276, Apr. 15, 1983.)

Pathologic cell loss is caused mostly by surgery, perforating injuries of the anterior segment, and acute increase of pressure. Cell density, as well as variation in size and morphology, can be examined by specular microscopy. Pump function and permeability may be determined by pachymetry and fluorophotometry.

Specular microscopy reached its significance through the introduction of newer techniques of cataract surgery, especially implantation of intraocular lenses (IOL) and phacoemulsification of the lenticular nucleus. Some researchers investigated the cell loss after intraocular extraction with and without implantation of an IOL; in the group with IOL implantation a cell loss of 34% to 70%, and therefore a high rate of severe corneal damage (10% bullous keratopathy), was observed. Since then many factors causing cell loss were discovered and with improvement of procedures the frequency of severe complications could be reduced. Routine preoperative endothelial examination is important for identification of patients at risk with predamaged corneal endothelium and for consideration of effects of the surgical method on the corneal endothelium.

Another important use of specular microscopy is the assessment of the donor's cornea. The transparency depends on the function of the donor's endothelial cells, which depends on the time period between death of donor and enucleation of bulbi, the storing method used until surgery, and surgical techniques. Postoperatively, the cell loss is higher than normal and is even more so when the cornea comes from an eye bank where it has been frozen.

Although specular microscopy is the most popular method of examination, it permits only indirect conclusions. Pachymetry and fluorophotometry will, as complementary methods, attain greater clinical importance by determining more accurately and earlier functional disturbances of the endothelium.

6. Glaucoma

Automated Perimetry
JACOB T. WILENSKY, M.D.

Eye and Ear Infirmary
University of Illinois, Chicago

Glaucoma has traditionally been defined by the diagnostic triad of elevated intraocular pressure, cupping of the optic nerve head, and characteristic visual field loss. For many years, however, the intraocular pressure level has been given paramount attention. There are still many ophthalmologists in practice who were taught during their residency that any intraocular pressure greater than 22 mm Hg or 24 mm Hg indicated the presence of glaucoma and necessitated the immediate institution of treatment. The occurrence of low-tension glaucoma presented a troubling dilemma. Moreover, epidemiologic studies conducted by different investigators during the 1960s clearly showed that there were many older patients with intraocular pressures above this "magical" value who had no evidence of glaucomatous damage to their eyes. As a result, the concept of ocular hypertension was developed. Although this is a controversial term, it clearly indicates the view that there is no one absolute intraocular pressure level that can be used to delineate the boundary between the presence or absence of glaucoma. Thus, glaucoma cannot be managed solely on the basis of tonometry.

In the 1970s a number of observers called greater attention to the optic nerve head and the changes that occur due to glaucoma. Features such as vertical elongation of the cup and asymmetry of cupping between the 2 eyes were brought to our attention as signs that could differentiate glaucomatous disks from those of normal patients who had large physiologic cups. Moreover, it was shown that patients could suffer progressive enlargement of the cups at a time when no glaucomatous visual field defects could be detected by kinetic perimetry. As a result, a greater emphasis has been placed on examination of the optic nerve head and recording the configuration of the cups, either by recording a cup to disk ratio, making a drawing of the disk or, preferably, obtaining stereo disk photographs.

In the routine clinical management of glaucoma patients, perimetry generally has been used less than tonometry or ophthalmoscopy.

There are many reasons for this. It is a time-consuming, tedious examination that requires both a cooperative and alert patient and a knowledgeable and well-trained perimetrist. There are problems with the reproducibility and the reliability of the results, due both to the psychophysical nature of the test itself and to technical problems arising from the manner in which the visual field is measured. Separate space must be set aside for the perimetry equipment and the lighting in this area must be carefully regulated.

Evidence during the past few years suggests that this relative neglect of perimetry may be coming to an end. The development of both improved strategies for testing of the visual field as well as improved automated equipment for conductingg those tests have now made perimetry much easier to perform and more readily available for the private practice ophthalmologist. Static suprathreshhold screening programs have also been developed and refined during the past decade. Almost all of the new automated perimeters have programs of this type available, with different degrees of complexity and sophistication. With these programs, patients can be screened for the presence of significant visual field defects in a matter of 2 or 3 minutes per eye. Such testing can be performed by relatively unsophisticated minimally trained office personnel, yet have a fairly high degree of reliability due to the fixation monitoring devices built into the perimeters, the standardization of presentation of test stimuli, and the programs that select the size and intensity of the test stimuli.

At the other extreme, instruments such as the Octopus 201 and Squid computerized automated perimeters permit detailed quantification of visual field defects to a degree not practically available in the past. These perimeters can determine the threshold for detection of light at almost any given point in the entire visual field. These instruments are expensive and probably will not achieve widespread penetration within the ophthalmic community, but simpler, much less expensive instruments that can accomplish most of the same tasks as these more sophisticated machines are now beginning to appear on the market. If these instruments prove to be as effective and efficient as they are touted to be, then accurate quantitative perimetry will soon be available to the private practice ophthalmologist at an affordable price and without the need for a highly trained perimetrist. Thus, detailed quantitative visual field studies of most glaucoma patients appear to be a goal that can be achieved in the near future.

Unfortunately, while these instruments will improve the ability of the clinician to monitor the status of his or her glaucoma patients, they will not necessarily simplify clinical decision-making. Although computer programs have been devised that analyze serial visual fields in an attempt to detect progression of visual field loss, none have yet really achieved a high degree of reliability. It is almost paradoxical that the improved sensitivity of testing of the visual field that can be achieved with the most sophisticated automated perimeters has made us aware of many of the spontaneous and seasonal fluctuations that occur in the visual field, unrelated to the disease process itself. In learning this, we have been made aware that interpretation of visual field changes is an extremely difficult and complex task and simply looking at a group of threshhold levels or isopter plots is not sufficient to determine whether pathologic changes have occurred. Thus, while automation may have made perimetry both more available and more accurate, it has simultaneously made its interpretation more difficult. This is a burden, however, that we can bear, and I think that the availability of improved perimetry ultimately can only help improve our management of patients with glaucoma.

6–1 **Argon Laser Trabeculoplasty in Secondary Forms of Open-Angle Glaucoma.** Alan L. Robin and Irvin P. Pollack (Johns Hopkins Hosp., Baltimore) conducted a pilot study of the usefulness of argon laser trabeculoplasty (ALT) in types of glaucoma other than primary open-angle. The technique of Wise and Witter (1979) was used in performing ALT on 55 eyes of 14 male and 32 female patients aged 13 to 86 years (mean, 52 years) who had secondary forms of glaucoma. All were candidates for conventional glaucoma surgery because of poor control of intraocular pressure (IOP) with maximal medical antiglaucomatous therapy. The 46 patients were followed up for 4 to 27 months (mean, 8 months).

Mean IOP was 34 mm Hg before ALT and 22 mm Hg after ALT. There was no significant correlation between preoperative and postoperative IOP levels for individual patients. Forty eyes (73%) had sufficient lowering of IOP after ALT to avoid conventional surgery, and 21 (53%) of these successfully treated eyes achieved IOP control with fewer medications. All patients had low-grade uveitis lasting up to 1 month after ALT and 33% experienced anterior synechiae formation, but no major complications occurred.

The response to ALT varied with the type of glaucoma. Angle-recession, uveitic, and congenital glaucoma responded poorly, with 11 of 16 such eyes (69%) requiring further surgery and only 1 of the remaining 5 being able to discontinue any of the preoperative medications.

In eyes that were either aphakic or had had filtering surgery, ALT produced satisfactory control of IOP provided preoperative medication levels were continued. Of 18 such eyes, 17 (94%) did not need conventional filtering surgery after ALT, but in only 6 (33%) could the number of medications be reduced.

In eyes with pigmentary glaucoma, pseudoexfoliation glaucoma, or glaucoma after iridectomy for angle closure, ALT lowered IOP and permitted reduction of antiglaucomatous medications. Of 19 such eyes, 16 (84%) required no further surgery, in 13 of the 16 (81%)

(6–1) Arch. Ophthalmol. 101:382–384, March 1983.

fewer antiglaucomatous drugs were needed, with 2 patients being able to discontinue all antiglaucoma medications.

▶ [All the patients treated had transient uveitis, although there were no long-term problems. It thus seems reasonable to continue studying the effects of laser trabeculoplasty on all types of glaucoma.] ◀

6–2 **Effect of Trabecular Photocoagulation on the Aqueous Humor Dynamics of the Human Eye.** Richard F. Brubaker and Thomas J. Liesegang (Mayo Found.) report the findings in 17 patients who received argon laser trabeculoplasty in one eye for either chronic simple glaucoma or open-angle glaucoma and exfoliation syndrome. The 10 men and 7 women in the study were aged 56 to 79 years. All patients had failed to gain satisfactory control from medical measures and were candidates for filtration surgery. No eye had a pretreatment intraocular pressure exceeding 34 mm Hg. Fluorescence studies were performed before and after trabeculoplasty.

Mean intraocular pressure decreased from 21 to 14 mm Hg 3 months after trabeculoplasty. Mean tonographic C value increased from 0.11 to 0.18 μl/minute/mm Hg. Apparent resistance to aqueous outflow decreased from a mean of 14.2 to 9.2 minutes/mm Hg/μl after treatment. Intraocular pressure decreased by 6 mm Hg or more in 9 treated eyes. These patients had noticeable improvement in tonographic C value or apparent resistance to aqueous outflow, or both. They had higher initial intraocular pressures than the nonresponders. More responders had exfoliation syndrome.

Laser trabeculoplasty appears to act by improving the outflow of aqueous humor, probably through improvement in canalicular outflow, in patients with chronic simple glaucoma or open-angle glaucoma with pseudoexfoliation. Gross perforation into Schlemm's canal seems unnecessary to produce sustained improvement in outflow in these cases.

▶ [In this careful study of aqueous humor dynamics before and after laser trabeculoplasty, the authors showed that there is an increase in outflow following the treatment. We still do not know the mechanism by which this occurs, however. It is probably not by punching holes in the meshwork and canal of Schlemm.] ◀

6–3 **Argon Laser Photocoagulation of Trabecular Meshwork in Open-Angle Glaucoma.** Adverse rises in intraocular pressure may occur with conventional laser photocoagulation of the trabecular meshwork in its pigmented portion. Therefore, it was proposed that it might be better to induce scarring on the anterior nonpigmented trabecular meshwork where drainage would be less affected. R. I. Kellen and W. H. G. Douglas (Univ. of Witwatersrand, Johannesburg, South Africa) evaluated the results of argon laser photocoagulation in 22 eyes of 17 patients with open-angle glaucoma. Seventeen eyes had primary open-angle glaucoma, 3 were aphakic, and 2 had pigmentary glaucoma. The average age was 68 years. All patients

(6–2) Am. J. Ophthalmol. 96:139–147, August 1983.
(6–3) S. Afr. Med. J. 64:557–558, Sept. 28, 1983.

had uncontrolled intraocular pressure despite maximally tolerated medical treatment; the maximal pressure was 29 mm Hg. A continuous-wave laser was used in outpatients to produce about 50 burns of 50-μm spot size in the anterior nonpigmented trabeculum. Exposure time was 0.1 second, and the power setting ranged from 0.75 to 1.5 watts.

The average fall in intraocular pressure was 6.1 mm Hg. The response at 4 weeks was a good indicator of the pressure at 6 months. The aphakic eyes responded well. Drug therapy was discontinued in 3 patients. Intraocular pressures of 17 mm Hg or below were achieved in 41% of all treated eyes. Peripheral anterior synechiae developed in 3 eyes but did not appear to be significant. Six eyes had a transient postoperative pressure rise, which in 2 eyes exceeded 9 mm Hg; however, none of these eyes had a final decrease in the visual field. A significant field loss occurred in 1 instance without a rise in intraocular pressure. Mild iritis occurred in 3 eyes that were effectively treated with topical steroids.

Laser photocoagulation of the nonpigmented trabecular meshwork can be used to produce a modest decrease in intraocular pressure in patients with open-angle glaucoma without causing serious complications in most cases. It is an outpatient procedure. Further studies are needed to establish the best means of applying the laser burns.

▶ [This is an important article since it clearly lists the many complications of laser trabeculoplasty, not least of which is the postoperative elevation in pressure.] ◀

▶ ↓ In the following 2 articles, the authors have studied the effectiveness of using fewer burns for laser trabeculoplasty. Fifty burns seem to have the same effect and indeed even 25 burns given in 2 doses seems to work. Long-term follow-up, however, is necessary to be certain the pressure-lowering effects are sustained. ◀

6–4 **Influence of the Number of Laser Burns Administered on Early Results of Argon Laser Trabeculoplasty.** To examine the influence of the number of laser burns administered on the postoperative intraocular pressure of patients with open-angle glaucoma, Robert N. Weinreb, Jon Ruderman, Richard Juster, and Jacob T. Wilensky (Univ. of Illinois Eye and Ear Infirm., Chicago) conducted a prospective, randomized, double-masked study on 40 patients. Twenty patients assigned to group 1 were treated with 50 burns to the nasal half of the trabecular meshwork (180 degrees), whereas in 20 patients in group 2 the entire circumference of the trabecular meshwork (360 degrees) was treated with 100 burns. The burns were equally spaced, using power of 800 mW, burn size of 50 μm, and duration of 0.1 second.

All patients were examined 1 week and between 6 and 8 weeks after operation. Mean corrected 2-month change in intraocular pressure (table) was -9.20 ± 6.43 mm Hg in group 1 and -6.95 ± 5.74 mm Hg in group 2, a difference that was not statistically significant.

(6–4) Am. J. Ophthalmol. 95:287–292, March 1983.

CORRECTED 2-MONTH CHANGES IN INTRAOCULAR PRESSURE
Changes in Intraocular Pressure (mm Hg)

Subgroups	Group 1 (180 degrees)	Group 2 (360 degrees)	Groups 1 and 2
A	−13.33 ± 5.81	−10.50 ± 7.37	−12.20 ± 6.38
B	−5.82 ± 4.85	−5.43 ± 4.36	−5.60 ± 4.49
A and B	−9.20 ± 6.43	−6.95 ± 5.74	−8.08 ± 6.12

(Courtesy of Weinreb, R.N., et al.: Am. J. Ophthalmol. 95:287–292, March 1983.)

Groups 1A and 2A included patients whose corrected intraocular pressure decreased or remained unchanged during the 8-hour period after laser trabeculoplasty. Groups 1B and 2B included patients whose corrected intraocular pressure increased during this period. In each group the intraocular pressure was lowest after 2 months in those patients in whom it was not increased during the immediate postoperative period (group 1, P < .006; group 2, P < .07).

Inflammation in groups 1 and 2 was minimal and in most instances absent after the first postoperative week. Synechiae appeared to be more common and extensive in patients in group 2; typically they were small and reached only to the scleral spur.

The similar responses in groups 1 and 2 suggest there is no advantage to administering 100 burns to the entire trabecular meshwork in an initial treatment session. It seems prudent to treat the least amount of trabecular tissue necessary for an acceptable result and 50 burns given during an initial session to one half the trabecular meshwork are often sufficient.

6–5 **Low-Dose Trabeculoplasty.** In an effort to reduce the incidence of increased intraocular pressure (IOP) in the immediate posttrabeculoplasty period, Jacob T. Wilensky and Robert N. Weinreb (Univ. of Illinois, Chicago) treated 21 eyes (18 patients) with open-angle glaucoma by using just 25 laser burns, rather than 50 or 100 burns. With the use of a continuous-wave argon laser, 900 mW of power, a duration of 0.1 second, and a 50-μm spot size, 25 laser burns were evenly scattered over 1 quadrant (90 degrees) of the trabecular meshwork. Sixteen eyes later received a second 25-burn treatment over an adjacent quadrant. All glaucoma medication was continued after operation.

At 4 weeks after treatment, IOP in the 21 eyes was decreased 2 to 11 mm Hg (average, 6.86 mm Hg). Of the 16 eyes undergoing a second treatment because IOP was still unsatisfactory, 13 had a further decrease in IOP of 1 to 8 mm Hg, 2 had no change, and 1 had an increase of 1 mm Hg after 4 weeks, for an average additional decrease

(6–5) Am. J. Ophthalmol. 95:423–426, April 1983.

of 3.56 mm Hg. In 5 of these 16 eyes, the decrease in IOP was greater after the second treatment than after the first. The IOP of 2 patients increased 10 mm Hg or more in the first few hours after ttreatment, showing that significant increases in IOP can still occur with this low-dose regimen.

Additional study is needed to determine whether low-dose and divided-dose regimens reduce the incidence of complications from laser trabeculoplasty and whether the reduction in IOP persists as long as it does in eyes receiving more laser burns.

▶ ↓ Half of this year's articles are on laser trabeculoplasty, and the 10 chosen include techniques, summaries of results, and side effects. The latter are just beginning to emerge but are becoming more and more important as we learn about the effects of coagulating the trabecular meshwork.

In the following 4 articles from the United States and Western Europe, more than 200 eyes are reported. The follow-up averages from 7 months to 2 years and the pressure-lowering effects are highly variable but usually less than 10 mm Hg. It is clear from these articles the type of glaucoma and the indications are still in a state of flux. The conservative view is to use laser only in those patients who would otherwise require surgery. It is likely, however, that indications will broaden as we learn more about the effects and side effects. ◀

6–6 **Argon Laser Trabeculoplasty** was performed by Paul R. Lichter (Univ. of Michigan, Ann Arbor) in 50 eyes in 42 consecutive male and female outpatients, aged 33 to 85 years (average, 63 years), with open-angle glaucoma with definite glaucomatous optic disk and visual field damage. The procedure was done with the patient under topical anesthesia using the technique of Wise and Witter (1979). The blue-green argon laser was directed at the posterior trabecular meshwork. Using 1 W of energy, a 50-μ spot size, and a 0.1-second duration, approximately 100 laser applications, evenly spaced, were made covering 360 degrees around the angle, with care taken to avoid inadvertent treatment of the iris or ciliary body. Postoperatively, the patients continued all antiglaucoma medication and added 1% prednisolone acetate drops to the eye 4 times daily. Follow-up was for as long as 13 months (average, 7 months).

Mean intraocular pressure (IOP) in the 50 eyes was 24.08 mm Hg before laser treatment, 21.72 mm Hg at the first posttreatment visit (average, 5½ days), 15.32 mm Hg at an average of 6½ weeks, 13.33 mm Hg at its lowest point (average, about 12 weeks), and 16.02 mm Hg at the latest examination (average, 6½ months). Although mean IOP reduction from baseline to the latest examination was 30%, some eyes showed reductions of more than 60%.

Of the 12 eyes having a higher IOP at 5 days than at baseline, 10 had a lower-than-baseline IOP at 6 weeks. A successful result (i.e., IOP reduced at 6 weeks by ≥20% from baseline IOP) was achieved in 37 of the 50 eyes (74%). Only 3 eyes had a higher IOP at 6 weeks than at baseline. Nearly all of the 12 eyes with diagnoses other than primary open-angle glaucoma were benefited.

(6–6) Trans. Am. Ophthalmol. Soc. 80:288–301, 1982.

Results of tonography, performed in many eyes but probably valid in only 11, suggested that laser treatment improved the facility of outflow. Other than minimal ocular irritation, there were few side effects of the procedure. Although all 50 eyes had been considered in need of filtering surgery, only 4 had such surgery. Thus, the procedure was successful in that it avoided incisional surgery in 92% of the eyes.

Laser treatment should be considered in any open-angle glaucomatous eye before resorting to filtering surgery, even in eyes with IOP of ≥40 mm Hg. Randomized, controlled trials are needed to determine if other methods are superior to that of Wise and Witter.

6–7 **Four-Year Experience With Argon Laser Trabecular Surgery in Uncontrolled Open-Angle Glaucoma.** Arthur L. Schwartz and Joel Kopelman (Washington Hosp. Center, Washington, D.C.) reviewed the results of argon laser angle treatment (ALT) in 89 consecutively treated phakic eyes with clinically uncontrolled open-angle glaucoma and a baseline intraocular pressure exceeding 19 mm Hg. Eighty-two eyes in 72 patients were evaluable.

Diagnosis was primary open-angle glaucoma in 66 eyes, exfoliation syndrome in 9, pigment dispersion syndrome in 4, and angle-recession glaucoma in 3. All patients underwent ALT as an alternative to standard filtering surgery. An average of 100 burns was applied to the anterior to midpigment trabecular meshwork band by using a 50-μ spot size, an exposure time of 0.1 second, and a power setting of 750 to 1,250 mW. Five eyes had the base of the iris treated in 1 quadrant

Fig 6–1.—Average pressure change versus time in treated *(T)* eyes. (Courtesy of Schwartz, A.L., and Kopelman, J.: Ophthalmology (Rochester) 90:771–780, July 1983.)

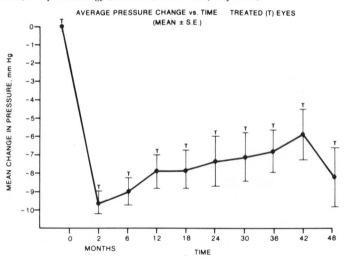

with low-power argon laser burns to contract the iris and open the angle.

Maximal reduction in mean pressure in the treated eye, 9.7 mm Hg, occurred after 2 months. The pressure-lowering effect diminished slowly from 2 to 42 months after the procedure (Fig 6–1). The reduction in pressure was more noticeable in patients with higher baseline pressures. A pressure reduction of more than 3 mm Hg was achieved with a stable visual field or optic nerve cupping, or both, in 77% of the treated eyes. Average follow-up was 21 months. The best response to ALT was in eyes with exfoliation. Older patients tended to do better. Six of 10 patients had a good outcome in both treated eyes. Peripheral anterior synechiae formed in 32% of eyes but did not compromise the final outcome. The pressure rose by 5 mm Hg or more in 9% of treated eyes in the first 3 weeks, compared with 26% of untreated eyes, despite continued medical treatment.

About 75% of the eyes with uncontrolled open-angle glaucoma in this series responded to argon laser trabecular surgery. The risk-benefit ratio of this procedure is excellent, compared with that of filtering surgery. Presently ALT is recommended for patients with open-angle glaucoma uncontrolled by maximally tolerated medical treatment. Studies are continuing to determine the best treatment parameters for ALT.

6–8 **Laser Trabeculoplasty in Open-Angle Glaucoma.** Laser trabeculoplasty is used increasingly to reduce the intraocular pressure in open-angle glaucoma. Christina Raitta and Ilkka Lehto (Univ. of Helsinki) evaluated the results of the procedure in 72 patients having 81 eyes treated for open-angle glaucoma 6 and 12 months after treat-

PRESSURE-REDUCING EFFECTS OF ARGON LASER TRABECULOPLASTY

Before treatment

average pressure	all patients mmHg		POAG mmHg		Gl. Caps mmHg	
lowest	22.3		20.7		22.7	
highest	30.8		26.4		32.9	

After six months follow-up:

	all patients		POAG		Gl. Caps	
	mmHg	%	mmHg	%	mmHg	%
lowest	15.8	29	17.2	17	17.1	25
highest	20.7	33	21.6	18	23.8	28

After one year follow-up:

	mmHg	%	mmHg	%	mmHg	%
lowest	17.1	23	17.7	15	16.7	26
highest	22.1	28	21.8	17	22.8	31

(6–8) Acta Ophthalmol. 61:673–677, August 1983.

ment. Laser treatment was indicated for poor pressure control despite maximal local treatment and acetazolamide therapy. Ocular hypertension was not an indication. Thirty-nine eyes had primary open-angle glaucoma, 34 eyes had capsular glaucoma, 5 eyes had chronic congestive glaucoma after iridectomy, and 3 eyes had other forms of secondary glaucoma. The complete chamber was coagulated with an argon-krypton laser, using a mean of 107 spots 0.05 to 0.1 mm in size at an energy setting of 1 to 2 W and a time of 0.2 second.

Only 6 of 32 eyes with primary open-angle glaucoma had a pressure reduction after 6 or 12 months, and 70% of the eyes showed no effect. Similar results were obtained in patients with chronic congestive glaucoma. The results were better in those with capsular glaucoma, especially thoose with an average peak pressure of 33 mm Hg (table). Three patients had complications possibly related to treatment, but none had visual field loss as a result. One patient had central vein occlusion in the treated eye 8 months after laser trabeculoplasty.

Laser trabeculoplasty led to somewhat lesser pressure reductions in these eyes than in others reported previously. All patients required medical treatment postoperatively, and 8 had surgery for glaucoma control. The greater pressure reduction obtained in eyes with capsular glaucoma might be related to the higher baseline pressures in these eyes, or to increased pigmentation of the trabecular meshwork. Laser trabeculoplasty can be a useful means of treating glaucoma, especially in high-pressure eyes. The intraocular pressure should be monitored closely for 2 to 3 days after the procedure.

6–9 **Argon Laser Trabecular Surgery in Primary Open-Angle Glaucoma.** M. Görne and D. Utermann (Hamburg, W. Germany) present data on 30 phakic eyes with primary open-angle glaucoma treated by argon laser trabecular surgery (Wise's technique).

The 19 patients in the study had a median age of 59.8 years. Mean intraocular pressure without low-pressure glaucoma was reduced from 28.8 to 18.8 mm Hg. The average reduction of pressure postoperatively was 10.0 mm Hg. In 4 eyes with low-pressure glaucoma the tension fluctuated an average of 14.9 mm Hg after coagulation. The mean observation time was 7.2 months. Therapy failed in 3 cases of pigmentary glaucoma. In the case of Rieger's syndrome the reduction of 10 mm Hg was insufficient for complete regulation of pressure and 0.5% timolol maleate drops had to be administered twice. There were no appreciable complications.

In 5 eyes a temporary increase of pressure was observed which was reduced with acetazolamide and normalized in 21 days at the latest. In all other cases the lowered pressure took effect within 24 hours. Thomas et al. (1982) coagulated 300 eyes within 2 years. Forty-seven (15.6%) were not regulated; all others were normalized with addi-

(6–9) Klin. Monatsbl. Augenheilkd. 182:125–128, February 1983.

tional local antiglaucomatous therapy. Histologic examination of the effectiveness of the trabecular coagulation according to Wise was done by Rodrigues (1982). Trabeculectomy was performed in 22 patients at 3, 6, and 18 hours, 1 week, 2, 8, and 12 months after laser coagulation of the trabeculae. Changes ranged from fibrinous exudation and decayed cells 3 hours postoperatively to complete proliferation of the trabeculae in the focal area 2 and 8 months later.

According to this study laser coagulation is recommended for patients with primary angle glaucoma if tension fluctuates up to 30 mm Hg and in patients with beginning turbidity of the lens. In most cases reduced pressure is established for at least 2 years and long-term results are not yet available. This surgery is especially recommended in so-called low-pressure glaucomas to improve the circulation in the papillary area. More extended case studies are needed before laser coagulation in aphakic glaucoma can be recommended. Apparently the treatment is not indicated in pigmentary glaucoma.

6–10 **What Happens to the Optic Disk and Retina in Glaucoma?** Douglas R. Anderson (Univ. of Miami) describes the spectrum of optic disk changes in glaucoma. There is a fair degree of individual variation in the distribution of axon loss within the optic nerve. The classic finding is loss of axons in bundles, which produces a notch in the affected sector of the disk, usually somewhat temporal to the inferior pole. A defect in a "nerve fiber bundle" field results. When one or

Fig 6–2.—All 3 scotomas could escape detection if central field were checked with pattern of 49 points. (Courtesy of Anderson, D.R.: Ophthalmology (Rochester) 90:766–770, July 1983.)

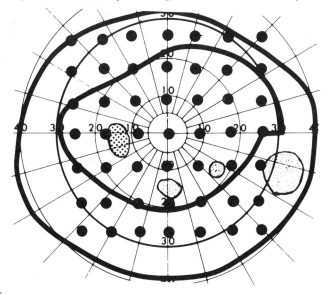

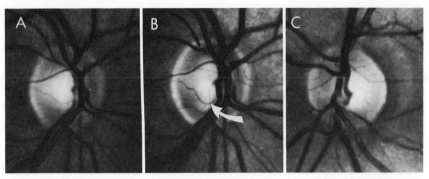

Fig 6–3.—A, right eye disk of patient with bilateral elevation of intraocular pressure in 1970. **B,** same disk in 1981, showing progressive enlargement of cup, bared circumlinear vessel *(arrow)*, and asymmetry with left eye. **C,** disk of left eye in 1981. (Courtesy of Anderson, D.R.: Ophthalmology (Rochester) 90:766–770, July 1983.)

several adjacent bundles are completely destroyed, the dense field defect may be small and well confined (Fig 6–2). Axonal loss also can be rather diffuse, involving scattered axons within many bundles across the entire cross section of the optic nerve. As a result the excavation enlarges concentrically (Fig 6–3). A concentrically enlarged optic cup may be difficult to distinguish from a larger than average physiologic cup. A greater than 50% loss of axons may be necessary for the excavation to reach a clearly abnormal size.

The best means of recognizing concentric enlargement of the optic cup as pathologic is to have a previous record of the disk. The exact size and configuration of the disk should be documented, preferably photographically, in all persons considered to be at particular risk of developing glaucomatous damage. The change in visual function also is rather subtle when axons are lost diffusely across the entire retina. Up to 50% of the axons may be lost diffusely before there is even a 0.5-log unit depression in visual sensation. A generalized depression of the fields can be recognized as glaucomatous when there is asymmetry between the 2 eyes.

Hopefully, more accurate methods of visual field screening will make it possible to distinguish pathologic changes in visual function from nonglaucomatous states such as macular change, lens opacity, and physiologic change accompanying aging. Complaints such as dimming of vision in one eye should be investigated.

▶ [In this well-thought-out article, the author helps us look for subtle optic disk changes in glaucoma and also warns us that our screening of visual fields may miss early functional loss. In the last 10 years there has been a great deal of work done on the pathogenesis of glaucomatous optic nerve disease, but so far the process remains an enigma. The experimental information has not helped us with our patients so we must rely on careful observation.] ◀

▶ ↓ The following 3 articles from Canada and England reinforce the experience in the United States that timolol maleate therapy is effective and well tolerated. Approximately 70% of patients achieved control and the only caution was for individuals with asthma or heart disease. The author of the third article presents persuasive evidence that there is little or no difference between 0.25% and 0.50% solutions, so that if the patient requires further medication, changing to the latter will most likely not be helpful. It is also important to note that a significant number of patients using timolol had a gradual pressure rise over the years. We must watch our patients carefully and be prepared for the possibility of the need for additional treatment. ◄

6–11   **Timolol: 4-Year Follow-Up Study.** Some studies of the β-blocker timolol have questioned its long-term benefit in lowering intraocular pressure. S. Markowitz and J. D. Morin (Univ. of Toronto) report findings from a 4-year study of 25 patients aged 38 to 76 with open-angle glaucoma who received timolol therapy. All had intraocular pressures of 22 mm Hg or higher without treatment. One drop of 0.25% timolol maleate was instilled in each affected eye once a day. Higher concentrations up to 0.5% twice daily were used if necessary to reduce the intraocular pressure to 21 mm Hg or less.

Timolol was effective, but the intraocular pressure tended to drift slightly upward over time (table). The course was similar regardless of the baseline intraocular pressure at the end of the first follow-up period, but subsequently an upward drift was more apparent in eyes with pretreatment pressures above 30 mm Hg. One trabeculectomy was performed. Acuity lessened by 1 or 2 lines from baseline in 40% of eyes examined after 2 years of timolol therapy, and after 4 years the acuity was lower than at 2 years in 37% of eyes. In 2 patients arcuate field defects developed during treatment and paracentral scotoma developed in 1; another patient had enlargement of a preexisting field defect. In 6 patients slight enlargement of the optic cup developed during follow-up; 4 of these had pretreatment intraocular pressures of 30 mm Hg or higher. The only complaint was occasional eye soreness. Blood pressure and pulse rate were unaffected by timolol therapy.

CHANGES IN INTRAOCULAR PRESSURE (IOP) DURING THERAPY WITH TIMOLOL MALEATE IN PATIENTS WITH GLAUCOMA (FOLLOW-UP PERIODS LASTING FOR 1, 1, AND 2 YEARS, RESPECTIVELY)

	Time of examination (no. of eyes)		
Change in IOP	End of first follow-up period (72)	End of second follow-up period (37)	End of third follow-up period (49)
Reduction to < 22 mm Hg, % of eyes	83	77	71
Decrease from pretreatment value, mean ± standard deviation (SD), mm Hg	9.0 ± 2.2	8.2 ± 2.3	7.3 ± 1.8
Increase from start of follow-up period % of eyes	75	49	65
Mean ± SD, mm Hg	4.0 ± 1.6	2.7 ± 1.8	3.6 ± 1.2

(Courtesy of Markowitz, S., and Morin, J.D.: Can. J. Ophthalmol. 18:278–280, October 1983.)

(6–11)   Can. J. Ophthalmol. 18:278–280, October 1983.

Timolol maleate maintained control of the intraocular pressure through 4 years in 71% of eyes with open-angle glaucoma in this series, but an upward pressure drift was apparent in some instances. Adverse effects were fewer than with certain other antiglaucoma agents, but caution is necessary in treating patients with asthma, bradycardia, or congestive heart failure.

6-12 **Chronic Open-Angle Glaucoma Treated With Timolol: Four Year Study—Timolol and Open-Angle Glaucoma.** Most previous studies of timolol have involved patients initially receiving other antiglaucoma therapy. Gordon M. Maclure (Middlesbrough, England) evaluated topical timolol therapy in 82 new patients with chronic primary open-angle glaucoma who were followed up for as long as 4½ years. Nine patients had been treated for glaucoma several months to years previously before defaulting. Timolol was used twice daily in 0.25% or 0.5% solution. A total of 154 eyes were treated in 49 men and 33 women aged 31 to 88 years; the age peak was 61 to 80 years.

Sixteen patients were withdrawn from the study. Timolol alone controlled the intraocular pressure in 9 of the 10 patients who died and in 4 of the 6 who failed to return. Pressure in 20 patients was not controlled by timolol alone. Forty-six patients received timolol alone, and pressure was controlled in 21 of them by 0.25% solution. Only a slight reduction in blood pressure was observed. Corneal sensitivity was unchanged.

More than 67% of the evaluable patients in this study with chronic open-angle glaucoma had pressure controlled by timolol alone.

6-13 **Blind Randomized Noncrossover Long-Term Trial Comparing Topical Timolol 0.25% With Timolol 0.5% in Treatment of Simple Chronic Glaucoma** was conducted by K. B. Mills (Manchester, England). Sixteen mean and 14 women (mean age, 70 years) with changes of the optic nerve head and visual field seen in open-angle glaucoma were randomly assigned to have either 0.25% or 0.5% timolol applied topically twice a day to each eye. Patients were examined at 1, 3, 6, 9, and 12 months.

Thirteen eyes (22%) in 8 patients (27%) required additional antiglaucoma medication to maintain an intraocular pressure (IOP) below 23 mm Hg after a minimal interval of 6 months; 5 of these patients were receiving 0.5% timolol and 3 were receiving 0.25%. After 12 months of topical timolol use, mean reduction in IOP from pretreatment values was 6.4 mm Hg (24%) in eyes receiving the 0.25% dose and 5.0 mm Hg (19.4%) in eyes receiving the 0.5% dose. When reductions in IOP at each follow-up interval were statistically significant, the significance always favored the 0.25% dose of timolol. Side effects were few. One patient had occasional hallucinations and 2 had temporary tinnitus.

(6–12) Trans. Ophthalmol. Soc. UK 103:78–83, 1983.
(6–13) Br. J. Ophthalmol. 67:216–219, April 1983.

In the 70% of patients in whom the reduction in IOP was sustained throughout the trial, there was little clinical significance in results produced by 0.25% and 0.5% timolol. This suggests that 0.25% timolol should be the preferred initial treatment. If this proves ineffective either early or late, then alternative or additive therapy should be considered in preference to the common clinical practice of changing the concentration of timolol to 0.5%. This report also confirms the existence and importance of long-term drift, or loss of control with continuous long-term treatment with topical timolol.

6–14 **Results of Iridectomy in Narrow-Angle and Open-Angle Glaucoma: A Retrospective Study.** W. Weder and M. Zeidler (Univ. of Marburg/Lahn, W. Germany) analyzed the results of a retrospective study involving the regulation of intraocular pressure (IOP) and loss of function. Between 1970 and 1975, 166 iridectomies were performed in patients with primary glaucoma. Follow-up examinations were performed between 6 weeks and 6 months, 12 months, 1.5 to 2.5 years, and 3 to 4 years after surgery in patients whose IOP was not adequately regulated.

Sixteen percent of the total number of cases required a second fistulating operation because of a progressive loss of visual field or inadequately stabilized IOP under additional pharmacotherapy. Hypotonia was rare. Of the eyes with acute narrow-angle glaucoma with an open iridocorneal angle by definition, which underwent surgery for the first time, 30% had an IOP of more than 21 mm Hg with or without additional tension-lowering medication (10% between 22 and 24 mm Hg; 10% greater than 24 mm Hg). The results for eyes operated on for the second time were better because of the prophylactic iridectomies in this group. Out of the total number of eyes operated on for the first time (narrow-angle and open-angle glaucoma) IOP was regulated by iridectomy alone in 54% after 1 year and in 33% after 2 years. In 33% of the cases the iridocorneal angle was occluded; in 66% an open angle was found. With regard to the iridocorneal angle in these 33%, it was found that 50% of the cases of narrow-angle glaucoma were regulated without further medication, but only 20% of the open-angle cases could be regulated. An analysis showed that regulation was better when the previous tension level had been high, while preoperative lower tension levels, between 20 and 25 mm Hg, often remained elevated after surgery. Loss of visual field after iridectomy occurred 1.6 times more in patients with open-angle glaucoma.

Results of a different study showed that not all narrow-angle glaucomas can be permanently regulated by means of basal iridectomy. In addition, another study showed that no specific surgical technique could be recommended in primary chronic glaucoma, and peripheral iridectomy was not the treatment for this condition. Both findings

(6–14) Klin. Monatsbl. Augenheilkd. 183:159–165, September 1983.

coincide with results of this study. Results showed that, after various fistulating surgical techniques, an average of 80% of eyes with chronic simple glaucoma were regulated, which would not have been possible with simple basal iridectomy. However, iridectomy is a relatively simple operation that may be indicated and recommended in cases of advanced age, contraindicated anesthesia, general severe illnesses, and when surgery is necessary only as a palliative measure or to offer the opportunity for administering mixed drops containing epinephrine postoperatively to patients with narrow-angle glaucoma.

▶ [This is an interesting article because the authors were able to study, albeit retrospectively, the effect of iridectomy on a series of patients who evidently had a diagnosis of open-angle glaucoma, as well as on angle-closure mechanism patients. In fact, 20% of the open-angle patients actually did not require further medication for control. One wonders if surgery affected patient compliance. Of the angle-closure mechanism patients, only 50% had control after 2 years and it thus seems reasonable to recommend careful and continual follow-up of angle-closure patients even after initially effective surgery.] ◀

6–15 **Developing Bleb: Effect of Topical Antiprostaglandins on the Outcome of Glaucoma Fistulizing Surgery.** A reduction in inflammation after trabeculectomy might improve the functional results of the procedure. Clive Migdal and Roger Hitchings (London) undertook a prospective comparison of topical antiprostaglandin therapy with placebo in a series of 30 patients followed up for a year after standard filtering operations for chronic simple glaucoma. Patients who had had previous eye operations and those with uveitis were excluded, as were patients given systemic corticosteroid therapy. Patients received either 0.5% indomethacin topically or the sesame oil placebo starting an hour before operation and then 3 times daily for a month, with 1% prednisolone 4 times daily and 1% atropine twice daily. Fourteen eyes were treated with indomethacin and 16 with the placebo.

Vision was reduced after operation in both groups. After 1 year acuity was at the preoperative level in 13 eyes, was improved in 8, and had declined in 8. All patients except 1 in the study group had normal intraocular pressures without further operation by 9 months. Four patients had transient pressure elevations to greater than 21 mm Hg in the first 3 postoperative months. Only 2 patients, 1 in each group, had poor intraocular pressure control on the water-drinking test at the end of the study. Intraocular inflammation resolved within 3 months in both groups of patients. Bleb development was similar in the 2 groups, although there were more cystic blebs in the control group.

Antiprostaglandins would appear to have no important role in the management of patients undergoing fistulizing operations for chronic simple glaucoma. There seems to be little relationship between the appearance of the fistulizing bleb and its functional reserve, as assessed by tonography, the water-drinking test, and intraocular pressure measurements.

(6–15) Br. J. Ophthalmol. 67:655–660, October 1983.

▶ [We continue to look for methods of improving fistualization surgery. Topical indomethacin, however, did not help patients in this prospectively studied series. The authors also make the important point that it is difficult to equate bleb function with its morphology. Indeed one might conclude that there are no simple yet reliable tests of bleb function.] ◀

6–16 **Two-Stage Neodymium-YAG Laser Trabeculotomy.** Paul A. Weber, Richard H. Keates, E. Mitchell Opremcek, Frederick M. Kapetansky, and Carol Szymanski (Ohio State Univ., Columbus) describe a procedure for the management of glaucoma that combines nonpenetrating trabeculectomy with neodymium-yttrium-aluminum-garnet (Nd:YAG) laser trabeculotomy to create a through-and-through filtration under a scleral flap without actually entering the anterior chamber. Two cases are reported in which the technique was successfully applied.

Man, 37, was first seen 1 year prior to the current surgery with pigmentary glaucoma. At that time, glaucoma treatment consisted of 0.5% timolol and 0.1% dipivalyl epinephrine solutions, applied twice daily to both eyes, and methaxolamide, 50 mg three times daily. His vision was 20/20 J-1 OD and 20/80 J-7 OS. External examination showed an afferent pupillary defect OS, and slit-lamp examination revealed pigment on the endothelium and midperipheral iris transillumination slits OU. Applanation tensions were 23 OD and 25 OS. Gonioscopy demonstrated grade-IV angles OU with heavy pigmentation of the meshwork and many iris processes. Bilateral argon-laser trabeculoplasty was performed, followed by a second procedure 3 weeks later. The intraocular pressure (IOP) stayed in the low teens for 10 months, but then increased to 24 OU with the same pretreatment medications. One year after the initial examination, the patient's vision was 20/20 OD and 20/40 OS. The optic disks showed no change. Visual fields were unchanged in the right eye and improved in the left.

A two-stage Nd:YAG trabeculotomy was performed in February 1983. Applanation tension, measured 4 hours after the nonpenetrating trabeculectomy, was 16. A very low filtration bleb was evident. The anterior chamber retained its preoperative depth and had no flare, and only a rare cell was observed. Gonioscopy showed the nonpenetrating trabeculectomy site actually lying anterior to the trabecular network. Six applications of the Nd:YAG laser, adjusted to the 8-millijoule setting, were applied to this site, with each application producing tissue disruption. The IOP immediately fell to 0 and the bleb increased in size. Thirty minutes after laser application, the IOP remained at 0. On the day after the procedure, vision was 20/200 and a good filtration bleb was observed. The anterior chamber remained very deep and no inflammatory reaction was observed. Applanation tension was 4. No choroidal detachment was observed. Four weeks after the procedure, vision was 20/60. An excellent avascular filtration bleb was observed, and the anterior chamber was deep and quiet. Applanation tension was 8. High-magnification gonioscopy showed a definite opening at the site of the Nd:YAG laser application.

The 2 cases reported demonstrate the feasibility of creating adequate filtration under a scleral flap without penetrating the anterior

(6–16) Ophthalmic Surg. 14:591–594, July 1983.

chamber. Long-term studies are being conducted to determine to what extent the theoretical advantages of this procedure are realized in actual practice.

▶ [The authors have devised a two-stage fistualization operation without iridectomy in an attempt to decrease surgical complications. A Krasnov sinusotomy (unroofing Schlemm's canal) is performed under a scleral flap. Several hours to a day later the trabecular meshwork is penetrated with a Nd:YAG laser. We shall have to wait and see what the long-term results will be. The major problem in fistualization surgery is scarring of the sclera and conjunctiva, and it is not clear how this procedure addresses that problem. Nonetheless if there really are few complications the two-stage method may prove to be useful.] ◀

6–17 **Long-term Results of Valve Implants in Filtering Surgery for Eyes With Neovascular Glaucoma.** Theodore Krupin, Paul Kaufman, Alan I. Mandell, Stuart A. Terry, Robert Ritch, Steven M. Podos, and Bernard Becker performed filtration surgery with a pressure-sensitive, unidirectional valve implant in 79 eyes with neovascular glaucoma. The device consisted of an open Supramid tube (outside diameter, 0.58 mm) sealed to a Silastic tube with a slit valve (Fig 6–4). The supramid tube was inserted at the corneoscleral limbus 1 to 4 mm into the anterior chamber. The Silastic portion was located under a scleral flap.

Intraocular pressure (IOP) was less than or equal to 24 mm Hg postoperatively in 53 of 79 eyes after a mean follow-up period of 23.7 ± 10.9 months. Of these 53 eyes, 27 required no medication; their mean IOP was 14.7 ± 6.0 mm Hg after a mean follow-up period of 25.0 ± 10.9 months. Medical therapy was required postoperatively in 26 eyes. This consisted of topically administered timolol or epinephrine (or dipivefrin); 5 patients also received orally administered car-

Fig 6–4.—Glaucoma valve consists of an open Supramid tube *(1)* that is placed in the anterior chamber and is cemented to a Silastic tube *(2)*. The end of the Silastic tube is sealed and contains horizontal and vertical slits *(arrow)* that function as the valve. Horizontal sidearms *(3)* are attached to provide suture fixation. The sidearms and Silastic end are placed outside the eye, under a scleral flap. (Courtesy of Krupin, T., et al.: Am. J. Ophthalmol. 95:775–782, June 1983.)

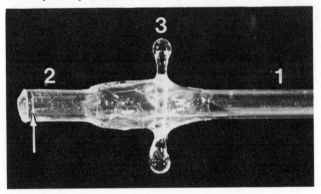

(6–17) Am. J. Ophthalmol. 95:775–782, June 1983.

bonic anhydrase inhibitors. The mean postoperative IOP in these eyes was 16.9 ± 5.3 mm Hg after 22.2 ± 10.5 months of follow-up. Additional surgery was required in some of the 53 successfully treated eyes. In 10 eyes, external bleb scarring with increased IOP occurred 1 to 11 months postoperatively. In 2 eyes, pupillary block developed after initial valve implantation. This was treated successfully by laser iridectomy. Five eyes showed growth of fibrovascular tissue on the internal portion of the device, which was also treated by laser. The glaucoma valve implant failed to keep IOP below 24 mm Hg in the remaining 26 eyes. External bleb scarring in the unsuccessful cases occurred 3 weeks to 20 months postoperatively. A comparison of preoperative and postoperative visual acuities in the 53 successfully treated eyes demonstrated an overall decrease. Cataracts were successfully removed in 3 eyes with functioning valve implants by planned extracapsular extraction. Mortality during long-term follow-up was high: 12 of 53 successfully treated patients and 5 of 26 unsuccessfully treated patients died.

▶ [The authors report the results of their multicenter study of a valve implant with an average follow-up period of approximately 2 years. Their implant appears to have solved the problems of fixation and obstruction of the internal segment, but the complication of external bleb scarring and obstruction remains similar to that in other types of fistualization surgery.] ◀

6–18 **Optic Disk and Visual Field Correlations in Primary Open-Angle and Low-Tension Glaucoma.** Richared A. Lewis, Sohan S. Hayreh, and Charles D. Phelps (Univ. of Iowa, Iowa City) attempted to confirm Levene's impression (1980) that the degree of visual field loss for a given amount of optic disk cupping is less in low-tension glaucoma than in primary open-angle glaucoma. Review was made of the findings in 127 eyes with primary open-angle glaucoma and 71 with low-tension glaucoma. No patient had other disorders that affected the visual fields. Those with low-tension glaucoma had intraocular pressures consistently below 23 mm Hg. Visual fields were assessed by Goldman perimetry. Stereoscopic photos of the optic disks were examined independently by 3 observers.

The proportion of eyes with mild, moderate, and severe field losses was similar in the 2 groups, but the average amount of field loss was slightly greater in the eyes with primary open-angle glaucoma (32.6 versus 26.7 sectors). None of the observers overpredicted visual field loss more in low-tension glaucoma than in primary open-angle glaucoma; each of them tended to do the opposite. Average frequency of overprediction was 33% for the group with open-angle glaucoma and 26% for the group with low-tension glaucoma. Respective frequencies of underprediction were 15% and 24%.

Optic nerve damage in glaucoma probably has a multifactorial pathogenesis. High intraocular pressure is certainly the chief factor

(6–18) Am. J. Ophthalmol. 96:148–152, August 1983.

in some cases, but other factors probably are equally or more important when the intraocular pressure is normal or only slightly increased. The present findings fail to support the view that optic disk damage in primary open-angle glaucoma differs from that in low-tension glaucoma.

▶ [We do not understand low-tension glaucoma although our failure is mostly based on a lack of understanding of the pathogenesis of the optic disk changes in primary open-angle glaucoma. The authors of this article have shown that the optic disk changes in the 2 diseases have a similar appearance. That doesn't mean, of course, that the pathogenesis is the same for both diseases. A great deal more work needs to be done on the pathogenesis of glaucomatous optic nerve disease.] ◀

6–19 **Relationship of Patient Age and Tolerance to Carbonic Anhydrase Inhibitors.** C. Eric Shrader, John V. Thomas, and Richard J. Simmons (Boston) gained a clinical impression that younger glaucoma patients tolerate carbonic anhydrase inhibitors better than older patients. Data were reviewed on 222 patients given these drugs for control of primary or secondary glaucoma. Use of the prescribed dose for 6 weeks or longer was taken to indicate tolerance if no symptoms occurred during treatment or if treatment was ended for unrelated reasons. Average patient age was 60 years; 31 patients were aged 40 and younger.

Forty-eight percent of patients tolerated carbonic anhydrase inhibitors, and another 17% continued to receive long-term treatment, despite mild symptoms, when a therapeutic adjustment was made. Treatment was continued by 77% of the patients aged 40 and younger and by 61% of older patients, a significant difference. Average durations of treatment in patients who continued were 2.9 years for those aged 40 and younger and 2.6 years for older patients. Most patients with side effects related to treatment had gastrointestinal symptoms or malaise. Malaise and depression were more frequent effects in patients aged 65 years and older.

The risk of operative complications exceeds that from carbonic anhydrase inhibitor therapy, and the chance of successful filtration is less in younger than in older patients. Initially successful operation may later fail, leaving few therapeutic alternatives. Argon laser trabeculoplasty is less safe and effective in younger glaucoma patients. These patients tolerate carbonic anhydrase inhibitors better than older patients, and it should be considered unless there are specific contraindications.

▶ [We are all familiar with the long list of complications of carbonic anhydrase inhibitors. The authors of this article, however, ask us to reexamine their use in young people mainly because the alternatives are so unsatisfactory. Indeed, laser trabeculoplasty has been disappointing in young patients and fistualization surgery has many serious, long-term complications.] ◀

6–20 **Effect of Physical Activity on Intraocular Pressure of Glaucomatous Patients.** A. Shapiro, E. Wolf, I. Ferber, and S. Merin

---

(6–19) Am. J. Ophthalmol. 96:730–733, December 1983.
(6–20) Eur. J. Applied Physiol. 52:136–138, November 1983.

(Hadassah Univ., Jerusalem) noticed that some patients with chronic simple glaucoma reported frontal headache and nausea while performing planned physical exercise. Intraocular pressures therefore were recorded in 12 patients, aged 40 to 69 years, with simple open-angle glaucoma who were referred for exercise in a rehabilitation clinic. Tests were done 48 hours after withdrawal of all medications. Ergometric exercise was performed up to a 75-W load. A significant reduction in intraocular pressure during exercise was observed at loads of 25, 50, and 75 W.

Normal subjects show a reduction in intraocular pressure during exercise that is proportional to the workload, and a similar decrease in pressure also occurs in patients with chronic simple glaucoma. The pressure fall seen in the authors' patients was significant even when the effects of repeated applanation measurements and of diurnal variations were taken into account. It seems likely that both patients and physicians sometimes attribute symptoms that can normally occur during exercise to glaucoma. Chronic simple glaucoma does not contraindicate physical activity.

7. Lens

Cataract Surgery

EDWARD COTLIER, M.D., AND
WARREN FAGADAU, M.D.

Yale University, New Haven

At a time when a reappraisal of outpatient cataract surgery is under way, R. M. Ingram, D. Banerjee, M. J. Traynar, and R. K. Thompson reviewed a series of 501 cataract extractions performed under local anesthetic as day-cases![1] Forty percent of the patients had no living spouse, but half of these lived with relatives or a friend. The other half (20% of total) lived alone, although four out of five of them had some support from neighbors, friends, or at-home help. All patients were visited at home by a trained nurse the day after surgery. About 75% of the patients were not affected by the operation or the few hours spent in the hospital, and the same number felt fit and active the following day; 77% of the patients said they would have been able to return to the hospital for examination on the day following surgery.

Beginning February 9, 1978, studies of intraocular lenses (IOL) were begun under Investigational Device Exemption (IDE) approved by the FDA to determine the safety and effectiveness of IOL as a medical device for the correction of aphakia.[2] Because of the "new model" IOL being developed and tested, studies should continue to evaluate the long-term safety of these prosthetic devices. Clinically significant sight-threatening complications, such as hyphema, secondary glaucoma, macular edema, and pupillary block, developed in a higher percentage of anterior chamber and iris fixation IOL cases.[2] Clinically significant "persistent" complications present at the 12- to 14-month follow-up visit, such as corneal edema, secondary glaucoma, and macular edema, developed more frequently in the anterior chamber and iris fixation lens cases. Surgical problems were reported more frequently for anterior chamber lenses (14% vs. 9% for the other IOL). Posterior capsular rupture for the anterior chamber lens and vitreous loss for the anterior and posterior chamber lenses were associated with a statistically significant reduction in visual acuity. If an eye had 20/40 or better before secondary anterior chamber lens implantation, there was a 10.4% chance of having less than 20/40 best corrected vision after secondary lens implantation.[2]

Along these lines, Jack T. Holladay, John E. Bishop, Thomas C. Prager, and J. Warren Blaker (University of Texas at Houston) have succinctly summarized the various design characteristics of an "ideal intraocular lens."[3] Independent of location, the lens must be stable in its fixation so that no intraocular lens movement occurs; lengthening the support loops of the posterior chamber lens to 14 mm for large eyes and the flexible anterior chamber lenses have helped minimize this problem. The ideal intraocular lens should have neutral buoyancy (i.e., a specific gravity of 1.0) to eliminate inertia of the lens with ocular movement. The diameter of the lens optic should be large enough to accommodate all rays entering the pupil. The optical resolution of a lens is most commonly measured in line pairs per mm (1 p/mm), and an intraocular lens with a resolution of 100 l p/mm has been adopted as an industry standard. The ideal intraocular lens should be located in the posterior chamber to achieve a more nearly iseikonic image, and have a minimal resolution of 100 l p/mm when measured in air. Lens optic should be biconvex, with the posterior surface being approximately three times more powerful than the anterior surface to minimize spherical aberrations, internal reflections, and lens-iris contact.

H. Richard McDonald and A. Rodman Irvine described a characteristic macular lesion observed in 6 patients who underwent extracapsular cataract extraction with posterior chamber lens implantation.[4] Despite the fact that aphakic cystoid macular edema was described prior to the use of the operating microscope, some recent authors have speculated that a large percentage of modern cases of aphakic cystoid macular edema are related to phototoxicity from the illumination source of the operating microscope. The finding of maculopathy, however, should force all clinicians to heed recent laboratory studies warning of potential dangers of the illuminating systems in ophthalmic instruments; this necessitates study of more effective filters for our ophthalmic instruments, and forces us to reexamine our surgical techniques in relation to their potential for retinal photic and thermal toxicity.

David K. Berler and Robert Peyser (Washington Hospital Center) analyzed 310 cataract operations that were randomly distributed between 2 operating rooms, each containing a microscope with different light intensity. Of 133 patients in the study, 71 were operated on under high-intensity light, and 62 were subjected to lower illumination in the operating room. Age and high-light intensity were the only factors that could be related to reduced visual acuity (20/40 or worse) during the 6 months after cataract surgery.[5]

Straatsma, Pettit, Wheeler, and Miyamasu (UCLA) have undertaken a prospective evaluation of extracapsular cataract extraction with posterior chamber intraocular lens implantation in 229 patients, of whom 20 (9%) were diabetic, with and without nonproliferative retinopathy.[6] To test for statistically significant differences between diabetic and nondiabetic cases, the 234 eyes of 229 patients were adjusted on a random basis to include only one surgical eye of each of the 229 patients. No statistically significant differences were observed in either operative or postoperative complications.

Wade Faulkner (Mobile, Ala.) used the laser interferometer to test 137 eyes to determine whether preoperative interference visual acuity tests could accurately predict postoperative Snellen visual acuities.[7] Several easily recognizable clinical conditions make the interferometer test unreliable. Those that produced false positive responses included serous detachment of the sensory epithelium of the macula, cystoid macular edema, visual field cuts through fixation, amblyopia, macular holes or cysts, geographic atrophy of the pigment epithelium of the macula, and early postoperative retinal detachment. Those that produced false negative responses were mature cataracts and testing without pupillary dilation.

References

1. Ingram, R.M., Banerjee, D., Traynar, M.J., et al.: Day-case cataract surgery. *Br. J. Ophthalmol.* 278–281, 1983.
2. Stark, W.J., Jr., Worthen, D.M., Holladay, J.T., et al.: The FDA Report on intraocular lenses. *Ophthalmology* 90:311–317, 1983.
3. Holladay, J.T., Bishop J.E, Prager, T.C., et al.: The ideal intraocular lens. *CLAO Journal* 9:15–19, January 1983.
4. McDonald, H.R., and Irvine, A.R.: Light-induced maculopathy from the operating microscope in extracapsular cataract extraction and intraocular lens implantation. *Ophthalmology* 90:945–951, 1983.
5. Berler, D.K., and Peyser, R.: Light intensity and visual acuity following cataract surgery. *Ophthalmology* 90:933–936, 1983.
6. Straatsma, B.R., Pettit, T.H., Wheeler, N., et al.: Diabetes mellitus and intraocular lens implantation. *Ophthalmology* 90:336–343, 1983.

7–1 **Experimental and Clinical Evaluation of Lens Transparency and Aging.** Sidney Lerman (Emory Univ., Atlanta) notes that the normal human lens is a precisely formed structure containing about 65% water and 35% organic matter, the latter being mainly (greater than 90%) structural proteins. The lens becomes encapsulated at the 13-mm embryonic stage and is consequently divorced from a direct blood supply for life. It provides the investigator with an organ that exists in an environment analogous to a single-cell type of tissue culture system and can be reproduced in vitro. Since the cornea and lens are transparent one can directly monitor morphological and biochemical aging changes in vivo. Recent developments now permit monitoring of certain molecular changes as well.

Laboratory studies have demonstrated enhanced fluorescence in the ocular lens associated with aging and psoralen ultraviolet A (PUVA)

(7–1) J. Gerontol. 38:293–301, May 1983.

therapy, and presumptive PUVA cataracts have been reported. A new method, UV slit-lamp densitography, now provides an objective and reproducible method for monitoring at least one parameter of lens aging, lens fluorescence (Fig 7–1). Preliminary studies in patients exposed to above ambient levels of UV radiation or to photosensitizing agents, or both, show an enhancement of lenticular fluorescence. In vivo UV slit-lamp densitography provides a useful diagnostic and prognostic screening method to identify lens photodamage due to excess UV exposure (occupational or accidental). Cortical opaque areas

Fig 7–1.—Densitometric analyses of lenses in patients aged *(from top)* 26, 37, 44, and 71 years shows increasing fluorescence levels with age and in nuclear sclerosis and correlation with increased in vitro fluorescence analyses on whole lenses derived from eye bank eyes and surgical specimens. (Courtesy of Lerman, S.: J. Gerontol. 38:293–301, May 1983.)

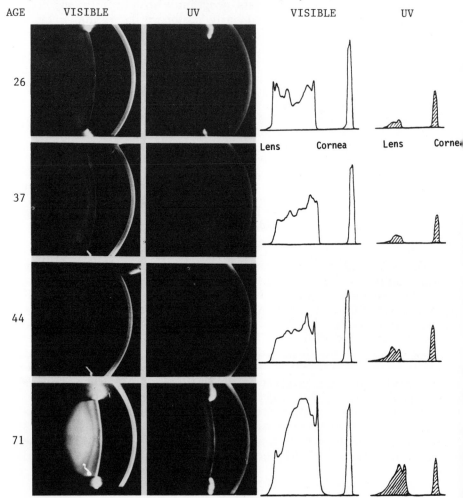

AGE   VISIBLE   UV   VISIBLE   UV

are also a common finding in older patients. In vitro nuclear magnetic resonance (NMR) (human and animal lenses) and in vivo (animal) experiments currently in progress are rapidly elucidating the physicochemical basis for the development of light scattering areas in the cortex of the aging lens. Thus, it is now feasible to use biophysical methods, in particular optical spectroscopy and NMR analyses, to delineate and monitor specific age-related measurements in the ocular lens in vivo as well as in vitro.

7–2   **Epidemiology of Senile Cataracts: A Review** is presented by M. Cristina Leske and Robert D. Sperduto. More than 25% of those aged 65 to 74 years may have lens opacities that reduce vision to 20/25 or worse. In the Framingham study the prevalence of lens changes that resulted in acuity of 20/30 or worse was reported as 18% in this age group. Lens extraction is one of the most common operations performed in adults, and it has increased in frequency in recent years.

The cause of senile cataract is unknown, but it is closely associated with increasing age and also is related to diabetes and elevated blood pressure. The role of inadequate nutrition remains unclear. Environmental factors that have been implicated include radiation exposure and a variety of topical and systemic drugs, including steroids. A role for microwave radiation in the development of senile cataract has not been established. It is possible that familial factors are important in senile cataract development.

A reproducible, standardized in vivo classification of the type and severity of cataract is badly needed. Photographic methods may aid the development of an objective classification scheme. Data on the incidence and prevalence of cataracts in the general population and on the magnitude of resulting visual impairment are incomplete. Further studies of risk factors are needed, as are controlled clinical trials to evaluate various treatment measures.

▶ [This is a fine review that emphasizes the important problem of the lack of a classification based on morphology. Indeed, it is difficult to obtain standardized morphological information with current photographic instruments. It may be that newer biomicroscopes and photographic techniques will solve the problem.] ◀

7–3   **Increased Mortality Among Elderly Patients Undergoing Cataract Extraction.** Robert P. Hirsch and Bernard Schwartz (Boston) compared age-specific and sex-specific mortality retrospectively in patients undergoing cataract extraction with that in patients having other elective surgical procedures. The study group included 167 patients aged 50 years or more who had a cataract extracted between January 1, 1970, and December 31, 1979; the control group included 824 patients who underwent elective cholecystectomy, hemorrhoidectomy, inguinal herniorrhaphy, spinal fusion, a procedure for trigeminal neuralgia, or varicose vein stripping and ligation. Followup of patients began 90 days after hospital discharge to exclude

(7–2)   Am. J. Epidemiol. 118:152–165, Aug. 1, 1983.
(7–3)   Arch. Ophthalmol. 101:1034–1037, July 1983.

from statistics any deaths directly related to the experience of surgery.

With reference to years of follow-up, analysis of mortality was so constructed that it is an estimate of the number of deaths per person-year. Age-specific mortality for men is shown in Figure 7–2 and that for women in Figure 7–3. Allowing for age, sex, race, and diabetes, there was a significant difference in mortality between the cataract patients and controls, but mortality was not significantly influenced by sex, race, or the presence of diabetes. The findings suggest that patients who undergo cataract extraction experience excess mortality largely as a result of diseases other than diabetes. It is possible that cataracts might be related to another distinct group of fatal diseases. As few deaths resulted from any specific cause, it was necessary to compare broad categories: heart disease, cancer, and arteriosclerosis. No significant differences for any of the 3 groups were observed.

Fig 7–2 (top).—Age-specific mortality among men undergoing cataract extraction *(shaded columns)* and in male controls *(open columns)*.

Fig 7–3 (bottom).—Age-specific mortality among women undergoing cataract extraction *(shaded columns)* and in female controls *(open columns)*.

(Courtesy of Hirsch, R.P., and Schwartz, B.: Arch. Ophthalmol. 101:1034–1037, July 1983; copyright 1983, American Medical Association.)

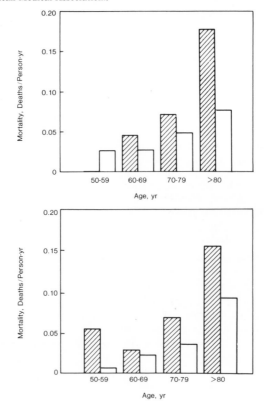

The origin of senile cataracts seems to be a component of a systemic process rather than a discrete ocular phenomenon. This process does not seem to be strongly related to the high frequency of diabetes observed among patients undergoing cataract extraction.

▶ [The authors conclude that senile cataract is part of a general, life-shortening, disease process. Patients considered for cataract surgery should have a good general physical examination as well as a reasonable probability of survival to benefit from the improved vision.] ◀

7–4 **Comparison of Two Interferometers for Predicting Visual Acuity in Patients With Cataract.** B. L. Halliday and J. E. Ross compared the two commercially available instruments, Rodenstock Retinometer and Haag-Streit Visometer, which are currently used to project interference grating on the retina.

In the first part of the study the authors compared the effect of a range of plus and minus 10 diopters of defocusing on Snellen visual acuity with and without a pinhole, with the same amount of defocusing on retinal acuity by using the interferometers in 2 normal subjects. In the second phase of the study 50 consecutive cataract patients operated on at Oxford Eye Hospital were tested. Ages ranged from 49 to 92 years. Twenty-two eyes in these 50 patients were

Fig 7–4.—Visual acuity *(decimal scale)* is plotted against added refraction (amount of defocusing) from emmetropia. Results are shown for Snellen *(solid circles)*, Snellen with pinhole *(open circles)*, visometer *(solid squares)*, and laser interferometer *(solid triangles)* visual acuities. In every case the eye was fully dilated and cyclopleged. (Courtesy of Halliday, B.L., and Ross, J.E.: Br. J. Ophthalmol. 67:273–277, May 1983.)

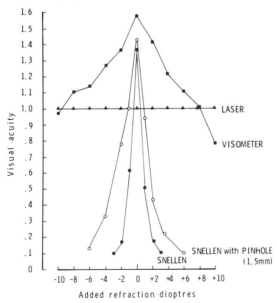

(7–4) Br. J. Ophthalmol. 67:273–277, May 1983.

aphakic or had a clear lens; the clear-lens eyes were used as controls to check instrument calibration. In the 50 cataractous eyes preoperative retinal acuity was compared, by using both interferometers, with postoperative Snellen acuity to see if the latter correlated well with the preoperative prediction.

Results from the first part of the study (Fig 7–4) showed both instruments could produce good retinal visual acuity in the presence of a marked degree of spherical ametropia. In the second part of the study it was found that in any 1 subject almost identical readings were obtained from the Visometer when used in either the green or white positions. Best Snellen acuity was plotted against Retinometer and Visometer retinal acuity for the 22 eyes with no medical opacities. Good correspondence was obtained. Postoperative Snellen acuity (achieved) was plotted against the preoperative retinal visual acuity (predicted) for the Retinometer and the Visometer. For any given eye similar predicted acuities were obtained from the two interferometers. However, the achieved acuity was often different from the predicted acuity.

Although the interferometers can project gratings through severe cataract and ametropia, visibility of the gratings is affected by cataract, and the grating acuity does not in any case correspond with postoperative Snellen acuity. These interferometers have little practical use in preoperative assessment and any surgeon relying on them would seriously misjudge the visual potential of many patients.

▶ [One would hope the manufacturers would continue to conduct research to develop an instrument that does work.] ◀

7–5 **Day-Case Cataract Surgery.** This report by R. M. Ingram, D. Banerjee, M. J. Traynar, and R. K. Thompson (Kettering, England) concerns 292 patients, 276 of whom had 501 day-case cataract extractions; the other 16 were hospitalized for reasons not directly connected with cataract surgery.

TABLE 1.—OPERATIVE AND POSTOPERATIVE
COMPLICATIONS

Complications	No. of eyes
Operative	
Extracapsular extraction	16
Extracapsular extraction+vitreous loss	1
Vitreous loss	14
Postoperative (to date)	
Iris prolapse	4
Retinal detachment	2
Panophthalmitis	0

(Courtesy of Ingram, R.M., et al.: Br. J. Ophthalmol. 67:278–281, May 1983.)

(7–5) Br. J. Ophthalmol. 67:278–281, May 1983.

TABLE 2.—PREFERENCES AS TO HOSPITALIZATION OR
DISCHARGE HOME POSTOPERATIVELY

	Male	*Female*	*Total*
Preferred home	78 (78%)	106 (73·6%)	184 (75·4%)
Preferred hospital	5 (5%)	26 (18%)	31 (12·7%)
Indifferent	17 (17%)	12 (8·3%)	29 (11·9%)
Totals	100	144	244

(Courtesy of Ingram, R.M., et al.: Br. J. Ophthalmol. 67:278–281,
May 1983.)

METHODS.—A detailed interview with the patient is conducted at the time surgery is advised. On the day of operation, the history is rechecked; pulse and respiration rates and blood pressure are measured, and urinalysis is done. Lashes are cut. At operation, the retrobulbar and facial nerves are injected with 2% lidocaine plus epinephrine, and cocaine drops are placed in the eye. Ab externo incision under a limbus-based conjunctival flap is followed by lens removal, usually with a cryoprobe. No intraocular lenses are inserted. Virgin silk corneoscleral sutures and 6–0 plain catgut sutures are used. Eight percent pilocarpine drops (round pupil) or 1% atropine (keyhole pupil) and neomycin drops are instilled. The eye is covered with a pad. Reasonably free mobility is allowed immediately postoperatively, with nursing supervision. The first dressing is applied 3 to 4 hours after operation. Plain dark or aphakic glasses are tried. Instructions are given for continuing care, and the patient is discharged at about 5:00 PM. During a home visit by a trained nurse on the day after the operation, the eye is inspected and bathed; 1% atropine drops and a combined prednisolone and neomycin preparation are instilled. Outpatient clinic visits are scheduled for 1 week, 3 to 4 weeks, and 7 to 8 weeks postoperatively; on the last visit, refraction and prescription of glasses complete the procedure.

Operative and postoperative complications are listed in Table 1. At the third postoperative outpatient clinic visit the patients are asked to complete a questionnaire concerning their reactions to the procedure. Most preferred the day-care procedure to hospitalization (Table 2).

With respect to the two complications most relevant to day-case surgery, iris prolapse and panophthalmitis, the advantages of hospitalization appear to be marginal. A home visit by an appropriately trained nurse is essential after day-case surgery to detect ocular complications that require immediate attention, and to demonstrate the best way to instill eyedrops, as well as to reassure the patient and relatives. All of the patients believed that 1 home visit was necessary, but that additional visits were not required.

▶ [Affluent middle-class patients may very well prefer and indeed do better postoperatively at home than in the hospital. There are a large number of patients, however, especially in the inner cities of the United States, who would have no one to help them at home even if they could obtain the transportation. One would think it desirable to assess carefully the postoperative environment before making a final decision about the type of postoperative care needed.] ◀

7–6 **Planned Extracapsular Cataract Extraction.** Interest in extracapsular cataract extraction has increased with evidence that maintenance of the posterior capsule may reduce posterior segment complications. Extracapsular cataract extraction also can decrease such anterior segment complications as the entrance of vitreous into the anterior chamber. Additionally, the procedure avoids creating problems where future surgery may be indicated, such as in penetrating keratoplasty or a filtering glaucoma operation. William S. Harris (Dallas) uses hand-held instruments rather than machines such as the phacoemulsifier. Senile cataracts make particularly suitable cases wherever intraocular lens insertion is anticipated. Patients with severe myopia and those with a family history of retinal detachment should have an intact posterior capsule after cataract surgery, as should glaucoma patients who may require filtering surgery and patients with a marginally functional cornea.

Ultrasonography should be performed preoperatively if an intraocular lens is to be used. Topically applied antibiotics and orally administered antiprostaglandins are used preoperatively. A soft eye is produced with an osmotic or a pressure device. Surgery is carried out using an operating microscope with coaxial illumination. The anterior capsulotomy is performed with the Visitec cystotome or a bent 23-gauge needle, and the nucleus is removed by the dialing-out technique. Cortex is removed by irrigation and aspiration. The capsule is polished and cleaned using the Graether collar-button iris retractor. After which, a posterior chamber lens is implanted, and a peripheral iridectomy is done using the DeWecker scissors and McPherson forceps. The wound is closed with a running suture of 10–0 nylon. No conjunctival closure is used. Antibiotic is injected into Tenon's space superiorly and steroid is injected inferiorly.

Primary posterior capsulotomy is done rarely, and only where there is obvious posterior capsule opacity in the visual axis. Secondary capsulotomy simplifies the primary implant procedure and reduces retinal and anterior segment complications. Secondary posterior capsulotomy is performed when a decrease in vision requires it, but not before 1 year has elapsed. Pars plana posterior capsulotomy can safely be performed in the office with good visual results.

▶ [This is a carefully written review of one surgeon's technique. It is a reflection on our time and rapidly changing technology that just a year after such a review was written, the YAG Laser has completely changed the treatment of the posterior capsule. The author was performing pars plana posterior capsulotomies in his office with a knife, but he has no doubt by now substituted the laser.] ◀

▶ ↓ In the following article the author recommends partial anterior vitrectomy at the time of cataract surgery in children because of eventual opacification of the posterior capsule. As discussed above, the YAG laser may change this procedure too, although there is a problem of patient cooperation. Use of general anesthesia and laser energy delivery in a recumbent patient are still serious problems. ◀

(7–6) Ophthalmologica 187:74–82, 1983.

7–7 **Posterior Lens Capsulectomy During Primary Cataract Surgery in Children** is preferable to lens aspiration techniques, according to a report from Marshall M. Parks (Washington, D.C.). After lens aspiration in these patients, the intact posterior lens capsule gradually becomes translucent, interfering with development of the fixation reflex and determination of the optimal aphakic optical correction. This often causes unequal visual inputs into the two retinocortical systems of the infant, producing intractable amblyopia during the weeks or months before secondary surgery is performed to open the clouded posterior lens capsule.

Removal of all but 2 mm of the peripheral posterior lens capsule with a vitreous suction cutter leaves a clear pupil. Anterior vitrectomy places the vitreous face posterior to the plane of the iris. As a result, formation of posterior synechia and development of iris bombe are unlikely, making iridectomy unnecessary. The pupil remains active, centered, and dilates well with a mydriatic, affording accurate retinoscopy and a complete view of the fundus by indirect ophthalmoscopy. In addition to reducing the risk of amblyopia, removing the posterior lens capsule during primary cataract surgery avoids the need for secondary surgery, with its attendant risks and costs.

Recently, continuous-wear soft contact lenses have been applied at the completion of surgery. The power varies with the age of the patient from approximately 35 + diopters (D) for those younger than age 1 month to 20 + D at age 3 months. Refraction is started within the first few days after surgery. To insure that maximally focused images continue to be projected onto the retina throughout the critical period, adjustments in lens power are made frequently to overcorrect the refractive error by +1 to +3 D.

Cystoid macular edema reportedly occurs more often after vitreous removal than when the posterior lens capsule is left intact. However, amblyopia at this time may be a greater risk to final visual acuity than cystoid macular edema.

▶ ↓ In the following two articles, the authors discuss cataract extraction in patients with diabetic retinopathy. It would appear that not only cataract surgery but also intraocular lens implantation are safe in eyes with only minimal background diabetic retinopathy. We have found that it is easy to photocoagulate through an intraocular lens. New lenses may be manufactured to absorb the shorter wavelengths and this may cause a problem in the future. In eyes with proliferative disease, however, the retinopathy is made worse by cataract surgery. Indeed, the incidence of rubeosis iridis and secondary glaucoma is significantly increased. Panretinal photocoagulation should be performed before, if possible, or if not, immediately following, lens extraction. ◀

7–8 **Experience With Intraocular Lens Implants in Patients With Diabetes.** John G. Sebestyen and M. Zafer Wafai (Boston) reviewed the outcome of intraocular lens implantation in 16 women and 13

(7–7) Ophthalmology (Rochester) 90:344–345, April 1983.
(7–8) Am. J. Ophthalmol. 98:94–96, July 1983.

men aged 60 years and older, all diabetic. The cataracts were unilateral or, if bilateral, the best corrected acuity differed markedly in the 2 eyes. Intracapsular cryoextraction was performed in 26 eyes and planned extracapsular extraction in 3 eyes. Twenty-three anterior chamber lenses, 3 iris-supported lenses, and 3 posterior chamber lenses were implanted.

No surgical complications occurred. Transient elevations in intraocular pressure in a few patients with angle-supported anterior chamber implants were readily controlled. Final acuities were determined by the extent of fundus abnormality. Twenty patients had acuity of 20/40 or better. In 2 patients, active background retinopathy developed leading to significant macular edema after uneventful surgery; laser photocoagulation was successful in these patients. In another, rubeosis iridis and neovascular glaucoma developed 15 months postoperatively without activation of the retinopathy. Four patients had senile macular degeneration leading to visual impairment.

Intraocular lens implantation after cataract extraction appears to be no more hazardous in diabetic patients than in other individuals if limited to patients with no retinopathy or only minimal background retinopathy. The advantages of intraocular lens implantation make it an option in selected diabetic patients.

7-9 **Neovascular Glaucoma and Vitreous Hemorrhage Following Cataract Surgery in Patients With Diabetes Mellitus.** Lloyd M. Aiello, Martin Wand, and Gwen Liang reviewed the results of intracapsular cataract extraction in 154 diabetic patients operated on in 1969 to 1976 at the Joslin Diabetes Center, Boston. The fellow eye was not operated on for at least a year after initial cataract surgery. No patient had laser photocoagulation in either eye within a year after cataract surgery. Active proliferative diabetic retinopathy, with or without vitreous hemorrhage, was present in 15 operated-on and 31 unoperated-on eyes. Quiescent proliferative retinopathy was present in 31 operated-on and 20 unoperated-on eyes. The 100 female and

TABLE 1.—PATIENTS WITH PREOPERATIVE ACTIVE
PDR WHO DEVELOPED RUBEOSIS AND NEOVASCULAR
GLAUCOMA AFTER OPERATION

	Yes	No	Total
Oper. eye	6 (40%)	9	15
Unoper. eye	0	31	31
Total	6	40	46

$P < .001$.
PDR = proliferative diabetic retinopathy.
(Courtesy of Aiello, L.M., et al.: Ophthalmology (Rochester) 90:814–820, July 1983.)

(7–9) Ophthalmology (Rochester) 90:814–820, July 1983.

TABLE 2.—Patients With Preoperative Active
PDR Who Developed Vitreous Hemorrhage
After Surgery

	Yes	No	Total
Oper. eye	3 (20%)	12	15
Unoper. eye	2 (6.5%)	29	31
Total	5	41	46

PDR = proliferative diabetic retinopathy.
(Courtesy of Aiello, L.M., et al.: Ophthalmology (Rochester)
90:814–820, July 1983.)

54 male patients had an average age of 65 years. About 65% of the patients had insulin-dependent diabetes.

Both vitreous hemorrhage and rubeosis iridis-neovascular glaucoma were 3 times more frequent in patients with insulin-dependent diabetes than in the others. Rubeosis iridis and neovascular glaucoma occurred in 8% of operated-on eyes and in less than 1% of unoperated-on eyes, a significant difference. The incidence was significantly increased only in eyes with existing active proliferative diabetic retinopathy (Table 1). Vitreous hemorrhage was twice as frequent in operated-on eyes. One fifth of the operated-on eyes with active proliferative retinopathy developed vitreous hemorrhage after operation (Table 2). The difference was significant, however, only in eyes without active proliferative retinopathy at the time of cataract surgery.

Diabetic patients with active proliferative diabetic retinopathy have a high risk of acquiring rubeosis iridis and neovascular glaucoma after intracapsular cataract extraction. Panretinal photocoagulation of active proliferative retinopathy should be carried out in a diabetic patient who is starting to develop a cataract. When an advanced cataract is already present and adequate panretinal photocoagulation is precluded, cataract surgery should be carried out and panretinal photocoagulation should be performed within a few days after surgery. A number of high-risk eyes have been successfully managed in this way without development of neovascular glaucoma or vitreous hemorrhage after operation.

7–10 **Bilateral Intraocular Lens Implantation.** Henry M. Clayman, Norman S. Jaffe, Mark S. Jaffe, and Susan M. Luscombe (Univ. of Miami) reviewed the data on 373 patients who had bilateral intraocular lens implantations, representing about 20% of a group of patients who received posterior chamber intraocular lens implants in 1978 to 1981. All posterior chamber lenses were of the "J-loop" Shearing type, while the iris-fixed lenses were chiefly Binkhorst iris clip lenses. Ex-

(7–10) Ophthalmology (Rochester) 90:321–323, April 1983.

tracapsular extractions were done in 59% of first eyes and 99.7% of second eyes. Eighty-seven percent of patients gained vision of 6/12 or better in the first eye, 90%, in the second eye. The main cause of lesser vision in both first and second eyes was senile macular choroidal degeneration (Table 1). Repeat surgery was necessary in 12%

CAUSES OF VISION LESS THAN 20/40				
	Cases 1st Eye		Cases 2nd Eye	
Cause	No.	Percent	No.	Percent
Senile macular degeneration	19	(39.6%)	11	(30.5%)
Cystoid macular edema	8	(16.6%)	5	(13.9%)
Other maculopathy*	6	(12.5%)	6	(16.7%)
Keratopathy†	5	(10.4%)	5	(13.9%)
Glaucoma	3	(6.3%)	2	(5.5%)
Ischemic optic neuropathy	0	(0.0%)	1	(2.8%)
Amblyopia	4	(8.3%)	1	(2.8%)
Unknown	3	(6.3%)	5	(13.9%)
Total	48	(100.0%)	36	(100.0%)

*Includes macula hole, macular pucker, and diabetic maculopathy.
†Includes one case of postradiation keratopathy.
(Courtesy of Clayman, H.M., et al.: Ophthalmology (Rochester) 90:321–323, April 1983.)

SURGICAL REINTERVENTION*		
Surgery	Cases 1st Eye	Cases 2nd Eye
Discision	18	3
Reposition IOL	5	1
Wound dehiscence	1	3
McCannel Suture	2	0
Retinal Detachment	4	1
Iridectomy	2	0
Paracentesis	1	0
Washout	1	0
Keratoplasty	7	2
Removal IOL	0	2
IOL Exchange	1	2
Iris suture removal	1	0
Pupillary membrane	1	0
Total	44	14
Percent/series	11.8%	3.75%

*IOL, intraocular lens.
(Courtesy of Clayman, H.M., et al.: Ophthalmology (Rochester) 90:321–323, April 1983.)

of first eyes, chiefly for secondary cataract. The second eye was reoperated on in 3.7% of cases (Table 2). Most patients went 1 to 3 years between surgical procedures; the interval was less than 3 months in 4% of cases.

Bilateral intraocular lens surgery is recommended. With modern posterior chamber lenses, most complications and reoperations result from the cataract operation rather than from the presence of an intraocular lens within the eye. Iatrogenic complications have been minimal with increased experience in extracapsular techniques. In nearly all instances, the interval between procedures on the 2 eyes was 6 months or longer. Unilateral lens implant surgery often fulfills the patient's immediate visual needs.

► [The authors make the important point that monocular lens implantation results in such good visual rehabilitation that the patient can wait 6 months or more for bilateral surgery. A study of the visual rehabilitation from monocular versus bilateral cataract surgery with intraocular lens implantation would be of interest.] ◄

► ↓ In the following article, however, the authors make it clear that at least in monocular aphakia, implantation results in better stereopsis than does contact lens correction. ◄

7–11 **Quality of Stereopsis in Unilateral Aphakia Corrected With Contact or Intraocular Lenses** is discussed by C. Huber, U. Meier, and F. Hess (Univ. of Zurich, Switzerland). Subjective aniseikonia was measured in patients with unilateral aphakia, which was corrected with a contact lens or an intraocular lens (IOL), by means of a test generated by a microcomputer and shown on a television screen. The results were compared with the calculated aniseikonia. The calculated optical aniseikonias were between 1% and 7% for patients with implanted lenses and between 4% and 16% for patients with contact lenses.

The major result of this study was derived from subjective measures of stereopsis. An aniseikonia of as much as 6% was compatible with excellent stereoacuity measured by random dot tests. In subjective stereotests, stereoacuity was found to be much better in the IOL cases. However, the result should not be overestimated; a high-grade stereopsis in itself is seldom necessary. This physiologic function can only be tested in the laboratory or examined under isolated testing situations. Under normal circumstances the stereopsis is evaluated together with the haziness of the picture and the parallax. This explains why patients with contact lenses are not disturbed by the poorer stereopsis. The authors' results show a great number of cases with normal stereoptic vision after lens implantation. The rate of the still-tolerated aniseikonia after lens implantation is 5% to 6% when measured by the degree of stereopsis.

The comparison of stereopsis in both groups should neither be used as argument for implantation preference nor for considering calcula-

(7–11) Klin. Monatsbl. Augenheilk. 182:379–382, May 1983.

tion of aniseikonia unnecessary before lens implantation. Relative to long-term correction, attention must be drawn to the fact that patients with unilateral aphakia often stop wearing their contact lenses because the advantage of binocular vision is not worth the annoyance of the lenses. The major advantage of the IOL is that it is always worn and that a sensory adaptation to the changed vision is easier to achieve. In myopic patients with unilateral cataract it is necessary to sacrifice emmetropic vision and maintain 5% aniseikonia rather than risk extensive aniseikonia developing in cases corrected with contact lenses. A planned increase of a preexisting myopia to achieve absolute iseikonia does not seem justified. Aniseikonia calculation should be included in preoperative assessment of unilateral aphakia, especially in axial myopia.

▶ ↓ With more than a million intraocular lenses implanted the procedure has obviously become enormously popular with patients and ophthalmic surgeons. Indeed most, if not all, training programs teach their residents the procedure. We seem to be at the point of debating only how complicated an eye disease needs to be to exclude implantation surgery; neither glaucoma, diabetes, nor retinal detachment, seems to be a contraindication.

In half of the articles in this chapter, the authors discuss intraocular lenses. In the first 5 papers, the staggeringly large numbers implanted in just the past few years are reviewed. The most recent trend is for use of posterior and anterior chamber lenses. One would hope that the anterior chamber lens is not being used when "something goes a little wrong" preventing posterior chamber implantation. Intraocular lens implantation is only a few decades old and experience with the "latest" lens invariably only a few years. Perhaps the patient should be prepared for contact lens use if the surgery does not go perfectly smoothly. The author of one of the following articles concludes with a line from Dickens, "It is a far far better thing I do than I have ever done before." It may be helpful to recall that shortly after uttering the line, the character had his head chopped off. Let us continue to maintain a cautious approach to intraocular lens implantation to avoid the possibility of a similar fate. ◀

7–12 **FDA Report on Intraocular Lenses.** Walter J. Stark, David M. Worthen, Jack T. Holladay, Patricia E. Bath, Mary E. Jacobs, George C. Murray, Eleanor T. McGhee, Max W. Talbott, Melvin D. Shipp, Nancy E. Thomas, Roger W. Barnes, Daniel W. C. Brown, Jorge N. Buxton, Robert D. Reinecke, Chang-Sheng Lao, and Scarlett Fisher (Johns Hopkins Med. Institutions, Baltimore, Md.) reviewed data collected in a 4½-year period on more than 1 million implanted intraocular lenses. More than 400,000 lenses were implanted in the last year of the study. Detailed review was made of 45,543 cases. The numbers of different types of lenses implanted are shown in Figure 7–5. The use of posterior chamber lenses and anterior chamber lenses has increased recently. In the most recent 6-month period, posterior chamber lenses accounted for 48% of all procedures, and anterior chamber lenses for 45%.

In the detailed review, 84.8% of study eyes had 20/40 or better vision after 1 year of follow-up. The results were best for iridocapsular and posterior chamber lenses and worst for iris fixation lenses. In the

(7–12) Ophthalmology (Rochester) 90:311–317, April 1983.

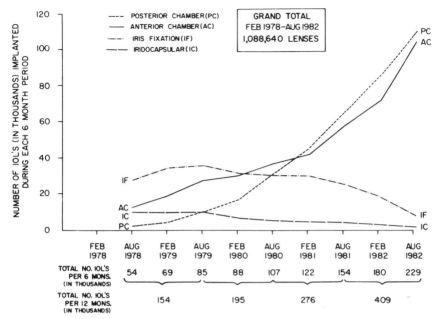

Fig 7–5.—Number of intraocular lenses *(IOLs)* (in thousands) plotted for each 6-month period since the FDA study began in February 1978. (Courtesy of Stark, W.J., et al.: Ophthalmology (Rochester) 90:311–317, April 1983.)

best cases, 90% to 94% of eyes achieved 20/40 or better acuity. Surgical problems were most frequent with anterior chamber lenses. Such problems tended to reduce the final acuity. The overall visual results of secondary intraocular lens implantation were similar to those of primary lens implantation. The visual outcome was adversely affected by advancing age.

The current trend in the United States is toward implantation of anterior chamber or posterior chamber intraocular lenses. Seventeen commercial types of lenses from 7 manufacturers have been recommended as being safe and effective.

7–13 **Trends in Cataract Surgery and Intraocular Lenses in the United States** are reviewed by Walter J. Stark, M. Cristina Leske, David M. Worthen, and George C. Murray. Cataracts currently are the second leading cause of blindness in the United States. Rates of cataract surgery have increased greatly in recent years, partly because of the extensive use of intraocular lenses for aphakic correction. Cataract surgery is done most often in patients aged 65 and older. National studies indicate that the percentage of intraocular lens implantation was 1.7 times higher in 1981 than in 1979. It was esti-

(7–13) Am. J. Ophthalmol. 96:304–310, September 1983.

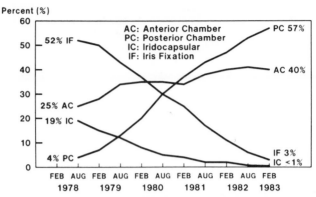

Fig 7–6.—Percentage of all intraocular lenses implanted shown by class for each 6-month period. (Courtesy of Stark, W.J., et al.: Am. J. Ophthalmol. 96:304–310, September 1983.)

mated that some 640,000 cataract operations were done in the United States in 1982, and an estimated 496,000 intraocular lenses were implanted in a similar period, representing more than 65% of all cataract operations. More than 50% of all lenses implanted in 1978 were iris fixation lenses; 57% of those implanted in a 6-month period in 1982 and 1983 were posterior chamber lenses and 40% were anterior chamber lenses (Fig 7–6).

One reason for the recent rise in cataract surgery may be the improved quality of vision obtained when an intraocular lens is implanted, especially in elderly patients. More than 70% of all cataract operations in the United States presently are associated with intraocular lens implantation.

7–14 **Update of the Intraocular Lens: Experience at the Wilmer Institute** was reviewed by Walter J. Stark and A. Edward Maumenee (Johns Hopkins Hosp.). Between 1975 and 1982, 3 different approaches to intraocular lens (IOL) implantation were used. Morcher four-loop lenses sterilized by the wet pack method were used in 200 eyes in the first 3 years of the series, and four-loop lenses sterilized by the dry pack method were used in 103 eyes in the next 2½ years. Subsequently, 547 Shearing-type and Sinskey-type posterior chamber lenses sterilized by the dry pack method were implanted. Mean ages of the patients were similar in the 3 groups, averaging 72 years. The mean follow-up ranged from 14 months for patients given posterior chamber IOLs to 76 months for those treated earliest.

Operative complications were generally minimal and were similar in the 3 groups. In more than 5% of eyes given Morcher lenses corneal edema developed. Retinal detachment and symptomatic retinal holes developed in up to 3.5% of patients in all groups. Cystoid mac-

(7–14) Ophthalmologica 187:65–73, 1983.

ular edema with reduced acuity was least frequent in the group given posterior chamber lenses. Although acuities cannot be compared directly because of differing follow-up periods, a significant decrease in acuity occurred in eyes with four-loop Binkhorst lenses. This is only partly explained by the onset of senile macular degeneration.

A cautious approach to IOL implantation is appropriate. Encouraging short-term results have been obtained with the Shearing-type posterior chamber IOLs in conjunction with extracapsular cataract extraction, but the longest meaningful follow-up of these lenses in the United States is only about 4 years, and potentially significant modifications in loop design and curvatures have been made during this time.

7–15 **Effects of Shearing Posterior Chamber Intraocular Lens on Corneal Endothelium.** Data on a consecutive series of 67 patients (70 eyes) with senile cataract were studied by Stanley P. Azen, Arthur Hurt, Douglas Steel, James Wilson, Jan Reinig, Jonine Bernstein, Meenu Bedi, and Ronald E. Smith (Univ. of Southern California, Los Angeles) to evaluate the decrease in corneal endothelial density and other complications after cataract extraction and insertion of intraocular lenses. Each patient underwent standard extracapsular cataract extraction with insertion of a Shearing posterior chamber lens. Capsulotomy was performed during surgery or during the follow-up period when clinically indicated. Most patients had 9 postoperative follow-up examinations. Complete endothelial photography was done preoperatively, and at 6 months, 1 year, and 2 years postoperatively.

There was a significant average decrease of 11% ± 1% in central cell density 1 month after surgery ($P < .001$). The decrease in superior cell density was 20% ± 2% ($P < .001$) and in inferior cell density

	Outcome*		
Variable	Good (No. = 57)	Poor (No. = 13)	P
Age (yrs)	71.9	78.1	.006
Preoperative cell density (cells/mm²)			
Central	2,441	2,488	.36
Superior	2,618	2,482	.14
Inferior	2,389	2,363	.40
Corneal thickness (mm)	0.54	0.53	.32
Immediate change in corneal thickness (mm)	0.008	0.013	.36
Preoperative superior cell density adjusted for age (cells/mm²)	2,647	2,377	.04

EFFECT OF VARIABLES ON FINAL OUTCOME

*Good outcome was defined as cell density loss of less than 30%; poor outcome was defined as cell density loss of 30% or more.

(Courtesy of Azen, S.P., et al.: Am. J. Ophthalmol. 95:798–802, June 1983.)

(7–15) Am. J. Ophthalmol. 95:798–802, June 1983.

5% ± 2% (P < .005) 2 months after surgery. Complications included corneal edema in 1 patient requiring a corneal transplant, a sterile nonhealing ulcer in 1 patient necessitating a conjunctival flap, and secondary glaucoma in a third patient. Visual acuities of 20/20 to 20/40 were found in 34 patients 2 years after surgery. None had cystoid macular edema, but dry macular degeneration and optic atrophy were identified as causes of poor visual acuity.

A poor outcome of surgery (central density loss ≥ 30%) was significantly correlated with low preoperative superior endothelial cell density (table). Older patients were more likely to have poor results than younger patients. During the 2-year follow-up there was no progressive damage to the endothelium caused by the Shearing posterior chamber lens. Unlike damage caused by some iris clip lenses, endothelial trauma due to posterior chamber lenses appears to occur only at the time of surgery and is not progressive.

7–16   **Lens Implantation: Lessons Learned From the First Million** are discussed by Robert C. Drews (Washington Univ., St. Louis). A survey of various types of intraocular lenses points up the many problems that can result from a lack of quality control. The Ridley lenses, which were too heavy, and the Dannheim lenses, with flexible loops that moved in the chamber angle and provoked inflammation, are examples. Barraquer lenses were rapidly abandoned as being insufficiently stable.

Pseudophakodonesis produces both lens dislocation and corneal dystrophy. The latter appears to be due to intermittent touch and a critical loss of endothelial cells that is exacerbated by preexisting endothelial dystrophy or surgical damage, or both. Complications have resulted from incomplete polishing of a small portion of the lens, emphasizing the importance of attention to all aspects of lens quality. At one time Rayner was the only company not making metal loop intraocular lenses.

Progressive biodegradation of nylon and polypropylene has been demonstrated. The question of whether polymethylmethacrylate can be biodegraded remains open. Some sterile hypopyons occurring in patients given lenses sterilized with ethylene oxide might have been avoided with standard sodium hydroxide sterilization.

Well over 10,000 ophthalmologists currently are performing lens implantation. The procedure has been firmly established in the visual rehabilitation of cataract patients and is unquestionably worthwhile.

(7–16)   Trans. Ophthalmol. Soc. U.K. 102:505–509, 1982.

8. The Uvea

The Promise of Cyclosporine

HOWARD H. TESSLER, M.D.

Eye and Ear Infirmary
University of Illinois, Chicago

Corticosteroids have been the mainstay of therapy for patients with ocular inflammatory disease. For severe ocular inflammatory disease that is resistant to or inadequately controlled by corticosteroids, immunosuppressive therapy with chemotherapeutic agents such as chlorambucil and azathioprine has been useful. Most physicians are reluctant to use chemotherapeutic agents, however, because of potential long- and short-term toxicity. Such toxicity includes neoplasia, bone marrow depression, secondary opportunistic infection, and sterility. Cyclosporine is a new chemotherapeutic agent that probably offers increased safety and efficacy.

Cyclosporine is produced by fungi found in soil samples in Wisconsin and Norway. It is water-soluble and seems to be a specific inhibitor of cell-mediated immunity (T cell). Cyclosporine's effects are reversible in that the T cells are not killed. Conventional chemotherapeutic immunosuppressive agents indiscriminately destroy all rapidly dividing cells (T cells, B cells, sperm).[1]

It is believed that cyclosporine inhibits the functioning of helper T cells by interfering with the production of interleukin-2 (IL-2), a lymphokine normally produced after exposure to specific antigens or mitogens. In addition, cyclosporine may inhibit other T-cell lymphokines such as interferon and interleukin-3. Suppressor T lymphocytes seem to be resistant to cyclosporine.[2-4] It has been observed that at pharmacologic doses natural killer cells are not affected by cyclosporine alone.[5] This is important to know because natural killer cells probably play a major role in immune surveillance against infectious agents and neoplasia.

Cyclosporine is a cyclic molecule of 11 amino acids, including an unusual D form and another hitherto unknown amino acid. The molecular action of cyclosporine is unknown.[1] Cyclosporine is dissolved in olive oil and ethanol for oral administration and in ethanol alone for intravenous injection. Cyclosporine is predominantly metabolized in the liver, with excretion into bile.[3]

Cyclosporine also kills parasites by interfering with an enzyme in the schistosome that degrades hemoglobin. A derivative of cyclosporine may be able to suppress schistosome without being immunosuppressive. Cyclosporine also may be effective for use in cases of chloroquine-resistant malaria.

The most widespread current usage of cyclosporine is in the promotion of renal graft survival without concomitant bone marrow suppression.[6, 7] In one study, graft survival was 80% after 1 year when cyclosporine and prednisone were used, as opposed to 64% with conventional immunosuppression by azathioprine, prednisone, and other agents.[7] Another recent study using cyclosporine alone had a 72% 1-year graft survival compared with 52% in a group treated with azathioprine and corticosteroids.[8] Whether cyclosporine is best used alone or combined with corticosteroids is controversial, however.

Toxic effects of systemic cyclosporine included nephrotoxicity, hepatotoxicity, hirsutism, tremors, central nervous system toxicity, seizures, gingival hyperplasia, hypertension, hemolytic anemia, thrombocytopenia, and lymphoma. Cytomegalovirus infections occur in 3% of cases treated with cyclosporine vs. 33% managed with standard immunosuppressive therapy.[1] Nephrotoxicity occurs in 10% to 15% of patients and usually can be controlled by reducing the dosage of cyclosporine. Similarly, hepatotoxicity can be managed by dosage reduction. Most other side effects are either minor or rare.[1]

Controversy exists over the potential for the induction of neoplasia with cyclosporine usage. The incidence of lymphoma in 3,000 patients treated with cyclosporine was 15 (0.5%). The rate of neoplasia with conventional immunosuppression has been reported to be between 2% and 11%.[9]

Cyclosporine may be beneficial in treating certain autoimmune diseases. Preliminary data imply its possible usefulness in Graves' ophthalmopathy, dermatomyositis, and type 1 diabetes mellitus.[10-12]

Cyclosporine has been effective in improving the survival of rabbit corneal grafts when given intravenously, subconjunctivally, and topically.[13-15] Nussenblatt and colleagues have recently demonstrated that cyclosporine effected an improvement in 15 of 16 patients with various types of uveitis resistant to conventional corticosteroids and immunosuppressive therapy.[16] These patients had diseases such as Behçet's disease, pars planitis, vitritis, sarcoid, sympathetic ophthalmia, Vogt-Koyanagi-Harada syndrome, and birdshot choroidopathy. In many of these patients the improvement in visual acuity was outstanding. Renal toxicity, which occurred in 5 of the 16 patients, was controlled by lowering the cyclosporine dosage. Cases of hepatotoxicity were also reversed in this manner.

Unfortunately, clinical experience with cyclosporine for ocular conditions has been limited. No double-masked studies have been completed to illustrate its clinical effectiveness. In spite of this, cyclosporine seems to be an effective immunosuppressive agent. Many of the serious drawbacks of classical immunosuppressive therapy appear to be avoided with cyclosporine. Reduced systemic effects may be achieved in ocular disease by administering cyclosporine topically and periocularly. Finally, cyclosporine may herald a new type of antiinflammatory agent that more specifically modulates the immune response. If this is true, we may no longer need to suppress the whole immune system to treat ocular inflammatory disease.

References

1. Kolata, G.: Drug transforms transplant medicine. *Science* 221:40, 1983.
2. Macek, C.: Cyclosporine's acceptance heralds new era in immunopharmacology. *JAMA* 250:449, 1983.
3. Abramowicz, M.: Cyclosporine—a new immunosuppressive agent. *Medical Letter* 25:77, 1983.
4. Bunjes, D.: Studies on the mechanism of action of cyclosporine A in murine and human T-cell response in vitro. In White, D. J. G. (ed.): *Cyclosporine A*. Amsterdam, Elsevier Biomedical Press, 1982, pp. 261–80.
5. Nussenblatt, R.B., Rouk, A.H., Wacker, W.B., et al.: Treatment of intraocular inflammatory disease with cyclosporine A. *Lancet* 2:235, 1983.
6. Calne, R.Y., Rolles, K., White, D.J.G., et al.: Cyclosporine A initially as the only immunosuppressant in 34 recipients of cadaveric organs: 32 kidneys, 2 pancreases, and 2 livers. *Lancet* 2:1033, 1979.
7. Canadian Multicentre Transplant Study Group: A randomized clinical trial of cyclosporine in cadaveric renal transplantation. *N. Engl. J. Med.* 309:811, 1983.
8. European Multicentre Trial Group: Cyclosporine in cadaveric renal transplantation: One year follow-up of multicentre trial. *Lancet* 2:968, 1983.
9. Cyclosporine and neoplasia. Editorial. *Lancet* 1:1083, 1983.
10. Weetman, A.P., Ludgate, M., Mills, P.V., et al.: Cyclosporine improves Graves' ophthalmopathy. *Lancet* 2:485, 1983.
11. Zabel, P., Leimenstoll, G., and Gross, W.L.: Cyclosporine for acute dermatoyomsitis. Letter to the editor. *Lancet* 1:343, 1984.
12. Laupacis, A., Gardell, C., Dupre, J., et al.: Cyclosporine prevents diabetes in BB Wister rats. *Lancet* 1:10, 1983.
13. Hunter, P.: Corneal graft rejection: A new rabbit model and cyclosporine. *Br. J. Ophthalmol.* 66:292, 1982.
14. Kana, J.S., Hoffman, F., Buchon, R., et al.: Rabbit corneal allograft survival following topical administration of cyclosporine. *Invest. Ophthalmol. Vis. Sci.* 22:686, 1982.
15. Salisbury, J.D., and Gebhardt, B.M.: Suppression of corneal allograft rejection by cyclosporine. *Arch. Ophthalmol.* 99:1640, 1981.
16. Nussenblatt, R.B., Palestine, A.C., and Chan, C.: Cyclosporine A therapy in the treatment of intraocular inflammatory disease resistant to systematic corticosteroid and cytotoxic agents. *Am. J. Ophthalmol.* 96:275, 1983.

8–1 **Factors Related to the Initiation and Recurrence of Uveitis** are discussed by G. Richard O'Connor (Univ. of California, San Francisco). Uveitis consists of a large group of diverse disorders involving the uvea, retina, optic nerve, and vitreous body. Some form of tissue injury is responsible for all cases. In the case of viral infection, cytotoxic reactions directed against virus-infested cells are pathogenically important. The immune system can react with inappropriate violence against a relatively benign pathogen, producing a severe inflammatory disorder. Reiter's syndrome, especially the form associated with chlamydial infection, is an example. Uveal tract injury from the deposit of immune complexes is assumed to be an important mechanism of the initiation of uveitis in such disorders as serum sickness and lupus erythematosus. Acute inflammation can be induced by a number of mediators such as prostaglandins and the leukotrienes. Autooxidation may be an important element of inflammation, especially in conditions such as Behçet's disease that are characterized by increased leukotactic activity. Neurotransmitters are also implicated in the initiation of uveitis, especially those forms related to corneal trauma or chronic corneal infection. Histamine undoubtedly is important in the induction of changes in vascular permeability.

Certain forms of uveitis exhibit a strong tendency to recur. Latent organisms such as herpesvirus may sometimes be responsible. The breakdown of *Toxoplasma* cysts has been related to recurrent toxoplasmic retinochoroiditis. Factors associated with pregnancy could contribute to recurrences of this disease. Decreased cellular immunity accompanying aging could have a role in the recurrence of some forms of uveitis such as herpes zoster uveitis. Changes in permeability may be responsible for the perpetuation of uveitis through the action of immune complexes. Some believe that emotional stress can help precipitate some forms of uveitis. The hypothalamus seems to be important in stress-mediated inflammatory reactions. Neurotransmitters may constitute a link between emotional stress of cerebral origin and the immunologic events that lead to inflammation in target tissues. The thymus and spleen are innervated by both the adrenergic and the cholinergic nervous systems, and changes in their neuroendocrine environment influence the output of these organs.

▶ [This is a splendid treatise on a complex disease process and should be read in its entirety by both clinician and researcher.] ◀

8–2 **Photocoagulation for Choroidal Neovascularization.** Almost 90% of the severe visual loss in patients with senile macular degeneration (SMD) can be attributed to the neovascular form of the disease. Stuart L. Fine and Robert P. Murphy (Johns Hopkins Med. Institutions, Baltimore) discuss the various forms of SMD and the use of argon laser photocoagulation in its treatment as reported by the Senile Macular Degeneration Study (SMDS) Group.

(8–1) Am. J. Ophthalmol. 96:577–599, November 1983.
(8–2) Ophthalmology (Rochester) 90:531–533, May 1983.

The atrophic form of SMD is the most common and includes drusen and varying degrees of pigment epithelial disturbance; most patients do not progress beyond this stage. The exudative, or neovascular, form of SMD is characterized by more severe visual loss from subretinal serous or serosanguinous exudation from a choroidal neovascular membrane. The SMDS has reported that argon laser photocoagulation was effective in reducing the risk of severe visual loss by more than 60% in patients with the neovascular form of SMD. Sixty percent of the untreated eyes, but only 25% of the treated eyes, progressed to severe visual loss within 18 months of follow-up. Criteria for entry into this study required that the patient have a visual acuity of 20/100 or better and a new vessel membrane at least 200 μ from the center of the foveal avascular zone (FAZ). Because the argon blue-green laser has particular toxicity within 200 μ of the center of the fovea, the Krypton Photocoagulation Study, also supported by the National Eye Institute, is evaluating whhether krypton red laser photocoagulation can reduce the risk of visual loss in SMD patients with neovascularization within 200 μ of the FAZ.

Since laser treatment can reduce the risk of severe visual loss by more than 60%, earlier evaluation of SMD patients with acute visual symptoms will allow identification of a considerably higher proportion of eyes with extrafoveal neovascularization that is amenable to laser treatment. Patients with eyes at risk for the development of neovascular maculopathy should be taught to check their central field daily with an Amsler grid or a similar chart. Patients with untreatable eyes and treatment failures may be helped by the use of appropriate low-vision aids.

▶ [The authors report their extremely important demonstration that photocoagulation may reduce the risk of severe visual loss due to the exudative form of senile macular degeneration (SMD). It is important to note, however, that the exudative disease, while causing most of the visual loss, makes up only about 20% of the total number of patients with SMD. It is also necessary to point out that the study was only continued for 1½ years so that there is no long-term follow-up. Finally, a number of clinicians have been suggesting name changes for SMD because of the stigmata of senility. Proposals include "age-related" macular degeneration and "involutional" macular degeneration, among others.] ◀

▶ ↓ In the following 6 articles, the authors discuss choroidal melanomas. The debate concerning conservative care versus enucleation continues and, indeed, because of the nature of the disease, the answers may be slow in coming.

In the first article, the authors conclude that diagnosis may be improved by fluorescein angiography and, in opaque media, by ultrasonography. Computerized axial tomography would also be helpful and, most recently, magnetic resonance imaging has become an important diagnostic tool for the eye and orbit. Indeed, we have high hopes for future magnetic resonance spectroscopy for tissue diagnosis. ◀

8–3 **Incidence of Misdiagnosed and Unsuspected Choroidal Melanomas: A 50-Year Experience.** Frederick H. Davidorf, Alan D. Letson, Esther T. Weiss, and Elliot Levine (Ohio State Univ., Columbus) reviewed the eye pathology files covering 1931 through 1981 to

(8–3) Arch. Ophthalmol. 101:410–412, March 1983.

PREVIOUS STUDIES OF MISDIAGNOSED MALIGNANT MELANOMA

Source	Institution*	Interval Studied	Misdiagnosis, %
Ferry	AFIP, Washington, DC	1949-1962	19.0
Shields and Zimmerman	AFIP	1962-1969	20.0
Blodi and Roy	University of Iowa, Iowa City	1940-1966	6.3
Badtke et al	...	1955-1964	12.8
Howard	Columbia Presbyterian Medical Center, New York	1957-1965	8.0
Shields and McDonald	Wills Eye Hospital, Philadelphia	1962-1972	3.7
Robertson and Campbell	Mayo Clinic, Rochester, Minn	1954-1977	2.7
Charlin	L'Hôpital du Salvador, Santiago, Chile	1956-1971	17.3
Addison and Wakelin	University of Ottawa	1964-1973	3.4
Harry	University of London	1968-1972	11.3
Current study	Ohio State University, Columbus	1931-1981	3.5

*AFIP indicates Armed Forces Institute of Pathology.
(Courtesy of Davidorf, F.H., et al.: Arch. Ophthalmol. 101:410–412, March 1983; copyright 1983, American Medical Association.)

determine the percentage of misdiagnoses of uveal melanomas and of unsuspected melanomas in 3 separate time periods.

During the 50-year period, 395 eyes were enucleated for choroidal melanoma, and 369 of these (93%) had clear media. Of these, 13 (3.5%) contained lesions imitating malignant melanoma, usually retinal detachment (6 cases), hemorrhage (2), or metastatic carcinoma (2). Of the 26 enucleated eyes with opaque media, 8 were misdiagnosed (30.8%). The incidence of misdiagnosis decreased from 10.9% in 1931–1959 to 1.7% in 1960–1981.

Of 411 choroidal melanomas present on histologic examination, 37 (9%) were unsuspected. All had opaque media. The percentage of unsuspected melanomas decreased from 19.6% in 1931–1959, to 13.3% in 1960–1969, and finally to 2.4% in 1970–1981.

The percentage of misdiagnosed malignant melanoma is probably not as high as previously believed (table). The results confirm the reliability of indirect ophthalmoscopy, widely used since the 1960s, in the diagnosis of melanoma in the presence of clear media and the reliability of ultrasonography, used since 1970, in the diagnosis of melanoma in eyes with opaque media. Fluorescein angiography is also useful in eyes with clear media.

8–4 **Prognostic Factor Study of Disease-Free Interval and Survival Following Enucleation for Uveal Melanoma.** Johanna M. Seddon, Daniel M. Albert, Philip T. Lavin, and Nancy Robinson attempted to identify prognostic indicators of survival after enucleation in a series of 267 patients with a diagnosis of ciliary body or choroidal melanoma. The patients were identified from records of the Massachusetts Eye and Ear Infirmary in Boston. Melanoma metastases were present in 114 patients, and 23 had a second primary malignant

(8–4) Arch. Ophthalmol. 101:1894–1899, December 1983.

tumor. The median age at enucleation was 58 years for men and 59.5 years for women. The median follow-up interval was 17 years.

Overall, 89 patients remained alive at the end of the study, 4 of them with melanoma metastases. Of the 177 deaths, 110 were caused by melanoma metastases and 23 by metastases from other tumors. Of the metastases, 25% occurred within 1½ years of enucleation, 50% within 3½ years, and 75% within 8 years. The liver was involved in most instances. The median time from metastasis to death was 113 days. The significant prognostic factors identified by multivariate

UVEAL MELANOMA SURVIVAL DATA FOR CATEGORIES OF LEADING PROGNOSTIC FACTORS

	No. of Patients*	% Alive ± SE		
		5 Year	10 Year	15 Year
Number of Epithelioid Cells per High-Power Field				
None	70	85 ± 4	80 ± 5	71 ± 6
0.1-0.49	47	91 ± 4	86 ± 5	81 ± 6
0.5-1.9	65	77 ± 5	66 ± 6	60 ± 7
2.0-4.9	37	55 ± 8	38 ± 9	25†
≥ 5.0	40	41 ± 9	30†	20†
Necrotic	8	63 ± 17	17†	17†
Largest Dimension, mm				
1-7	40	92 ± 4	89 ± 5	85 ± 6
8-10	78	88 ± 4	78 ± 5	70 ± 6
11-13	58	80 ± 5	57 ± 7	50 ± 8
14-15	43	55 ± 8	40 ± 8	36 ± 21
16-18	23	39 ± 11	31†	24†
19+	9	22 ± 15	0	0
Location of Anterior Margin				
Posterior to equator	151	86 ± 3	76 ± 4	71 ± 4
Anterior to equator Without ciliary body involvement	45	69 ± 7	45 ± 9	21†
With ciliary body involvement	51	47 ± 7	39 ± 7	34†
Invasion to Line of Transection				
No	217	81 ± 3	69 ± 3	62 ± 4
Yes	32	41 ± 9	25 ± 8	21†
Pigmentation				
Minimal	68	85 ± 4	81 ± 5	71 ± 7
Moderate	96	74 ± 4	60 ± 5	55 ± 6
Heavy	89	68 ± 5	50 ± 6	46 ± 6

*Survival data based on melanoma-related deaths. Patients dying of other causes were considered to be censored observations and contributed survival data only until their time of death. Total number of patients for each variable might not add to 267, because some characteristics could not be determined for all patients.

†Five patients survived beyond the specific time period.

(Courtesy of Seddon, J.M., et al.: Arch. Ophthalmol. 101:1894–1899, December 1983; copyright 1983, American Medical Association.)

analysis included the number of epithelioid cells per high-power field; the largest tumor dimension, the location of the anterior tumor margin, invasion to the line of transection, and pigmentation of the tumor. Survival is related to the leading prognostic factors in the table. Favorable prognostic factors included fewer than 2 epithelioid cells per high-power field and a largest tumor dimension of 11 mm or less.

The largest tumor dimension was the best prognostic indicator in this series apart from the number of epithelioid cells per high-power field. The site of the anterior tumor margin was an important independent predictor of outcome.

▶ [It is evident from this article that histologic study of the tumor is most helpful for prognosis. This is certainly not a reason for enucleation, but its value should not be ignored.

8–5 **Survival in Metastatic Ocular Melanoma.** S. Rajpal, R. Moore, and C. P. Karakousis (Buffalo, N.Y.) reviewed the outcome in 46 patients seen from 1966 to 1980 with ocular melanoma. The choroid was the primary site in all but 2 of the 38 evaluable patients. The primary lesion was more than 10 mm in diameter in 22 patients. Thirty-eight patients had undergone enucleation of the primary melanoma; 3 were treated by exenteration, 1 by partial excision, and 4 by radiation or photocoagulation. Nine patients remained free of disease, 1 is alive with disease, and 1 died of other causes. In 35 patients metastatic disease was present or developed subsequently. The median time to recurrence was 28 months. The sites of metastasis are listed in the table. Fifteen patients with metastatic disease had surgical treatment.

The patients without metastasis had a median survival of 146 months, compared with 37 months for those with metastatic disease.

METASTASES IN OCULAR MELANOMA

Clinical incidence (35 Cases)

Organ	Initial organ involvement		Subsequent involvement		Total		Autopsy incidence (33 Cases)	
	No.	%	No.	%	No.	%	No.	%
Liver	16	45.7	9	25.7	25	71.4	24	72.7
Lung	6	17.1	8	22.9	14	40.0	17	51.5
Subcutaneous tissue skin	3	8.6	9	25.7	12	34.3	4	12.1
Bone	1	2.9	5	14.3	6	17.1	8	24.2
Lymph nodes	3	8.6	2	5.7	5	14.3	12	36.4
GI tract	1	2.9	4	11.4	5	14.3	9	27.3
Brain	1	2.9	1	2.9	2	5.7	8	24.2
Other	3	8.6	4	11.6	7	19.2	12	36.4

(Courtesy of Rajpal, S., et al.: Cancer 52:334–336, July 15, 1983.)

(8–5) Cancer 52:334–336, July 15, 1983.

The median survival after recurrence was 8 months. Patients with liver involvement had a median survival of only 2 months, compared with 19 months for those with lung involvement. Females appeared to live longer after recurrence than did males. Liver involvement carried a poor prognosis independently of sex and age. The disease-free interval did not influence subsequent survival significantly. Eight patients having all gross tumor resected had a mean survival of 2 years.

Ocular melanoma has a definite tendency to metastasize to the liver, and patients with hepatic metastases have a poorer prognosis than do those with involvement of other sites. Patients younger than age 50 years and women appear to do better than others with metastatic disease. Combined treatment (e.g., resection of tumor plus chemotherapy) appears to offer improved palliation, but this approach was used in patients having a relatively favorable prognosis.

▶ ↓ The authors of the final 3 articles in this series concerning choroidal melanomas discuss a spectrum of therapeutic modalities. There is a treatment for every philosophy. Tumors may be watched or treated with photocoagulation and cobalt plaques. Tumors may be treated with external beam radiation or, if enucleated, they may first be frozen to prevent metastases. The difficulty is in deciding not only when but if treatment should be initiated. We must use our own judgment while we wait for the results of definitive clinical studies.

8–6 **Choroidal Melanoma: Role of Conservative Therapy.** Clive Migdal (London) reviewed experience with cobalt plaque therapy and photocoagulation in a series of 99 patients seen between 1954 and 1978 with choroidal melanoma and followed up for at least 5 years. Mean age at presentation was 51 years. Most patients treated with plaques received circular cobalt applicators 5 to 15 mm in diameter, which were left in place long enough to deliver an average of 8,000 rad to the apex of the tumor. Xenon arc photocoagulation was usually carried out in a single stage.

Ninety patients received primary treatment with cobalt plaques and 15 with photocoagulation. Twenty-four patients required other treatment also. Twenty-three eyes were enucleated because of uncontrolled tumor growth or loss of vision. Forty-five patients had stable or improved visual acuity 5 years after treatment. Fifteen others had a reduction in vision of more than one line on the Snellen chart but better than 6/60. Vision was less than 6/60 in 23 patients, most of whom were treated with 10- or 15-mm plaques. Cataract developed in 29 patients, retinopathy in 16, vitreous hemorrhage in 6, and optic nerve ischemia in 8. Four patients had dry eyes, and 6 had other complications. Five patients died of metastatic melanoma, and 14 of other causes. No patients with tumors larger than 10 mm in diameter died of tumor. All tumor-related deaths occurred in patients with lesions posterior to the equator.

There appears to be a definite place for conservative measures such as cobalt plaque therapy and photocoagulation in the management of

(8–6) Trans. Ophthalmol. Soc. U.K. 103:54–58, 1983.

choroidal melanoma, but the indications for such treatment must be strictly observed. Plaques as large as 10 mm can be used for tumors no larger than 10 × 10 mm and no higher than 5 mm that are at least 3 mm from the optic disk or macula. Xenon-arc photocoagulation is suitable for tumors no larger than 10 × 10 mm and no higher than 2 mm that do not involve the macula.

8-7 **Helium Ion Therapy for Choroidal Melanoma.** Both the physical dose distribution of helium ion therapy and the biologic advantages of heavier charged particles recommend the trial of helium in the management of choroidal melanomas. Devron H. Char, William Saunders, Joseph R. Castro, Jeanne M. Quivey, Alexander R. Irvine, Robert D. Stone, J. Brooks Crawford, Michael Barricks, Lawrence I. Lonn, George F. Hilton, Ariah Schwartz, George T. Y. Chen, John T. Lyman, Michael Collier, Hector Sulit, Bradley R. Straatsma, and Anna Kaminski performed helium ion irradiation in 82 patients with choroidal melanoma seen from 1977 to 1982 in the Ocular Oncology

Fig 8–1.—Tumor thickness changes with respect to time after irradiation with 70 GyE of helium ion. (Courtesy of Char, D.H., et al.: Ophthalmology 90:1219–1225, October 1983.)

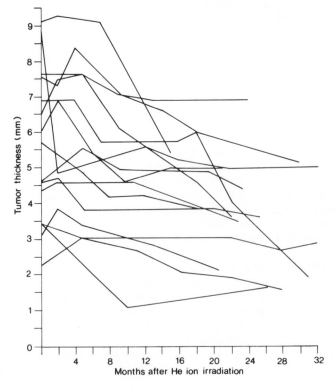

COMPLICATIONS OF TANTALUM RING PLACEMENT AND
HELIUM ION THERAPY

Lid epitheliitis/lash loss	50
Radiation vasculopathy of nerve or fovea	15
Cataract	6
Neovascular glaucoma	3
Vitreous Hemorrhage	1
Punctal occlusion	1
Loss of eye	6

(Courtesy of Char, D.H., et al.: Ophthalmology 90:1219–1225, October 1983.)

Unit at the University of California in San Francisco. The patients mean age was 62 years. Seven patients had small melanomas with confirmed growth, 24 had medium sized lesions, and 51 had large tumors. Thirty-two melanomas developed within 3 mm of the optic nerve or fovea. In recent patients, treatment planning was computerized. Most patients received a total tumor dose of 80 GyE in 5 fractions over 8 to 11 days. One patient was retreated. A 2-mm margin of normal tissue surrounding the lesion was treated.

Forty-eight patients were followed up for a year or longer after treatment, and 25 for more than 2 years. The tumor in all but 4 patients in the overall series remained stable or shrunk. All but 1 of those followed up for a year or longer had tumor regression, with a mean tumor shrinkage of about 30%. Changes in tumor thickness are shown in Figure 8–1. There were no significant differences in outcome whether 70 GyE or 80 GyE of helium ion irradiation was used. Acuity in 11 of 20 patients with acuities of better than 6/12 before treatment remained stable during follow-up 2 years and more after treatment. Complications are listed in the table.

Charged particle irradiation may be an excellent alternative treatment of choroidal melanoma. Comparable results have been achieved with proton beam irradiation. However, a number of complications occurred, and prospective trials are needed to determine the efficacy of this form of treatment in comparison with others. Currently, helium ion therapy can be used appropriately in patients with small, growing choroidal melanomas, in those with medium-sized or large melanomas and good vision, in those with tumor in an only functioning eye, and in those who refuse enucleation.

8–8 **Ocular Melanoma: Surgical Experience With "No Touch" Enucleation.** Enucleation is currently the standard treatment of ocular melanoma. About 50% of patients undergoing enucleation live for 15 years. R. Sloan Wilson (Univ. of Arkansas, Little Rock) has devel-

(8–8) South. Med. J. 76:202–204, February 1983.

oped an atraumatic technique, based on liquid nitrogen cryocoagulation surrounding the tumor, that immobilizes the blood supply until
the eye is removed. Conjunctival peritomy is performed gently, avoiding pressure on the eye. After rectus muscle transection and placement of a muscle stump fixation suture, the cryoring is placed gently
on the sclera overlying the tumor, and cryocoagulation is performed
in about 2 to 3 minutes. After which the optic nerve is transected,
and the procedure is completed. The author uses a glass sphere, but
simply closes Tenon's capsule rather than attempting to incorporate
the muscles. Electrocoaption of the overlying conjunctiva is then performed.

Demonstrable metastasis is infrequent at the time ocular melanoma is diagnosed. No-touch cryoenucleation is recommended for patients with tumors that grow or are larger than 8 to 10 mm in diameter or more than 2 mm in elevation, provided that there is a good
eye. If the tumor is in the only seeing eye, radiation therapy is considered. No-touch cryoenucleation has proved to be a simple and safe
technique and is a potentially life-saving measure. Posterior tumors
are readily managed by placing the cryoring as far to the posterior as
possible; the tumor will freeze even if it is not completely encircled.
The histologic features of the tumor do not appear to be altered by
cryocoagulation. No deaths have occurred in 5 years of experience,
and there have been no surgical problems. Discomfort appears to be
less with the no-touch cryoenucleation technique than with conventional enucleation. The sphere implants have not extruded.

8–9 **Ocular Presentation of Sarcoidosis in Children.** Ocular abnormalities reportedly are more frequent in sarcoidosis than other manifestations apart from hilar adenopathy and pulmonary changes, particularly in young children. Sudesh Kataria, G. Earl Trevathan,
James E. Holland, and Yash P. Kataria (East Carolina Univ., Green-
ville, N.C.) describe findings in a child with the insidious onset of
decreased visual acuity who was subsequently found to have systemic
sarcoidosis.

Boy, 14, had irritation and redness of the left eye and discomfort in bright
light for 3 months and decreased acuity and blurred vision for 4 days. A mild,
intermittent cough productive of scanty white sputum also was reported, as
well as increased fatigue. Finger-counting vision was observed on the left,
with distinct conjunctival hyperemia and an irregular, fixed pupil; the intraocular pressure was 22 mm Hg in the left eye and 17 mm Hg in the right
eye. Mutton-fat keratitic precipitates and anterior chamber flare were observed in the left eye. The iris showed vascularized nodular lesions and rubeosis iridis. Multiple posterior synechiae were observed. Slightly elevated
yellow-white lesions were present in the retinal periphery of the right eye.
Levels of serum immunoglobulins were elevated, and chest x-ray films
showed bilateral, diffuse, reticulonodular infiltrates. Results of lung function
studies suggested mild restrictive disease. A cervical node biopsy specimen

(8–9) Clin. Pediatr. (Phila.) 22:793–797, December 1983.

showed changes of sarcoidosis. The iris abnormalities and acuity improved with oral and topical steroid therapy. Steroid treatment was tapered, and examination at 6 months showed a best corrected acuity of 20/200 in the left eye. Extensive posterior synechiae were present, with anterior and posterior subcapsular cataractous changes but no inflammation.

Ocular involvement is noted in about 20% of children with sarcoidosis. All of those with suspected disease should have a complete ophthalmologic examination. Anterior segment changes are most frequent, usually in the form of chronic granulomatous uveitis. Cataracts can develop from either the chronic inflammation or from steroid therapy. Periphlebitis is the most common form of posterior segment involvement. Conjunctival biopsy is a safe, simple diagnostic procedure. Steroid therapy should be instituted if any vital organ is involved, and usually is effective in patients with ocular sarcoidosis. Chronic lesions, however, can produce serious ocular morbidity, including blindness.

▶ [The authors of this article make the reasonable point that all patients with suspected sarcoidosis should have a complete ophthalmologic examination and all patients with suspected ocular sarcoidosis should have thorough medical examinations.] ◀

8–10   **Clinical and Immunological Studies of Behçet's Disease** are reported by G. Richard and B. Dieckhues (Univ. of Münster, W. Germany). Behçet's disease is a chronic systemic disease characterized by various clinical inflammatory changes. In this study data on 8 patients with clinically diagnosed Behçet's disease were immunologically investigated. Although anterior uveitis is rarely a first presentation of Behçet's disease, it tends to be bilateral when it does occur and to involve both the anterior and posterior segments repeatedly. The diagnosis was established when, besides recurrent oral or genital ulcers, 2 more primary symptoms were found. The frequency of main symptoms (Table 1) and ophthalmologic alterations (Table 2) are shown. It is currently rare to observe a hypopyon due to early initiation of therapy. The patients' vision was generally good due to the cooperation of the dermatologic clinic and its early referral for treatment. Among the controlled 16 eyes, 7 had full vision, 8 had a visual

TABLE 1.—PRINCIPAL SYMPTOMS OF BEHÇET'S
DISEASE

Aphthous oral ulcers	8/8
Genital ulcers	7/8
Uveitis	3/6
Synovitis	3/7
Dermavasculitis	3/8
Meningoencephalitis	3/8

(Courtesy of Richard, G., and Dieckhues, B.: Ophthalmologica 186:141–150, 1983.)

(8–10)   Ophthalmologica 186:141–150, 1983.

TABLE 2.—Optic Symptoms in Behçet's Disease

Iridocyclitis	6/8
Synechiae	3/8
Hypopyon	3/8
Cellular vitreous infiltration	6/8
Complicated cataract	3/8
Macular edema	2/8
Retinal edema	4/8
Papilledema	3/8
Retinal exudate	2/8
Pigment changes of retina	5/8
Arterial occlusion or occlusive arteriopathy	1/8

(Courtesy of Richard, G., and Dieckhues, B.: Ophthalmologica 186:141–150, 1983.)

acuity of hand motions up to 0.2, and 2 eyes were blind. The antigen HLA-B5 can frequently be demonstrated in patients with Behçet's disease. Detailed serologic investigations, such as measles hemagglutination inhibition test plus complement fixation test (CFT), rubella hemagglutination inhibition test, hepatitis HBS antigen, adenovirus CFT, varicella zoster CFT, mumps CFT, herpes simplex CFT, anticytomegalovirus IgM and IgG, toxoplasmosis immunofluorescence, tuberculosis Middlebrock-Dubois, were unable to uncover a connection with past or present infections. Determinations of haptoglobin, lactate dehydrogenase, albumin, and ceruloplasmin showed no distinct abnormal conditions. Electrophoresis can indicate the duration of the illness. In 1 patient the results of the lymphocyte adherence inhibition test was abnormal.

Since the disease has a monosymptomatic beginning it generally takes several years to establish a final diagnosis. With early immunosuppressive treatment a severe, irreversibly impaired function can be prevented. In the late stages, recurrent vitreous hemorrhage complicates the course of the disease and can lead to blindness. Diminishing vision is mostly caused by edema of the retina, macula, and papilla.

A final assessment of therapeutic possibilities cannot be established at this time. Chlorambucil and azathioprine have been found to be beneficial. Cyclophosphamide has been used successfully but has possible teratogenic effects. At any rate early diagnosis is of major importance.

▶ [Uveitis associated with Behçet's disease is rare but serious since it usually involves both eyes and responds poorly to treatment. The author of this article points out that, while HLA-B5 may be demonstrated, little else is immunologically abnormal so that the diagnosis is difficult to confirm.] ◀

8–11 **Central Pigmentary Retinal Dystrophy and Its Angiographic Classification.** Hiroyuki Iijima, Osamu Okajima, Michika Okamoto,

(8–11) Jpn. J. Ophthalmol. 27:468–495, 1983.

and Tsuyoshi Tanino reviewed the findings in 21 patients with central pigmentary retinal dystrophy (PRD) seen in the Retina Clinic of the Tokyo University Hospital in a 3-year period. The diagnosis was based on the presence of acquired, progressive involvement of the posterior poles of both eyes, with black dots or bone corpuscle-like pigment present. No probable cause (e.g., inflammation, trauma, or intoxication) was evident.

The characteristic feature on fluorescein fundus angiography was a localized lesion in the posterior pole, in which granular hyperfluorescence due to damage of the retinal pigment epithelium was evident, with or without spotty or geographic hypofluorescence caused by atrophy of the choriocapillaris. Type 1 central PRD is characterized by annular or bow-shaped atrophy of the choriocapillaris around the vascular arcade in the posterior pole, with little disturbance of the foveal choriocapillaris. A typical example is shown in Figure 8–2. Type 2 PRD features round or irregular atrophy of the choriocapillaris in the center of the posterior pole, always including the foveal region, and a surrounding hyperfluorescent area with atrophy of the retinal pigment epithelium alone. Type 3 PRD features no atrophy of the choriocapillaris, but only granular hyperfluorescence in the posterior pole

Fig 8–2.—Fluorescein fundus angiography of the right eye of patient with type 1 central pigmentary retinal dystrophy. (Courtesy of Iijima, H., et al.: Jpn. J. Ophthalmol. 27:468–495, 1983.)

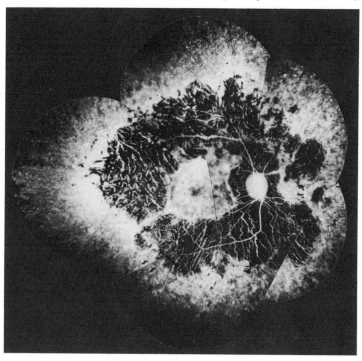

caused by damage to the retinal pigment epithelium. Patients with type 1 changes had fairly good vision in the fifth and sixth decades, whereas those with other types of PRD had poor acuity by the fourth decade of life. Deterioration of electroretinograph findings occurred rapidly at a young age in those with type 3 PRD. A familial occurrence of central PRD was evident in several instances. All patients had central or ring scotomas. Findings on electro-oculography were below normal in all 14 patients examined.

This classification is applicable to previously reported data on patients with central PRD. The disease is not a single clinical entity, and its nature and relationship to typical PRD require further study.

▶ [There is a wide range of patterns in the pigmentary retinal dystrophies. Indeed, the authors of this article emphasize the broad differences in the types affecting only the central retina. It is clear that careful pedigree information must be combined with ophthalmoscopy, fluorescein angiography, psychophysiology, and electrophysiology for diagnosis and the all important prognosis.] ◀

9. Vitreous

Intravitreal Antineoplastic Drugs

GHOLAM A. PEYMAN, M.D.

Eye and Ear Infirmary
University of Illinois, Chicago

Proliferative vitreoretinopathy (PVR)[1] is a disease process that occurs in long-standing detachments of the retina. It is clinically characterized by cloudiness of degenerated and contracted vitreous combined with various degrees of star-fold and membrane formation, leading to fixed retinal detachment. Histologic studies of the tissue involved in PVR[2, 3] have shown the presence of pigment epithelial cells, glial cells, and fibroblasts in membranes formed over and under the retina.

In the past, the preferred treatment has been the surgical combination of a buckling procedure and vitrectomy with dissection of the preretinal membrane. The success of this surgery has depended on the extent of retinal involvement, and the results have not been uniform or encouraging.[4] The inflexible retina resists reattachment, and cell proliferation then progresses to new membrane formation and further contraction of the retina.

Recent efforts have been directed toward the chemical inhibition of cell proliferation in PVR.[5-10] The drugs used in the studies have been antineoplastic agents employed in medicine for the treatment of metastatic cancer. They affect various phases in the cycle of cell growth. Antimetabolites such as 5-fluorouracil (5-FU) or methotrexate affect the S phase of the cell cycle. The 5-FU replaces the natural substrate uracil, thus inhibiting thymidine formation for DNA synthesis. Methotrexate inhibits the reduction of folic acid to tetrahydrofolic acid by binding to dihydrofolate reductase to prevent purine synthesis. Other antineoplastic drugs such as vincristine and etaposide affect cells in the M phase, or mitosis. However, some drugs such as doxorubicin do not specifically act in any one phase of the cell cycle.

To date, 10 antineoplastic drugs have been evaluated for their toxicity after injection into the vitreous cavity of rabbits.[5, 9, 10] Twelve agents also have been studied after their addition into vitrectomy infusion fluid.[11] A few of the more promising anticancer drugs have been investigated further in primate eyes.[12]

Tissue culture studies with pigment epithelial cells and fibroblasts have shown doxorubicin to be superior in the inhibition of cell proliferation over other antimetabolites and anticancer drugs.[13]

Although the concept of inhibiting cell proliferation in the vitreous cavity seems interesting, some practical problems exist with its clinical application. Clearance of the drugs from the vitreous is rapid.[14] Studies from our laboratory indicate that the half-life of 5-FU in normal vitreous is 90 minutes. In vitrectomized eyes, it is 45.6 minutes. If 5-FU is administered in combination with hyaluronic acid, the half-life is increased to 108 minutes. These data demonstrate the need for repeated intravitreal injections for the drug to be effective. However, this method of therapy would have some clinical limitations. Thus far, only a small clinical study in human beings has shown some success (60% of cases) in preventing or halting cellular proliferation in PVR.[15] Double-masked studies are needed to evaluate the concept of chemical inhibition of proliferating cells in the human eye. However, these will be difficult to design, considering the manifold manifestations of PVR and the different stages of retinal detachment in this disease process.

References

1. Hilton, G.F.: The terminology of the entity previously known as massive vitreous retraction. Presented at the XIII Meeting of the Jules Gonin Club, Cardoba, Argentina, March 1982.
2. Laqua, H., and Machemer, R.: Glial cell proliferation in retinal detachment (massive periretinal proliferation). *Am. J. Ophthalmol.* 80:602, 1975.
3. Laqua, H., and Machemer, R.: Clinical pathological correlation in massive periretinal proliferation. *Am. J. Ophthalmol.* 80:993, 1975.
4. Machemer, R.: Therapy of massive periretinal proliferation with closed vitrectomy. Presented at the XIII Meeting of the Jules Gonin Club, Cardoba, Argentina, March 1982.
5. Blumenkranz, M.S., Ophir, A., Claflin, A.J., et al.: Fluorouracil for the treatment of massive periretinal proliferation. *Am. J. Ophthalmol.* 94:458, 1982.
6. Blumenkranz, M.S., Norton, E.W.D.: A pharmacological approach to intraocular proliferative disorders. Presented at the XIII Meeting of the Jules Gonin Club, Cordoba, Argentina, March 1982.
7. Stern, W.H., Lewis, G.P., Erickson, P.A., et al.: Fluorouracil therapy for proliferative vitreoretinopathy after vitrectomy. *Am. J. Ophthalmol.* 96(1):33, 1983.
8. Stern, W.H., Guerin, C.J., Erickson, P.A., et al.: Ocular toxicity of fluorouracil after vitrectomy. *Am. J. Ophthalmol.* 96(1):43, 1983.
9. Kirmani, M., Santa, M., Sorgente, N., et al.: Drug treatment of MPP. *Invest. Ophthalmol. Vis. Sci.* 24:241, 1983.
10. Peyman, G.A., Greenberg, D., Fishman, G.A., et al.: Evaluation of toxicity of intravitreal antineoplastic drugs. *Ophthalmic Surg.* (in press).

11. Barrada, A., Peyman, G.A., Greenberg, D., et al.: Toxicity of antineoplastic drugs in vitrectomy infusion fluids. *Ophthalmic Surg.* 10(14):845, 1983.

12. Barrada, A., Peyman, G.A., Case, J., et al.: Evaluation of intravitreal 5-fluorouracil, vincristine, VP16, doxorubicin, and thiotepa in primate eyes. Unpublished data, 1983.

13. Fiscella, R., Peyman, G.A., Elvart, J., et al.: In vitro evaluation of cellular inhibitory potential of various antineoplastic drugs and dexamethasone. Unpublished data, 1983.

14. Case, J.L., Peyman, G.A., Barrada, A., et al.: Clearance of intravitreal ³H-fluorouracil. Unpublished data, 1983.

15. Blumenkranz, M., Hernandez, E., Ophir, A., et al.: 5-fluorouracil: New applications in complicated retinal detachment for an established antimetabolite. *Ophthalmology* 91(2):122, 1984.

▶ ↓ In the following 3 articles the authors describe abnormalities and methods of examination of the vitreous body and retina. In the first 2 articles, biomicroscopy is performed through a 58.6 diopter lens placed in front of the patient's eye. The images, while inverted, are large and, when coupled with intermittent eye movement, clearly show vitreous body detachments with considerable resolution. The authors of the third article use ultrasonography with surprisingly reliable results.

In the first article, the authors point out that the vitreous body is easier to see if the patient first makes rapid eye movement so that it is momentarily displaced. The dangerous eyes are in patients 50 years of age or older who complain of multiple, small floaters. In the second article, using the same technique the authors furnish persuasive evidence that vitreous traction contributes to macular breaks. The authors of the third article have clearly demonstrated the efficacy of and need for ultrasonographic assessment of the vitreous and retina prior to vitrectomy if the media are opaque. ◀

9–1 **Vitreous Floaters.** Kimio Murakami, Alex E. Jalkh, Marcos P. Avila, Clement L. Trempe, and Charles L. Schepens (Boston) reviewed the findings in 136 patients seen between 1979 and 1982 with the sudden onset of floaters. The 88 women and 48 men had an average age of 61 years. Twelve patients had symptoms in both eyes. None had a history of ocular disease, high myopia, or trauma. The vitreous of the symptomatic eyes and that of 114 asymptomatic fellow eyes were photographed using an El Bayadi-Kajiura lens mounted on a Zeiss-Jena slit-lamp camera. The entire vitreous cavity was observed before and after rapid vertical and horizontal ocular movements.

The floaters were located chiefly in the central field of vision. Many floaters were present in 24% of the affected eyes. Posterior vitreous detachment (PVD) was found in 83% of symptomatic eyes. Most of the others had a single floater or only a few floaters. Complete vitreous detachment was present in 123 eyes (table). Prepapillary opaque areas were solely responsible for symptoms in 38% of eyes with PVD. Vitreous hemorrhage was responsible for symptoms of many floaters in 17% of the eyes. Of symptomatic eyes with PVD, 18% had retinal breaks. Complete PVD was observed in 28% of the asymptomatic

| | Symptomatic Eyes | | | | Asymptomatic Eyes | | | |
| | PVD | | No PVD | | PVD | | No PVD | |
Patient's Age (Years)	(N = 123)	%	(N = 25)	%	(N = 32)	%	(N = 82)	%
Under 50†	3	14	19	86	0	0	15	100
50 or over‡	120*	95	6	5	32	32	67	68

*Includes 2 eyes with partial posterior vitreous detachment.
†Three patients had symptoms in both eyes.
‡Nine patients had symptoms in both eyes.
(Courtesy of Murakami, K., et al.: Ophthalmology (Rochester) 90:1271–1276, November 1983.)

eyes, with retinal breaks in 2 of them. All affected patients were aged 50 or older.

Vitreous biomicroscopy showed that, in patients aged 50 or older, PVD usually is responsible for the complaint of floaters. Numerous small floaters often are a result of vitreous hemorrhage, whereas a single floater is related most often to prepapillary opaque areas. Vitreous hemorrhage in these eyes is often associated with retinal breaks. Indirect ophthalmoscopy with scleral depression is recommended in patients with many floaters, especially those aged 50 years or older.

9–2 **Ultrasonographic Mapping of Vitreoretinal Abnormalities.** Nonophthalmoscopic methods are required to evaluate the intraocular structures before vitrectomy. Z. Nicholas Zakov, Louise A. Berlin, and Froncie A. Gutman (Cleveland) correlated the preoperative ultrasonographic mapping of vitreoretinal abnormalities with the surgical findings in 50 consecutive patients with media opacification precluding visualization of the fundus. Vitrectomy was performed after combined A-scan and B-scan ultrasonography was carried out. Forty-seven patients were involved in the study with the Ophthalmoscan and 10-MHz transducer, using the immersion technique, and 3 with the Ocuscan 200 and a 7.5-MHz transducer, using the contact technique. A sector transducer path was used to achieve maximal resolution. The mapping method is illustrated in Figure 9–1. Most eyes had vitreous opacities caused by diabetes.

The median time between ultrasonography and vitrectomy was 6 days. Retinal detachments, present at the time of operation in 32 eyes, included the macula in 13. Ultrasonography correctly predicted the position of the retina in 45 of the 50 eyes evaluated. There were 4 false positive readings and 1 false negative examination. Elevations of the macula were accurately predicted in 48 of the 50 eyes, with 1 false positive and 1 false negative result. Most false positive predictions resulted from incorrectly labeling membranes as retina. One

(9–2) Am. J. Ophthalmol. 96:622–631, November 1983.

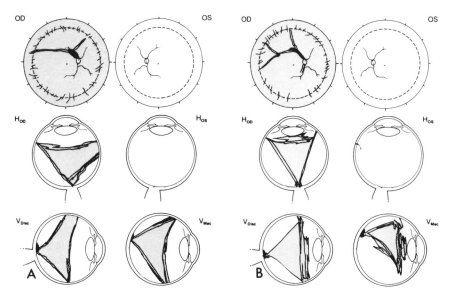

Fig 9–1.—Comparison of fundus drawings used in ultrasonographic prediction and surgical confirmation (in original drawings, speckled patterns were colored). **A,** previtrectomy, ultrasonography predicted a low traction retinal detachment *(blackened area)* localized to superotemporal arcade adjacent to the optic disk. Membranous partial posterior vitreous detachment and anterior vitreous membrane were also seen. **B,** at vitrectomy, the fundus had similar findings. Extent of retinal detachment and presence of membrane were in agreement. (Courtesy of Zakov, Z.N., et al.: Am. J. Ophthalmol. 96:622–631, November 1983.)

false negative study probably was caused by a long delay between sonography and operation. The circumferential extent of retinal detachments was accurately predicted in 43 eyes. Predictions of the position of the posterior vitreous face were correct in all 50 eyes. Errors were made in predicting the location and number of points of adherence between the posterior vitreous hyaloid and the retina in 11 eyes. Three giant traumatic tears were correctly identified, but their extent was not accurately described. Four subretinal and 4 subchoroidal hemorrhages were accurately described, as was a foreign body.

Ultrasonography is a highly accurate means of evaluating retinal detachments when performed shortly before vitrectomy. A systematic search should be made in all meridians in all extremes of gaze, and all membranes should be traced to their points of attachment. Kinetic techniques are useful.

9–3 **Biomicroscopic Study of the Vitreous in Macular Breaks.**
Schepens (1955) reported that macular breaks can result from vitreous traction, but subtle changes in vitreoretinal relationships near the posterior pole are difficult to detect by conventional methods. Marcos P. Avila, Alex E. Jalkh, Kimio Murakami, Clement L.

(9–3) Ophthalmology (Rochester) 90:1277–1283, November 1983.

Trempe, and Charles L. Schepens (Boston) examined the vitreous in 74 eyes with macular breaks by using the El Bayadi-Kajiura preset lens mounted on a slit lamp. All patients had full-thickness macular breaks, 15 of which were secondary to various causes and 59 of which were idiopathic senile breaks.

The 56 patients with 59 idiopathic senile macular breaks had an average age of 66 years. Posterior vitreous detachment (PVD) was found in 47.5% of the eyes. It was complete in 19 of the 28 affected eyes. Vitreous traction was evident from opercula or visible vitreous strands in 49% of the idiopathic cases. An operculum was seen in 17 of 31 eyes without PVD, 6 of the 9 with partiall PVD, and 5 of the 19 with a complete PVD. A complete PVD was seen in 10 of the 15 eyes with macular breaks secondary to various identified causes; 1 of these had an operculum. Opercula were found in 2 of 4 eyes with partial PVD. In 1 eye in the secondary group and 1 in the senile group, partial PVD caused traction at the edges of the macular break, resulting in retinal detachment.

Modern vitreous biomicroscopy permits the documentation of subtlee changes in vitreoretinal relationships. Vitreous traction appears to have a major role in the formation of macular breaks, and residual traction on the edges of macular breaks can cause retinal detachment. Since idiopathic senile macular breaks can be bilateral, careful evaluation of fellow eyes is necessary. If an El Bayadi-Kajiura present lens is unavailable, the fundus should be examined with a flat contact lens and slit lamp.

▶ ↓ In just a decade pars plana vitrectomy has become a routine surgical procedure for retinal specialists. The technique received its impetus from use in proliferative diabetic retinopathy with vitreous hemorrhage, but now more than 50% of the procedures are performed for other vitreous problems. The authors of the following 3 articles describe a broad range of indications and variable results. The diabetic eye continues to do less well although prior photocoagulation or endophotocoagulation, or both, has improved the prognosis to some extent. The major indication for vitrectomy in children was, not surprisingly, trauma. ◀

9–4   **Five Years Pars Plana Vitrectomy.** J. François, H. Verbraeken, and L. Vanhulst (Univ. of Ghent, Belgium) reviewed the results of 516 pars plana vitrectomies done in a 5-year period using Kloti's vitreous stripper. Follow-up ranged from 5 months to 5 years. The functional results are summarized in the table. About 40% of the patients with massive vitreoretinal retraction can be cured by vitrectomy and air injection. No endophthalmitis developed in this group, but phthisis bulbi occurred in 4 patients. If vitrectomy fails, silicone oil is used in selected patients. Diabetic patients without membranes, intravitreous proliferations, or retinal detachment improved after vitrectomy, but variable results were obtained in those with complications. Endophthalmitis occurred in 3 and phthisis bulbi in 3 of the diabetic patients. Nondiabetic vitreous hemorrhage was treated by

(9–4) Ophthalmologica 187:148–151, 1983.

FUNCTIONAL RESULTS

Indications	n 516	Visual acuity % of improvement
Massive vitreoretinal retraction	129	40
Diabetes	87	
Echography –	16	94
Echography +	71	30
Vitreous hemorrhage (non-diabetic)	61	62
Corneoscleral perforations (without IOFB)	57	37
Intraocular foreign bodies	34	33
Aphakic retinal detachments	33	88
Endophthalmitis	25	32
Congenital, juvenile cataracts	20	100
Chronic uveitis	18	72
Traumatic cataracts	17	94
Lens subluxations	11	73
Macular pucker	9	55

(Courtesy of François, J., et al.: Ophthalmologica 187:148–151, 1983.)

vitrectomy if present for 6 months with no tendency to resolve. Anatomical results usually were good, but macular function sometimes remained impaired by the underlying process.

Vision improved in 37% of the patients with corneoscleral perforation, but phthisis bulbi occurred in 14 and endophthalmitis in 2 patients in this group. A similar proportion of eyes with foreign bodies improved. Functional results in patients with aphakic retinal detachment were slightly improved by vitrectomy compared with the results achieved by classic retinopexy. Useful vision was obtained in 32% of patients with endophthalmitis after vitrectomy. Chronic posterior uveitis also is a very good indication for vitrectomy. Congenital and juvenile cataracts are effectively treated with the vitreous stripper, as are traumatic cataracts. Good results were obtained in eyes in which lens masses remained after intracapsular lens extraction. Lens subluxation is treated by vitrectomy only in patients younger than age 25 years. Satisfactory results were obtained in a number of patients with macular pucker, but not if the adhesion is so great that retinal holes may be produced.

9–5 **Prognostic Parameters in Pars Plana Vitrectomy.** The results of vitrectomy have varied widely in different reports, partly because

(9–5) Acta Ophthalmol. (Copenh.) 61:788–805, October 1983.

of varied indications for the procedure. Erik Scherfig, Jens Edmund, Steen Tinning, and Erik Krogh (Copenhagen) reviewed the results of 143 vitrectomies performed in 135 patients between 1976 and 1980. The 86 men and 57 women had a mean age of 50 years. All operations but 1 were done with general anesthesia. The Klöti macrostripper was used in all instances. An intravitreal fiberoptic illumination was seldom employed. Physiologic saline solution and Ringer's solution were used for infusion, without antibiotics. The average duration of operation was 2½ hours.

Sixty-two vitrectomies were done for diabetic patients. Sixteen procedures were followed by visual improvement of 2 steps or more and 24 by a comparable reduction in vision. There was an insignificant trend for poorer results to be obtained in older patients. No improvement occurred in patients with absent or doubtful light perception before operation. Few patients with visual impairment for more than 3 years improved. Age at onset of diabetes was not a prognostic factor, but patients with diabetes for less than 15 years were likelier to improve after vitrectomy. Results were comparable in phakic and aphakic patients. Only 1 of 17 eyes with an existing detachment improved after vitrectomy. Severe bleeding markedly compromised the outcome of vitrectomy in diabetic eyes.

Among 36 patients with rhegmatogenous detachment and vitreoretinal traction who underwent combined vitrectomy and external scleral operations, only 1 of 19 phakic patients had visual improvement, compared with 5 of 17 aphakic patients. Two and 6 patients, respectively, had reattachment of the retina. Among 25 patients with traumatic disorders, 7 of 8 without detachment had improved vision postoperatively, but none of those with detachment improved and 7 of the 17 had worse acuity after operation. Nine of 20 vitrectomies done because of other indications were followed by improved visual acuity and 3 by worsening vision. Eight of 14 eyes with vitreous hemorrhage of nondiabetic and nontraumatic origin improved after vitrectomy.

Primary vitreous hemorrhage in a diabetic eye can be observed for 3 months before vitrectomy is performed if no regression occurs. In traumatic cases, vitrectomy should be done after 3 to 10 days. Patients with infectious panophthalmitis should be operated on immediately after the diagnosis is made.

9–6   **Vitrectomy in Children.** Gary C. Brown, William S. Tasman, and William E. Benson (Thomas Jefferson Univ., Philadelphia) reviewed the results of 24 consecutive pars plana posterior vitrectomies performed in 23 patients younger than age 20 years from 1978 to 1982.Vitrectomy was done using a 3-incision technique in each case. The mean age at operation was 12 years. Surgery was done for vitreous hemorrhage or retinal detachment in 21 instances. Two eyes

SUMMARY OF UNDERLYING PATHOPHYSIOLOGIC
DISEASE ENTITIES IN 24 EYES

Intraocular foreign body	7
Scleral or corneo-scleral laceration	5
Retrolental fibroplasia	3
Blunt trauma	2
Diabetic retinopathy	2
Macular pucker	2
Ocular toxocariasis	2
Retinal capillary angioma	1

(Courtesy of Brown, G.C., et al.: Ophthalmic Surg. 14:1017–1020, December 1983.)

had macular pucker, 1 was affected by endophthalmitis, and in 1 there was a traumatic cyclitic membrane. The underlying pathophysiologic processes are listed in the table.

There were 16 retinal detachments preoperatively and 7 postoperatively. Intraoperative complications included iatrogenic retinal holes in 2 eyes. One of these patients had a friable, necrotic retina and later had the eye enucleated. Malignant hyperthermia occurred in 1 instance but was arrested. There was 1 postoperative rhegmatogenous retinal detachment. In 2 eyes late traction detachments of the retina occurred, and a second vitrectomy succeeded in 1 of these. Two eyes had macular pucker from inoperable subretinal macular folds. Rubeosis iridis developed in 2 eyes. Visual improvement occurred in 59% of the treated eyes. Only eyes with no light perception and 1 with bare light perception were eventually enucleated.

Trauma appears to be the leading cause of disorders necessitating vitrectomy in children. Improved visual acuity has been reported in up to 66% of eyes of unselected patients having pars plana vitrectomy. Complications are not unduly serious in view of the severity of the ocular disorders present in most cases. Poor visual results have been attributable to severe underlying pathologic conditions rather than to vitrectomy. Modern vitrectomy can restore or maintain vision in previously unsalvageable eyes of pediatric patients.

▶ ↓ In the following 3 articles the authors describe vitrectomy for vitreoretinal diseases other than diabetic retinopathy. ◀

9–7 **Vitrectomy for Nondiabetic Vitreous Hemorrhage.** Ray T. Oyakawa, Ronald G. Michels, and William P. Blase (Johns Hopkins Univ.) reviewed the results of pars plana vitrectomy in 94 eyes with nondiabetic vitreous hemorrhage operated on between 1974 and 1982. Patients with penetrating injury or rhegmatogenous retinal detach-

(9–7) Am. J. Ophthalmol. 96:517–525, October 1983.

BEST POSTOPERATIVE VISUAL ACUITIES

Postoperative Visual Acuities

Preoperative Condition	20/15 to 20/20	20/25 to 20/40	20/50 to 20/200	20/300 to 20/400	9/200 to 5/200	H. M. or L. P.*	No. of Eyes Improved
All eyes	10	37	26	11	3	7	88 of 94
Retinal branch vein occlusion	2	11	13	5	1	4	33 of 36
Blunt trauma	1	5	2	2	1	0	11 of 11
Cataract extraction	3	5	1	1	0	0	10 of 10
Subretinal neovascularization	0	1	1	3	1	3	6 of 9
Eales' disease	2	4	2	0	0	0	8 of 8
Terson's syndrome	1	3	0	0	0	0	4 of 4
Idiopathic	0	4	1	0	0	0	5 of 5
Miscellaneous	1	4	6	0	0	0	11 of 11

*H.M. = hand movements; L.P. = light perception.
(Courtesy of Oyakawa, R.T., et al.: Am. J. Ophthalmol. 96:517–525, October 1983.)

ment or traction detachment involving the macula were excluded. The most common causes of hemorrhage were retinal branch vein obstruction, blunt trauma, cataract extraction, subretinal neovascularization, and Eales' disease. The mean age at operation was 56 years. Three of the 91 patients had surgery on both eyes at different times. The mean follow-up was 19.5 months. The O'Malley Ocutome was used in most instances. Sixteen eyes were aphakic before vitrectomy and 28 others had lensectomy at the time of vitrectomy. Some early patients in the series had prophylactic peripheral retinal cryotherapy or scleral buckling. Transvitreal endophotocoagulation was done for neovascularization in 3 later patients.

Final visual acuity was improved in 88 of the 94 treated eyes, as defined by a gain of 5 lines or more on the Snellen chart. In 47 eyes a final acuity of 20/40 or better was achieved, and in 26 others a final acuity of 20/50 to 20/200 (table) was gained. Postoperative acuity often depended on the underlying abnormality. Most eyes with vitreous bleeding after cataract extraction or with Terson's syndrome had a good visual outcome, whereas most of those with subretinal neovascularization or choroidal hemorrhage had a poor outcome. Thirteen eyes had iatrogenic anterior retinal tears near the sclerotomy site and 5 had posterior retinal tears. One eye required a second reattachment procedure. Lens opacities developed in 16 of 50 phakic eyes. Three eyes had late retinal detachments. Recurrent vitreous hemorrhage and epiretinal membrane formation each occurred in 5 eyes. Phthisis bulbi and rubeosis iridis with secondary glaucoma developed in 3 eyes each.

Visual improvement can be expected after vitrectomy in more than 90% of eyes with nondiabetic vitreous hemorrhage, but the final visual acuity depends partly on the functional capacity of the macula, which often is influenced by factors related to the underlying disease. Major complications other than lens opacification were infrequent.

▶ [These eyes did relatively well and the incidence of induced retinal tears has decreased. Postoperative cataract formation, however, is still a major problem and it is unclear if it is due to trauma at the time of surgery or the absence of the vitreous body.] ◀

9–8 **Anterior Pars Plana Vitrectomy for Phakic Malignant Glaucoma.** The removal of vitreous through the pars plana now is a relatively safe procedure. Sakae Momoeda, Hideyuki Hayashi, and Kenji Oshima (Fukuoka Univ., Japan) report the successful use of anterior pars plana vitrectomy with lens extraction to treat 5 eyes of 4 patients with phakic malignant glaucoma.

TECHNIQUE.—The procedure is illustrated in Figure 9–2. The operation is performed with the patient receiving general anesthesia. The infusion pressure is maintained at 50 cm H_2O during surgery. The lens is extracted with a cryoprobe through a sector iridectomy. An Ocutome probe is then introduced into the vitreous cavity, and the anterior vitreous is removed. The anterior chamber is deepened by pushing the iris back with a spatula before closing the scleral and conjunctival wounds.

The anterior chamber deepened to its normal state after surgery in each instance, and no recurrent flattening was observed during a mean follow-up period of 18 months. Intraocular pressure was kept normal with pilocarpine drops postoperatively in 3 eyes, but an additional filtering operation was necessary in 2 eyes. Visual acuity was improved in all eyes postoperatively. Mild corneal endothelial damage was present for a few weeks, but gradually resolved. No serious complications were observed.

Anterior vitrectomy is the preferred treatment for malignant glaucoma if medical management is ineffective. When removal of the lens is indicated, this can be done through the pars plana with the vitrectomy instrument or through the limbus with the open-sky technique. Lenses with advanced nuclear sclerosis should be removed with the conventional intracapsular method through a limbal or corneal inci-

Fig 9–2.—Surgical procedures for phakic malignant glaucoma: **1,** lens extraction with cryoprobe through corneal incision; **2,** continuous suturing of corneal wound; **3,** anterior vitrectomy with Ocutome probe through pars plana; and **4,** iris is pushed backward with spatula to deepen anterior chamber. (Courtesy of Momoeda, S., et al.: Jpn. J. Ophthalmol. 27:73–79, 1983.)

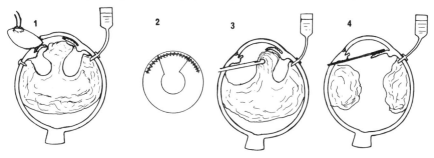

sion. The pars plana approach to anterior vitrectomy has several advantages over the anterior approach through a limbal incision. Retinal detachment and periretinal proliferation have been described after pars plana vitrectomy for malignant glaucoma, but no serious complications occurred in the present cases.

▶ [Partial anterior vitrectomy seems a superb treatment for malignant glaucoma. In this series, the lenses were removed, but, at least in theory, this should not be necessary. Indeed, a more conservative approach would be vitrectomy followed by a wait-and-see period.] ◀

9–9 **Vitrectomy in Inflammatory Diseases of the Posterior Segment** is discussed by S. Binder and H. Freyler (Univ. of Vienna). Indications for vitrectomy are clearing of optical media (including removal of preretinal membranes, pupillary membranes, pupillar formation after chronic inflammations, and loosening of anteroposterior tractions); gaining of material for causative proof or cytologic examinations; removal of the vitreous as an eventually effective autoimmune substance; the possibility of intravitreous antibiotic or corticosteroid therapy; and prevention of permanent intoxication of the retina through the inflamed, altered vitreous. Vitrectomy in inflammations of the posterior segment is performed to obtain examination material for diagnosis of uveitis, to clear optical media, and to prevent postoperative complications. With this technique the following steps should be considered carefully: (1) removal of all axial opaque areas in the vitreous chamber, especially the posterior segment; (2) the careful circumcision of all adhesions between the inner surface of the retina and vitreous; (3) the retaining of a retrolental vitreous bolster to protect the lens; and (4) the retaining of a preretinal vitreous segment in severe retinal exudations.

Eight patients with chronic endogenous uveitis, chorioretinitis, toxoplasmosis, and infective endophthalmitis underwent pars plana vitrectomy. All patients had a definite improvement in vision. Within the postoperative observation period of at least 6 months no complications were observed. However, the diagnostic aspect was unsatisfactory. Cytologic and histologic examinations of vitrectomy material showed no uveitis. Cultures to determine the etiology of the disease and serologic tests were negative.

The most favorable time for surgery in patients with chronic uveitis and endophthalmitis has yet to be determined when, in addition to clearing of optical media and gaining biopsy material, a therapeutic effect from the removal of the vitrous is expected. The most favorable time for vitrectomy is when within 2 to 3 days the clinical situation has become worse in spite of massive doses of antibiotics. There is general agreement that a long postponement of vitrectomy because of collection of pus in the vitreous chamber makes surgery more difficult if not impossible.

(9–9) Klin. Monatsbl. Augenheilkd. 183:86–89, August 1983.

In addition to improvement of vision in eyes with chronic endogenous uveitis, vitrectomy might also alter or diminish the severity, as well as the frequency of attacks.

▶ [Except in some cases of infective endophthalmitis, the use of vitrectomy in uveitis seems a little radical although indications are changing rapidly as we learn more about methods and side effects.] ◀

▶ ↓ In the following 2 articles the authors discuss the complications of vitrectomy in the worst cases for which it is done, diabetic retinopathy. All the eyes bled at the time of surgery and retinal tears were induced in 20%, but these complications were treated successfully. Vitreous hemorrhage was present in 75% of eyes after surgery but cleared, although a third had recurrent bleeding. Iris neovascularization was a serious problem in 34% of the aphakic eyes. It is evident that vitrectomy is still a complicated, relatively high-risk operation in diabetic patients, but it has been extraordinarily helpful for patients who would otherwise be blind. ◀

9–10 **Complications of Vitreous Surgery for Diabetic Retinopathy—*I*. *Intraoperative Complications*.** Ray T. Oyakawa, Andrew P. Schachat, Ronald G. Michels, and Thomas A. Rice (Johns Hopkins Univ., Baltimore) analyzed the incidence of intraoperative complications in 179 eyes undergoing pars plana vitrectomy for proliferative diabetic retinopathy.

Corneal epithelial defects occurred during surgery in 51 eyes (28%), 31 (61%) of which had an epithelial defect involving a fourth of the area of the cornea or less. Larger defects occurred in the remaining 20 eyes (39%). Almost all of these defects were inadvertent and rarely was the epithelium removed only to improve visualization. No intraoperative endothelial damage was observed. Removal of the lens was performed in 42 (25%) of 170 phakic eyes. Lens damage from the vitrectomy instrument occurred in 1 eye. Large fragments of lens material were accidentally displaced into the vitreous cavity in 3 eyes, but the displaced material was removed in each case without complications. Pharmacologic lens damage occurred in 2 eyes (1.1%). Two of the 51 aphakic eyes sustained accidental damage to the iris from the vitrectomy instrument. Some bleeding from fibrovascular tissue or from the inner retinal surface was common during dissection and removal of proliferative tissue, but was easily controlled in most cases by intraocular diathermy. However, the bleeding was severe enough in 7 eyes to require premature termination of the operation. Iatrogenic retinall tears occurred in 36 (20%) of the 179 eyes, of which 5 had 2 retinal tears and 1 had 4 tears. Of the 44 retinal tears, 15 (34%) were anterior to the equator and 11 of these 15 were near the sclerotomy through which the vitrectomy probe was introduced. The remaining 29 retinal tears (66%) were posterior to the equator, 19 of which were within a 15-degree radius of the fovea.

Except for peripheral retinal breaks, most pars plana sclerotomy complications can be avoided and most peripheral retinal breaks can be treated successfully during the same operation. The incidence of

(9–10) Ophthalmology (Rochester) 90:517–521, 522–530, May 1983.

posterior retinal tears can probably be reduced by additional refinements in surgical technique. Despite the possible complications, vitreous surgery is an effective treatment for severe proliferative diabetic retinopathy and provides partial visual improvement and a lasting beneficial effect in most cases.

II. Postoperative Complications.—Oyakawa, Schachat, Michels, and Rice analyzed the postoperative complications in 179 eyes following pars plana vitrectomy for proliferative diabetic retinopathy.

A final visual acuity of 5/200 or better, believed to be in the functional range, was achieved in 117 (65%) of the 179 eyes (table). The final vision was equal to or better than the preoperative level in 129 eyes (72%). Sixty-two eyes (35%) were regarded as visual failures. Fifty-one eyes showed corneal epithelial defects during the immediate postoperative period. The defect healed before discharge from the hospital in 48 (94%) of these eyes, although 22 required longer than 3 days to heal. Three patients had recurrent epithelial defects. Thus, corneal epithelial defects were observed in 6 patients at the first postoperative examination. Corneal opaque areas were rare, with only 11 eyes (8%) showing late corneal edema. The lens was retained in 128 eyes (75%). Of 114 eyes that were phakic at the time of the final examination, 17 (15%) showed mild opacification and 19 (17%) had moderate or severe lens opacification. Postoperative iris neovascularization (rubeosis iridis) was present at the final examination in 21 (32%) of 65 aphakic eyes and in 15 (13%) of 114 phakic eyes ($P = 0.012$). Twenty of these 36 eyes with rubeosis iridis also had extensive retinal detachment. An intraocular pressure greater than 21 mm Hg was observed in 31 (18%) of the 179 eyes, but only 12 (7%) had an intraocular pressure greater than 30 mm Hg at the final examination. Rupture of the sclerotomy site, with or without formation of a filtering bleb, did not occur. However, fibrovascular ingrowth from the sclerotomy site occurred in 10 eyes. This was localized in 3 eyes and diffuse in 7. In each case, diffuse fibrovascular ingrowth was associated with iris neovascularization and, in 6 of the 7 eyes, retinal detachment.

VITRECTOMY VISUAL RESULTS FOR DIABETIC RETINOPATHY		
Final Visual Acuity	Number of Eyes	Percent
20/20	6	3%
20/25–20/40	18	10%
20/50–20/200	59	33%
20/300–5/200	34	19%
<5/200	62	35%
	179	100%

(Courtesy of Schachat, A.P., et al.: Ophthalmology (Rochester) 90:522–530, May 1983.)

Some degree of vitreous hemorrhage was present in 134 (75%) of the eyes on the first postoperative day and cleared in an average of 6.2 weeks in phakic eyes and 5.4 weeks in aphakic eyes. Recurrent vitreous hemorrhage occurred in 52 eyes (29%). At the final examination, 24 eyes showed vitreous hemorrhage, of which 15 also had extensive retinal detachment and 12 also had rubeosis iridis. Twenty-eight eyes (16%) developed a new retinal detachment following surgery, of which 38% were treated successfully. Forty-five eyes (25%) were reoperated on. Most of these procedures were performed for repair of retinal detachment or removal of nonclearing vitreous hemorrhage (32 eyes; 71%). Phthisis bulbi developed in 6 eyes (3%) and 1 eye was enucleated.

The incidence of postoperative complications after vitrectomy for proliferative diabetic retinopathy is high. However, severe corneal complications have virtually been eliminated as a result of a better understanding of the pathophysiologic abnormalities of the diabetic cornea and by minimizing postoperative mechanical and pharmacologic damage. In about 75% of the cases, the lens is now retained, thereby reducing the incidence of postoperative iris neovascularization, but increasing the problem of postoperative vitreous hemorrhage. Postoperative retinal detachment is a major problem.

9–11 **Pars Plana Vitrectomy for Complicated Retinal Detachments.** Vitreous surgery now is being done for several types of complicated retinal detachment not effectively managed by scleral buckling alone. Clifford M. Ratner, Ronald G. Michels, Cheryl Auer, and Thomas A. Rice (Johns Hopkins Univ.) reviewed the results of such surgery in 514 patients whose average age was 44 years. Follow-up averaged 17 months and was at least 6 months in all patients. Proliferative diabetic retinopathy was present in 71% of the eyes. Traction detachment was treated in 72% of eyes, and in 28% there was a rhegmatogenous component. Giant retinal tears were present in 20 eyes.

	VITRECTOMY FOR NONDIABETIC RETINAL DETACHMENT		
Type of Retinal Detachment	Final VA 5/200 or Better	Retina Reattached	Total Cases
1. Traction detachment	21 (66%)	27 (84%)	32
2. Giant retinal tear	13 (65%)	13 (65%)	20
3. Opaque media	18 (43%)	21 (50%)	42
4. Posterior retinal hole	8 (80%)	9 (90%)	10
5. Proliferative vitreoretinopathy	21 (30%)	29 (42%)	69
6. Trauma	28 (62%)	29 (64%)	45

(Courtesy of Ratner, C.M., et al.: Ophthalmology (Rochester) 90:1323–1327, November 1983.)

(9–11)   Ophthalmology (Rochester) 90:1323–1327, November 1983.

Patients with retrolental fibroplasia were excluded. In 45 eyes detachment followed blunt or penetrating trauma.

The retina was completely reattached in 55% of eyes with detachments complicating proliferative diabetic retinopathy and partially reattached in another 32%. Successful visual results with a final acuity of 5/200 or better were obtained in 62% of diabetic eyes. Better visual results were associated with retention of the crystalline lens, an attached macula before operation, and a detachment limited to 25% or less of the retina. Iatrogenic retinal breaks compromised the outcome. The results obtained in other patients are shown in the table. All eyes with proliferative vitreoretinopathy had extensive epiretinal membrane proliferation and severe vitreoretinal traction.

Vitreous surgery is successful in most patients with complex retinal detachment that cannot be managed adequately by conventional methods of scleral buckling alone. Most failures are a result of biologic features of the disease. Results might be enhanced by improved timing of surgery and by pharmacologic methods of suppressing abnormal cellular proliferation.

9–12 **Early Vitrectomy in Proliferative Diabetic Retinopathy.** Partial vitreous separation with firm vitreous adhesion to fibrovascular proliferative material precedes catastrophic visual loss in patients with diabetic retinopathy, and early vitrectomy might preserve vision. Michael Shea (Univ. of Toronto) performed pars plana vitrectomy on 140 eyes of 115 patients seen between 1975 and 1982 with

FINAL VISUAL ACUITY IN PATIENTS WITH MODERATE OR SEVERE PROLIFERATIVE DIABETIC RETINOPATHY TREATED BY PARS PLANA VITRECTOMY

Grade of Initial Traction Retinal Detachment (TD)	Visual Acuity			
	≥ 20/40 (%)	20/50 to 20/100 (%)	20/200 to Hand Movements (%)	Less Than Hand Movements (%)
	All Patients			
TD0 (n = 71)	41 (57.7)	16 (22.5)	9 (12.6)	5 (7.0)
TD1-4 (n = 69)	23 (33.3)	25 (36.2)	10 (14.4)	11 (15.9)
Total (N = 140)	64 (45.7)	41 (29.2)	19 (13.5)	16 (11.4)
	Patients With Initial 20/40 or Better			
TD0 (n = 31)	24 (77.4)	4 (12.9)	3 (9.6)	0 (0)
TD1-4 (n = 10)	6 (60.0)	2 (20.0)	0 (0)	2 (20.0)
Total (N = 41)	30 (73.1)	6 (14.6)	3 (7.3)	2 (4.8)
	Patient With Initial 20/50 or 20/200			
TD0 (n = 40)	17 (42.5)	12 (30.0)	6 (15.0)	5 (12.5)
TD1-4 (n = 59)	18 (30.5)	22 (37.2)	10 (16.9)	9 (15.2)
Total (N = 99)	35 (35.3)	34 (34.3)	16 (16.1)	14 (14.1)

(Courtesy of Shea, M.: Arch. Ophthalmol. 101:1204–1205, August 1983; copyright 1983, American Medical Association.)

(9–12) Arch. Ophthalmol. 101:1204–1205, August 1983.

proliferative diabetic retinopathy and relatively good visual acuity. Most patients were insulin-dependent diabetics. The mean follow-up period after vitrectomy was 26 months. The final acuity is shown in the table. Nearly 75% of patients with initial acuity of 20/40 or better retained economically useful vision (20/40 or better), and another 15% retained socially useful (20/50 to 20/100) vision. Of the patients operated on when vision was below the economically useful level, about 43% gained such vision if no traction detachment was present, and 31% gained it even if detachment was present. The visual prognosis of patients with initially good vision but elevated neovascularization was substantially improved by vitrectomy.

Pars plana vitrectomy is best performed in patients with proliferative diabetic retinopathy when elevated neovascularization or partial vitreous detachment is present, and before substantial visual loss or traction detachment has occurred.

▶ [Unfortunately all the patients were operated so that there was no randomized control group. Nonetheless the results are impressive and it is hoped that the results of the National Eye Institute-sponsored early vitrectomy study will be available shortly.] ◀

9–13 **Effect of Lensectomy on the Incidence of Iris Neovascularization and Neovascular Glaucoma After Vitrectomy for Diabetic Retinopathy.** Thomas A. Rice, Ronald G. Michels, Maureen G. Maguire, and Ellen F. Rice (Johns Hopkins Univ.) examined 596 con-

Fig 9–3.—Survival curves showing cumulative incidence of iris neovascularization after vitrectomy for 3 groups of eyes in diabetic patients. (Courtesy of Rice, T.A., et al.: Am. J. Ophthalmol. 95:1–11, January 1983.)

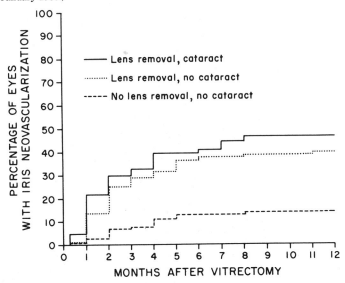

secutive eyes subjected to vitrectomy for complications of diabetic retinopathy to assess the effects of lens removal on the occurrence of postoperative iris neovascularization and neovascular glaucoma. None of the eyes had had previous vitreous surgery. The chief indications for vitrectomy were nonresolving vitreous hemorrhage, traction retinal detachment involving the macula, and rhegmatogenous retinal detachment.

The occurrence of iris neovascularization is shown in Figure 9–3. In the group with clear lenses, iris neovascularization was more frequent in patients who underwent lensectomy than in those who did not. Both severe retinal neovascularization and the absence of scatter retinal photocoagulation were associated with a higher rate of iris neovascularization. The estimated relative risk of neovascular glaucoma for eyes on which lensectomy was performed during vitrectomy was 4.6. Patients who did not undergo lensectomy had somewhat better visual results than the others.

These findings support the current practice of not removing a clear lens unless this is necessary to achieve essential goals of the operation. It is not concluded that preoperative scatter retinal photocoagulation should be used to reduce the incidence of iris neovascularization and neovascular glaucoma after vitrectomy, but the possibility deserves further consideration. It is possible that lensectomy with the removal of retrolenticular vitreous gel reduces the physical barrier to anterior diffusion of a vasoproliferative factor. Eyes that undergo extensive laser therapy preoperatively may have a lower level of vasoproliferative factor.

▶ [This study provides further evidence that removal of the lens during vitrectomy increases the incidence of iris neovascularization and glaucoma. It is not proved but there is some evidence that these eyes do better if photocoagulated before, during or immediately after (if possible) the vitrectomy.] ◀

9–14 **Electroretinogram and Electrooculogram of Eyes With Intravitreously Injected Silicone Oil.** The effect of intravitreously injected silicone oil on the electroretinogram (ERG) and electrooculogram (EOG) was investigated in clinical and in vitro conditions by D. Momirov, G. H. M. van Lith, and R. Živojnović (Erasmus Univ., Rotterdam). Experiments with 8 enucleated pig's eyes injected with 1 to 5.5 ml of silicone oil after removal of the same amount of vitreous showed that the oil in amounts up to 2 ml had little effect on the amplitude of the fundal potential; however, larger amounts of oil gradually decreased these amplitudes. Similar results were obtained in patients; in 5 eyes the potentials increased more than 2 times after removal of silicone, which means that the isolating effect of silicone resulted in a decrease of 40% to 50% in the potentials. This decrease is a purely physical effect, because the same reduction was observed in the enucleated pig's eye. The isolating effect of silicone was also

(9–14) Ophthalmologica 186:183–188, 1983.

checked in 6 patients by recording the ERG and EOG 1 day before and 3 to 6 days after removal of silicone.

Even if the isolating effect of silicone is taken into account, the ERG potentials of silicone-injected eyes are still lower than those from nonsilicone-injected eyes. The fact that retinal changes caused by the primary disease are usually greater in silicone-injected eyes than in those without indication for silicone application may account for this result. Furthermore, most of these eyes have been operated on more than once and have extensive chorioretinal scars.

The findings suggest that the standing potential is less influenced by the isolating effect of silicone. Originating in the retinal layers, it might progress along the choroid and sclera to the anterior side. No arguments could be found in favor of silicone retinopathy.

▶ [There is still controversy concerning possible toxic effects of silicone oil on the retina. The authors of this article did show that silicone oil in the vitreous cavity reduces electrophysiologic signals unrelated to any effect it might have on the retina. It is evident that a randomized clinical trial comparing silicone vitreous substitution with other methods used to augment retinal detachment repair is needed.] ◀

9–15 **Fluorouracil Therapy For Proliferative Vitreoretinopathy After Vitrectomy.** No solution has been found to the problem of continued epiretinal membrane formation after vitrectomy for proliferative vitreoretinopathy. Walter H. Stern, Geoffrey P. Lewis, Page A. Erickson, Christopher J. Guerin, Don H. Anderson, Steven K. Fisher, and James J. O'Donnell evaluated the use of fluorouracil as an inhibitor of epiretinal membrane growth and traction retinal detachment in the aphakic rabbit eye subjected to vitrectomy and the subsequent injection of tissue-cultured retinal pigment epithelial cells. Growth of cells on the inner retinal surface in this model leads to a funnel-shaped traction detachment of the medullary rays. Treated animals had 0.5 or 1.25 mg of fluorouracil injected into the gas-filled eye 2 hours after cell injection and then every 24 hours for 6 consecutive days.

Traction detachment was observed 2 weeks after the instillation of 200,000 cultured cells in all 12 control eyes and in 6 of 14 eyes treated with 0.5 mg of fluorouracil. At 4 weeks, 8 of the treated eyes had detachments. The height of the detachments was reduced in treated eyes. Where 400,000 cells were instilled and the higher dose of fluorouracil was given, traction detachments occurred only in control eyes 2 weeks after injection. At 4 weeks, all 5 treated eyes and all 8 control eyes had detachments; these were of similar height in the 2 groups.

Fluorouracil may prove useful in the treatment of proliferative vitreoretinopathy by delaying the onset of proliferation and permitting a stronger adhesion to develop between the sensory retina and the retinal pigment epithelium. The condition appears to be self-limiting, and use of fluorouracil might lead to an earlier onset of the stable

(9–15) Am. J. Ophthalmol. 96:33–42, July 1983.

phase. Fluorouracil could be used as an adjunct to scleral buckling, vitrectomy, the use of intraocular tamponade, and other anticontractile and antiproliferative drugs.

▶ [Epiretinal membrane formation after vitrectomy is a dreaded complication. Fluorouracil may inhibit this development and may become a valuable adjunct to vitreous surgery.] ◀

10. Retina

Pigmentary Photoreceptor Dystrophies: Progression as Monitored by Visual Field and Electroretinogram Testing

GERALD A. FISHMAN, M.D.

Eye and Ear Infirmary
University of Illinois, Chicago

The spectrum of diffuse pigmentary photoreceptor dystrophies includes several disorders such as retinitis pigmentosa, choroideremia, gyrate atrophy of the choroid and retina, and cone-rod dystrophy. The pathogeneses of these disorders are obscure and no known effective therapy is currently available.

Research efforts from different laboratories now allow investigators to chart the long-term course of photoreceptor deterioration better in at least some pigmentary photoreceptor dystrophies monitored by visual fields and electroretinography (ERG).

Inherent in the validity of any measurements is a firm knowledge of its short-term variability. This engenders an understanding of factors that contribute to this fluctuation, such as examiner idiosyncrasies; patient variability, stemming from individual attention spans or response times; or physiological features such as hormonal influences, diurnal variations, and others. It is surprising how relatively little data are available on the short-term variability of visual field testing not only in patients with photoreceptor dystrophies, but also in normal individuals. Without the knowledge of the limits of short-term variability in visual fields among patients with pigmentary photoreceptor dystrophies, the long-term progression cannot be monitored with any reliable accuracy.

Recently Ross, Fishman, Gilbert, and Anderson[1] obtained data on the variability of visual field measurements in 21 normal subjects and 26 patients with retinitis pigmentosa (RP). A Goldmann perimeter was used with a 4-3-II test target. Twenty RP patients and 15 normal subjects returned for a repeat field examination within a 2-month period. The 15 normal subjects had a mean variability of approximately 5% in the retinal area measured at 2 visits by the same examiner, with a range from 0 to 16%, considering each eye separately. For the RP patients, the mean intervisit variability in perimetric area by the same examiner was approximately 12% with a range from 0 to 50%. Since percent change would relate to some extent to the size of the initial visual field, we also determined significant (95% control limits) field change for intervisit variability in perimetric area. In absolute numbers, this was approximately 5 sq in. for normal subjects and approximately 7 sq in. for RP patients. These RP patients still had visual fields that were quantitatively substantive in most cases (16/26 had a total horizontal diameter of 80 degrees or greater in at least one eye to a 4-3-II test target). Nevertheless, the findings emphasize the importance of determining limits of field variability for patients and normal subjects before deciding that field loss is a measure of retinal photoreceptor deterioration.

While visual fields offer a subjective means of monitoring photoreceptor loss, the ERG can objectively assess changes in cone-rod function over time. To accomplish this accurately, however, it is necessary to know short-term (i.e., daily, weekly, or perhaps monthly) fluctuations in ERG amplitudes that are likely to occur independently of photoreceptor deterioration resulting from the patient's underlying disease.

As in the monitoring of visual fields, a relative paucity of data is available on the subject of short-term variability in ERG measurements. Because of different stimulus conditions, each laboratory monitoring a patient's progress would need to determine its own limits of short-term fluctuations in ERG measurements. We measured 3 normal individuals during 6 to 9 follow-up visits, and determined a tolerance of up to 30% in intraindividual short-term variability for a full-field single-flash white photopic b-wave for the 3 patients. The tolerance level was up to 20% in a combined cone and rod 30-minute full-field single-flash white scotopic b-wave response. Similar data are needed on patients with different diffuse pigmentary photoreceptor dystrophies who have variable degrees of ERG loss.

Data on visual field and ERG short-term variability have implications not only for monitoring long-term natural history, but also for assessing claims of improvement in visual function as the result of "therapeutic intervention." Before credibility can be assured, any claims of improved visual function must be accompanied by statements regarding the short-term variability of the testing procedure being used to monitor "therapeutic" outcomes.

Reference

1. Ross, D.F., Fishman, G.A., Gilbert, L.D., et al.: Variability of visual field measurements in normals and patients with retinitis pigmentosa. *Arch. Ophthalmol.* accepted for publication, 1984.

▶ ↓ There are 6 multicenter randomized controlled trials sponsored by the National Eye Institute as separate parts of the Macular Photocoagulation Study. The favorable results from the Senile Macular Degeneration study were reported last year. In the following 2 articles, the equally favorable results from the Ocular Histoplasmosis

Study and the Idiopathic Neovascularization Study are reported. It is important to point out that the neovascular membranes were all 200 to 2,500 µm from the center of the fovea in a select group of patients. Nonetheless, these are important studies of considerable benefit to some patients. ◄

10-1 **Argon Laser Photocoagulation for Ocular Histoplasmosis: Results of a Randomized Clinical Trial** are reported by the Macular Photocoagulation Study Group. The Ocular Histoplasmosis Study is a multicenter trial of argon laser photocoagulation for preventing severe loss of visual acuity in patients with ocular histoplasmosis and choroidal neovascular membranes 200 to 2,500 µm from the center of the foveal avascular zone. Patients with at least one atrophic scar and acuity of 20/100 or better in the study eye were admitted to the trial. Eyes with a peripapillary neovascular membrane were included only if treatment to cover the neovascular complex would spare at least 1.5 clock hours of the peripapillary nerve fiber layer adjacent to the disk. Photocoagulation was performed in 124 cases; 121 other patients were observed. The treatment method is illustrated in Figure 10–1. Modifications were permitted when the foveal edge of the complex was within 350 µm of the foveal center.

Fig 10–1.—Schematic of protocol treatment. **A,** noncontiguous 100-µm burns are used to outline neovascular complex. **B,** foveal edge is treated with overlapping 200-µm burns at duration of 0.2 second. **C,** perimeter of complex is treated with overlapping 200-µm burns at duration of 0.2 second. **D,** entire complex is treated with overlapping 200- to 500-µm burns at duration of 0.5 second. End point is uniformly white lesion that covers entire complex and extends to initial outline. (Courtesy of Macular Photocoagulation Study Group: Arch. Ophthalmol. 101:1347–1357, September 1983; copyright 1983, American Medical Association.)

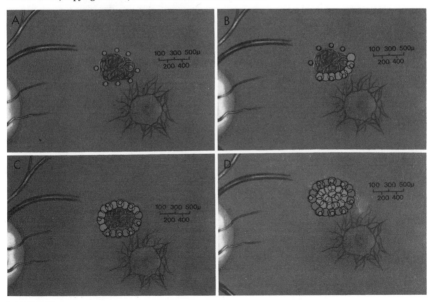

(10–1)   Arch. Ophthalmol. 101:1347–1357, September 1983.

At a median follow-up of 18 months, 34% of untreated eyes and 9% of treated eyes had lost 6 or more lines of visual acuity from baseline. Photocoagulation was advantageous in all subgroups of patients and at all follow-up intervals. More than 3 times as many untreated as treated eyes had an acuity less than 20/200 at the most recent follow-up visit. Complications occurred in 50 (41%) of the treated eyes. Seven of the 50 were among the 11 eyes with a decrease in acuity of 6 or more lines.

Argon laser photocoagulation reduces the risk of severe visual loss in eyes with histoplasmosis and a symptomatic choroidal neovascular membrane 200 to 2,500 μm from the center of the foveal avascular zone. Control patients are no longer being accepted because of the effectiveness of treatment. Krypton-red laser photocoagulation is under evaluation in patients with neovascular membranes within 200 μm of the center of the foveal avascular zone.

10–2 **Argon Laser Photocoagulation for Idiopathic Neovascularization: Results of a Randomized Clinical Trial** are reported by the Macular Photocoagulation Study Group. The Idiopathic Neovascularization Study is a multicenter trial of argon laser photocoagulation for preventing severe visual loss in eyes with a choroidal neovascular membrane (NVM) and no other clinically significant eye disease. Patients with a NVM of 200 to 2,500 μm from the center of the foveal avascular zone and a best corrected acuity of 20/100 or better were eligible for the trial. All had symptoms related to the NVM but no evidence of atropic scarring or significant drusen. The patients were aged 18 years and older.

Thirty-three patients were assigned to photocoagulation and 34 to a control group with no treatment. The most recent acuity findings

TABLE 1.—VISUAL ACUITY IN STUDY EYE AT
MOST RECENT FOLLOW-UP

	No. (%) of Eyes	
Visual Acuity	Treat-ment Group	No Treat-ment Group
20/20 or better	10 (33.3)	10 (30.3)
20/25 to 20/40	11 (36.7)	4 (12.1)
20/50 to 20/100	5 (16.7)	7 (21.2)
20/125 to 20/200	2 (6.7)	8 (24.2)
20/250 or worse	2 (6.7)	4 (12.1)
Total*	30	33

*P value for chi-square test with quantitatively ordered classes was .08.
(Courtesy of Macular Photocoagulation Study Group: Arch. Ophthalmol. 101:1358–1361, September 1983; copyright 1983, American Medical Association.)

(10–2) Arch. Ophthalmol. 101:1358–1361, September 1983.

TABLE 2.—CHANGE IN VISUAL ACUITY IN STUDY
EYE BETWEEN BASELINE AND MOST RECENT
FOLLOW-UP

No. (%) of Eyes

Change	Treatment Group	No Treatment Group
Increase or no change	21 (70.0)	17 (51.5)
2-5-line decrease	4 (13.3)	5 (15.2)
6-9-line decrease	4 (13.3)	7 (21.2)
Decrease of 10 or more lines	1 (3.3)	4 (12.1)
Total*	30	33

*P value for chi-square test with quantitatively ordered classes was .08.
(Courtesy of Macular Photocoagulation Study Group: Arch. Ophthalmol. 101:1358–1361, September 1983; copyright 1983, American Medical Association.)

are given in Table 1, and the changes in acuity in the study eye from baseline are shown in Table 2. Nearly 3 times as many untreated as treated eyes had acuities below 20/100 at the last follow-up examination. More treated eyes had an increase in acuity or no change, whereas more untreated eyes had large reductions in acuity from baseline. About 3 times as many untreated as treated eyes lost 6 or more lines of acuity after 1 year of follow-up. Comparable proportions of treated and untreated eyes had a lesion extending under the center of the foveal avascular zone after 1 year. Treatment was too extensive in 2 instances. In 3 eyes there was "runoff" into the center of the foveal avascular zone. One perforation of Bruch's membrane occurred. No hemorrhage exceeding 25% of the disk diameter was observed. Two treated eyes had acuity less than 20/200 at follow-up; both had minor hemorrhage produced by treatment.

Randomization of patients for this study has been stopped, and all eligible patients now are being treated. The current findings do not apply to patients with NVM secondary to such disorders as pathologic myopia, angioid streaks, and traumatic choroidal rupture.

10–3 **Choroidal Neovascularization in Fellow Eyes of Patients With Advanced Senile Macular Degeneration: Role of Laser Photocoagulation.** Progressive visual loss has been associated with the development of choroidal neovascularization in patients with senile macular degeneration, but successful photocoagulation of cho-

(10–3) Arch. Ophthalmol. 101:1194–1197, August 1983.

CHANGE IN VISUAL ACUITY IN 52 EYES TREATED WITH MONOCHROMATIC GREEN ARGON
LASER PHOTOCOAGULATION

Treatment Result	No. (%) of Eyes		
	Foveal	Juxtafoveal	Perifoveal
No change or improvement	18 (75)	4 (40)	14 (78)
Decrease	6 (25)	6 (60)	4 (22)
Total	24 (100)	10 (100)	18 (100)

(Courtesy of Jalkh, A.E., et al.: Arch. Ophthalmol. 101:1194–1197, August 1983; copyright 1983, American Medical Association.)

roidal neovascular membranes with the argon laser has been reported. Alex E. Jalkh, Marcos P. Avila, Clement L. Trempe, J. Wallace McMeel, and Charles L. Schepens (Boston) evaluated the effects of photocoagulation with the monochromatic green argon laser on 52 fellow eyes of patients with advanced disciform macular scars. All had acuities of 20/400 or worse in the affected eye and evidence of choroidal neovascularization seen on fluorescein angiography in the fellow eye. The locations of the neovascular membranes were foveal in 24 fellow eyes, juxtafoveal in 10, and perifoveal in 18. Fluorescein angiography was repeated a week after treatment, and further treatment was given if residual new vessels were found.

Closure of new vessels was seen in 88% of treated eyes, and vision stabilized or improved in 69% of eyes. Neovascularization was successfully closed in 96% of eyes in the foveal group, and good visual results were obtained in 75% of this group (table). All eyes in the perifoveal group responded to treatment, and vision stabilized or improved in 78% of cases. The outcome of treatment could not be related to age, sex, or the size of the choroidal neovascular membrane.

These results suggest that all perifoveal choroidal neovascular membranes in fellow eyes of patients with advanced disciform macular scarring should be treated with the monochromatic green argon laser. Treatment also is helpful in patients with juxtafoveal and foveal choroidal neovascular membranes. Patients with foveal membranes and an acuity of 20/70 or worse should be treated. The value of the krypton-red and krypton-yellow lasers in treating choroidal neovascular membranes is under study.

▶ [The authors of this article treated the fellow eye of all of the patients they saw with visual loss due to a disciform subretinal scar. These results were good but an important point is that they repeated the fluorescein angiogram 1 week following treatment so that any residual new vessels could be treated. These patients must be followed up frequently and carefully with fluorescein angiography because, while we don't have good data on the recurrence rate, it nonetheless appears to be relatively high.] ◀

10–4 **Senile Macular Degeneration: Review of Epidemiologic Features** is presented by Frederick L. Ferris III (Natl. Eye Inst., Bethesda, Md.). The risk of senile macular degeneration increases particularly after the fifth decade of life, and the disorder undoubtedly will become more prevalent over time unless successful means of preventing or treating it are discovered.

The primary site of the pathologic change resulting in drusen is unclear. Drusen may be ubiquitous in older persons when carefully sought, and it is unclear that the mere presence of asymptomatic drusen warrants a diagnosis of senile macular degeneration. Loss of retinal pigment epithelium also is associated with the disorder. It can occur focally, or it can be widespread and associated with decreased visual acuity. Hemorrhage or serous exudation from subretinal neovascular networks can lead to detachment of the retinal pigment epithelium or the retina, or both. Resolution of subretinal blood often leads to fibrovascular scarring, destruction of retinal structures and the pigment epithelium, and severe visual loss.

Fundus photographs are helpful in diagnosing senile macular degeneration. An attempt should be made to determine whether the reduction in vision can be explained by the degree of macular degeneration that is present.

Senile macular degeneration is a leading cause of blindness, and it may become the leading cause because of the rapid rise in prevalence in persons older than age 65 years. Women are affected more often than men. The disorder appears to be rare in black persons in the United States. A consistent association with hyperopia has been reported. An association with cigarette smoking has not been confirmed. A family history of senile macular degeneration may increase the risk.

The exudative form of senile macular degeneration is more likely to produce seriously impaired acuity than the atrophic form. Persons with exudative disease in one eye and drusen in the other are at a high risk of having exudative disease in the second eye. The only effective treatment has been photocoagulation, and only certain types of neovascular membranes associated with the exudative type of disorder are amenable to treatment.

▶ ↓ The authors of the following 2 articles describe their experience and treatment recommendations for patients with cystoid macular edema. When anterior segment vitreous tug is evident, cutting the strands noninvasively with a YAG laser seems reasonable. For cystoid macular edema without obvious vitreous tug, steroids and indomethacin may be helpful. Clinical trial data is needed but, more importantly, we need to discover the basic pathogenesis if we hope to rid ourselves of this frustrating surgical complication. ◀

10–5 **Clinical Experiences and Current Concepts of Cystoid Aphakic Macular Edema** are reviewed by Charles J. Campbell and

(10–4) Am. J. Epidemiol. 118:132–151, Aug. 1, 1983.
(10–5) Ocular Inflammation Ther. 1:5–9, Spring 1983.

Anita Anderson (Columbia Univ.). Cystoid aphakic macular edema is characterized by the presence of cystoid spaces in the outer plexiform and outer nuclear layers, inflammatory cells in the ciliary body, and retinal vasculitis. The presence of cyclitis and vasculitis suggests a degree of generalized inflammation. Miyake (1978) suggested that iris trauma results in the release of prostaglandins, breakdown of the blood-aqueous and blood-retina barriers, and the development of intraretinal vasculitis and cystoid macular edema. Clinical edema is comparably frequent after intracapsular and extracapsular cataract surgery, but complicated extracapsular extractions are more often followed by clinical cystoid macular edema than are complicated intracapsular operations. An intact posterior capsule may theoretically have some value in protecting the macula from the development of angiographic cystoid maculopathy. Fluorescein angiography may be diagnostically helpful when the pupil does not dilate fully or an intraocular lens is present.

Attempts at treatment have yielded widely varying results. A trial of steroids probably is warranted in the absence of systemic contraindications if the condition lasts longer than 3 to 4 months without evidence of remission. Indomethacin may be useful when given in higher doses, e.g., more than 25 mg/day. Anterior vitrectomy has shown promising results in patients with protracted, refractory disease. About 80% of all patients, however, have useful vision within 6 to 12 months without specific treatment. Every attempt must be made to minimize trauma to the other eye. Prophylactic indomethacin therapy may be worthwhile. Optimization of the vascular status in aged patients is helpful. Implantation of an intraocular lens does not seem to increase the chance of the disease developing, although it may make the diagnosis difficult.

10–6   **YAG Laser Treatment of Cystoid Macular Edema.** Leeds E. Katzen, James A. Fleischman (Univ. of Maryland), and Stephen Trokel (Columbia Univ.) treated 14 eyes (some aphakic and some with implanted intraocular lenses) with the neodymium-YAG laser for cystoid macular edema with vitreous incarceration in the corneoscleral wound. The 9 men and 5 women ranged in age from 54 to 79 years. Some patients had been unsuccessfully treated with topical steroids or ibuprofen.

Visual acuity and intraocular pressure was measured before operation and the configuration of the vitreous strand was noted. Topical anesthesia in eyedrop form was used. Vitreous strands were observed with slit-lamp biomicroscopy (Fig 10–2). After the helium-neon aiming beam was focused on the thinnest accessible distal portion of the strand, the laser was applied. Several patients required 2 or 3 treatment sessions of 50 to 200 laser applications each.

The laser was successful in breaking the corneovitreal adhesions in

(10–6)   Am. J. Ophthalmol. 95:589–592, May 1983.

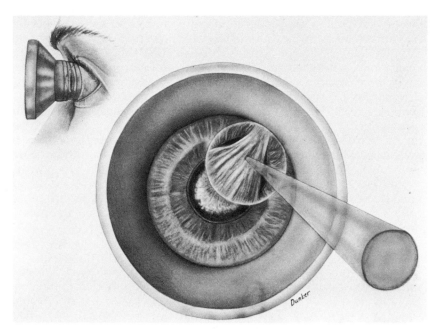

Fig 10–2.—Placement of Abraham contact lens on cornea enhances slit-lamp visualization of vitreous strand in anterior chamber. (Courtesy of Katzen, L.E., et al.: Am. J. Ophthalmol. 95:589–592, May 1983.)

every case. In all 14 eyes posttreatment visual acuities were better than pretreatment visual acuities. Ten eyes improved at least 3 Snellen lines and 12 eyes improved at least 2. Eleven eyes had visual acuities of 20/40 or better 1 to 9 months after treatment. Chronic cystoid macular edema of more than 1 year's duration appeared to respond less well to laser treatment. No significant treatment complications occurred at 1 week after treatment. In several patients laser shots inadvertently delivered to the corneal stroma and iris produced white opaque areas in the corneal stroma and small hemorrhages in the iris; in all cases these resolved spontaneously without sequelae.

The neodymium-YAG laser provides a noninvasive means of sectioning vitreous strands without thermal effects or any other discernible complications.

10–7 **Effect of One Year of Near Normal Blood Glucose Levels on Retinopathy in Insulin-Dependent Diabetics.** Serious diabetic complications have been related to failure to achieve normal blood glucose levels in insulin-dependent patients. Torsten Lauritzen, Kim Frost-Larsen, Torsten Deckert, and the Steno Study Group (Gentofte, Denmark) assessed the value of near normal glycemic control in pre-

(10–7) Lancet 1:200–204, Jan. 29, 1983.

venting progressive retinopathy in a series of 30 insulin-dependent diabetic patients with background retinopathy. Mean age was 34 years and mean duration of diabetes was 19 years. Study patients had continuous subcutaneous insulin infusion (CSII) with a portable infusion pump, while controls received conventional insulin injections, usually twice a day. Blood glucose level was measured every 2 weeks for 1 year, and retinal status was assessed every 6 months.

Patients receiving CSII had lower mean blood glucose levels than controls during the study year, although the frequency of hypoglycemia did not differ significantly in the 2 groups. One patient in each group was admitted with ketoacidosis. Hemoglobin A_{1C} levels were significantly lower than at baseline in the CSII-treated group only. Overall, more patients showed deterioration than improvement determined by fundus examination, but there was no significant difference in the 2 groups, and no differences between well-regulated and poorly regulated patients. Retinal function, reflected by oscillatory potential and macular recovery time, improved significantly in the CSII-treated group and deteriorated significantly in the control group.

Retinal morphology was not better preserved by improved glycemic control in this study of insulin-dependent diabetic patients, but retinal function was superior in patients managed by CSII than in those treated conventionally. Two of the 3 patients who had proliferative retinopathy were in the CSII group. Further studies are needed to define the association between retinal morphology and function and to determine the point at which progression of retinopathy can no longer be influenced by normalization of metabolite levels.

▶ [This is one of several studies that have been unable to show an improvement in retinopathy with use of the insulin pump, although there was some improvement in function. Perhaps long-term data will show different results, but, thus far, the results are very discouraging.] ◀

10–8 **Diabetic Rubeois and Panretinal Photocoagulation: Prospective, Controlled, Masked Trial-Using Iris Fluorescein Angiography.** It does not appear that the finding that panretinal photocoagulation or cryoablation of the retina can cause rubeosis to regress has been tested by prospective, controlled, masked studies. Peter R. Pavan, James C. Folk, Thomas A. Weingeist, Vernon M. Hermsen, Robert C. Watzke, and Paul R. Montague (Univ. of Iowa, Iowa City) used iris fluorescein angiography to evaluate the effect of panretinal laser photocoagulation in, a prospective, controlled, masked study of 35 eyes in 28 patients with diabetic retinopathy. Thirty-one of the eyes had high-risk characteristics and could not ethically be randomized to a "treatment" or "no treatment" group. Iris fluorescein angiograms were obtained 5 to 7 weeks apart. The eyes with rubeosis received either panretinal argon laser photocoagulation immediately after the first angiogram, delayed laser treatment, or no laser treat-

(10–8) Arch. Ophthalmol. 101:882–884, June 1983.

ment between angiograms. The rubeosis was considered to have improved if all 3 masked readers independently selected the angiogram last performed as demonstrating less severe rubeosis.

Only 2 (18%) of 11 eyes with severe rubeosis showed spontaneous improvement, whereas 11 (73%) of 15 eyes with severe rubeosis improved after laser therapy (P = .008). However, only 1 of 10 eyes with mild rubeosis treated by laser therapy showed improvement and 1 of 10 eyes with mild rubeosis showed spontaneous improvement without laser photocoagulation. The difference in the number of days between angiograms in the treated and untreated groups was not statistically significant. In addition, the number of laser burns received by the eyes with mild rubeosis and the number received by those with severe rubeosis did not differ significantly. Eyes with distinctively severe rubeosis usually showed a dramatic response to laser treatment.

Iris fluorescein angiography showed that eyes with severe rubeosis had a statistically significant response to panretinal laser photocoagulation when compared with nontreated controls. However, the low and insignificant response rate of eyes with mild rubeosis may indicate that the mild rubeosis did not regress significantly after laser therapy or that iris fluorescein angiography is relatively insensitive in detecting changes in rubeosis. Further studies evaluating the effectiveness of panretinal cryopexy or other treatments on rubeosis using iris fluorescein angiography are best performed if the patients with severe rubeosis are randomly examined separately from patients with mild rubeosis.

▶ [We have known for some years that panretinal photocoagulation has a beneficial effect on diabetic rubeosis, but it is surprising that the mild form of the disease was unaffected in this study.] ◀

10–9 **Prospective Follow-Up Study of Panretinal Photocoagulation in Preventing Neovascular Glaucoma Following Ischemic Central Retinal Vein Occlusion.** Photocoagulation of the fundus may help protect against neovascular glaucoma (NVG) in patients with central retinal vein occlusion (CRVO). L. Laatikainen (Helsinki) reviewed the results of panretinal photocoagulation in 10 women and 5 men, mean age 71, with recent CRVO and extensive retinal capillary closure observed on fluorescein angiography. All affected eyes had an ischemic type of CRVO with extensive capillary nonperfusion both centrally and peripherally in 3 or 4 retinal quadrants. Abnormal leakage of the iris vessels was observed in all 11 eyes examined. The intraocular pressure was elevated in 7 eyes at the time of diagnosis of CRVO (table). Two eyes had rubeosis iridis at the time of treatment. In 2 or 3 sessions of argon laser photocoagulation, about 2,000 burns having a 0.5-mm spot size were made over the entire postequatorial retina, sparing the center of the macula.

In none of the nonglaucomatous eyes did NVG or new iris vessels

(10–9)   Graefes Arch. Clin. Exp. Ophthalmol. 220:236–239, June 1983.

CLINICAL DATA ON PATIENTS WITH ISCHEMIC CENTRAL RETINAL VEIN OCCLUSION (CRVO)
TREATED BY ARGON LASER PHOTOCOAGULATION

Case no.	Sex Age	Pre-existing glaucoma	Time of photocoagulation after CRVO (months)	No. of burns	Central vision[b] Pre-treatment	Central vision[b] Latest	Intraocular pressure Pre-treatment	Intraocular pressure Latest	Other treatment	Follow-up (months)
1	M 64	–	2	1,500	CF 5 m	CF 3 m	15	16	–	50
2	M 75	–	6	900	CF 2 m	CF 4 m	15	13	–	16
3	M 66	–	3	960	CF 1 m	0.1	13	18	–	13
4	M 68	–	< 1	1,500	PL	HM	60	18	–	12
5	F 80	Capsular glaucoma[a]	6	1,200	CF 3 m	PL	29	29	Pilocarpine. adrenaline	36
6	F 68	Capsular glaucoma[a] < 1		750	CF 5 m	PL	44	62–23	Pilocarpine	39
7	F 78	Capsular glaucoma[a] < 1		1,850	CF 1 m	HM	33	23[d]	–	43
8	F 70	Chronic congestive glaucoma[a]	4	1,900	HM	HM	36	17	Trabeculectomy	11
9	F 62	–	< 1	1,850	HM	HM	19	19	–	52
10	M 78	–	2	2,200	CF 1 m	PL	33[c]	54	Cyclocryocoagulation	5
11	F 69	Capsular glaucoma	1	2,100	CF 1 m	CF 1 m	53	19	Trabeculectomy	5
12	F 65	–	3	900	CF 1 m	CF 2 m	15	16	–	20
13	F 73	Chronic simple glaucoma[a]	not known	2,400	CF 3 m	NPL	38	70[d]	Cyclocryocoagulation. retrobulbar alcohol	4
14	F 70	–	2	1,800	HM	HM	15	14	–	12
15	F 74	–	not known	1,100	CF 1 m	HM	16	17	–	9

[a]Glaucoma diagnosed at initial examination after development of central retinal vein occlusion.
[b]CF = counting fingers; HM = hand movements; PL = perception of light; NPL = no perception of light.
[c]Neovascular glaucoma developed before photocoagulation.
[d]Rubeosis iridis developed after photocoagulation.
(Courtesy of Laatikainen, L.: Graefes Arch. Clin. Exp. Ophthalmol. 220:236–239, June 1983; Berlin-Heidelberg-New York; Springer.)

develop, but in 2 of them new vessels were noted on the optic disk. Vision improved in 1 of the 7 eyes and deteriorated in another. An eye with acute angle-closure glaucoma improved after photocoagulation without further antiglaucoma medication. Four of the 8 glaucomatous eyes did not have rubeosis iridis nor did it develop. In 2 instances the pressure was subsequently controlled by trabeculectomy. Iris new vessels regressed in 1 of the 2 eyes in which rubeosis developed despite photocoagulation. Vision deteriorated in 5 glaucomatous eyes, and 7 of the 8 eyes had final vision worse than having ability to count fingers.

The likelihood of ischemic-type CRVO developing appears to increase with advancing age. Panretinal photocoagulation apparently can prevent iris neovascularization and NVG following ischemic CRVO, but treatment should be given before rubeosis iridis develops. If the angiogram is difficult to interpret because of retinal edema and large hemorrhages, abnormal leakage from the iris vessels, especially the radial ones, suggests extensive retinal vascular closure.

▶ [The author of this article treated all of her own patients, so the control group had to be from previous studies. Nonetheless, the patients did relatively well, which is probably further evidence of the effectiveness of panretinal photocoagulation in central retinal vein obstruction. The problem is that it is difficult to assess the amount of capillary nonperfusion when there are extensive retinal hemorrhages.] ◀

10–10 **Differential Diagnosis of Central Retinal Vein Obstruction.** Thomas P. Kearns (Mayo Clinic and Found.) clarifies the meaning of the term, "venous-stasis retinopathy," and the differential diagnosis of "retinopathy of carotid occlusive disease" and "retinopathy of central retinal vein occlusion." The differential features between these 2 entities are listed in the table.

Hemorrhages are more likely to develop on the disk in a patient with a vein occlusion than in a patient with carotid disease because disk edema is a major feature of a florid vein occlusion in its complete form and is never seen in retinopathy of carotid disease. In retinopathy of carotid disease the veins have an irregular caliber similar to that seen in diabetic retinopathy; however, this irregularity is never seen in central retinal vein occlusion. Hemorrhages, microaneurysms, and capillary dilatations are usually distributed evenly over the entire retina in central retinal vein occlusion, whereas these lesions are usually located in the midperiphery of the retina in carotid disease.

Retinopathy of carotid disease is linked to atherosclerotic changes; it occurs generally in older patients and is more frequent in men than in women (75% vs. 25%). The patient with retinopathy of carotid occlusive disease may have fluctuating or persistent blurring of vision; the latter often heralds complications such as rubeosis iridis and glaucoma, whereas the patient with central retinal vein occlusion never has intermittent blurring or loss of vision. Presence of both ischemic pain of the orbit and venous-stasis retinopathy is indicative of carotid occlusive disease. Such pain does not occur in patients with central retinal vein occlusion.

DIFFERENTIAL FEATURES OF RETINOPATHY OF CAROTID ARTERY OCCLUSIVE DISEASE AND RETINOPATHY OF INCOMPLETE OCCLUSION OF THE CENTRAL RETINAL VEIN

	Central Vein Occlusion	Carotid Occlusive Disease
Optic disc	Hemorrhages and new vessels may be present, disc edema may occur	Hemorrhages and new vessels not usually present, disc edema never occurs
Retinal veins	Engorged, dark, but regular in caliber	Engorged, dark, and irregular in caliber
Type and location of lesions	Hemorrhages, microaneurysms, and generalized capillary dilatations	Hemorrhages, microaneurysms, and capillary dilatations more likely in midperiphery
Age and sex of patient	Middle-aged men or women	Past middle age, men more common (75%)
Visual symptoms	Blurred vision, but vision is stable rather than episodic	Amaurosis fugax and blur from slow retinal adaptation
Associated ocular findings	Open-angle glaucoma, neovascular glaucoma as a complication	Retinal emboli, ischemic eye and orbital pain, neovascular glaucoma as a complication
Associated systemic findings	Hypertension	Atherosclerotic diseases and their manifestations
Retinal artery pressure	Always normal	Always low

(Courtesy of Kearns, T.P.: Ophthalmology (Rochester) 90:475–480, May 1983.)

(10–10) Ophthalmology (Rochester) 90:475–480, May 1983.

Low retinal artery pressure is the most important differentiating feature between retinopathy of carotid occlusive disease and incomplete central retinal vein occlusion. The mechanism of production of retinopathy of carotid disease is dependent on low perfusion pressure and its resulting ischemia and anoxia; therefore, the retinal artery pressure must be low; it is usually measured with an ophthalmodynamometer or in a neurovascular laboratory by oculopneumoplethysmography. The retinal artery pressure on the side with venous-stasis retinopathy of carotid disease is usually 50% of that measured on the opposite side; a finding of low retinal artery pressure excludes retinopathy of central retinal vein occlusion.

▶ [This is an important article because the author clears up part of the confusion concerning the term, "venous-stasis retinopathy." The term should clearly not be used for the retinopathy associated with carotid artery disease. Indeed, the simplest solution might be to abandon the term for both carotid artery disease retinopathy and that of retinal vein obstruction.] ◀

10–11 **Rupture of Retinal Pigment Epithelial Detachment in Senile Macular Disease.** Serous detachment of the retinal pigment epithelium is an early form of senile macular disease. Leila Laatikainen (Univ. of Helsinki) reports 3 cases in which senile pigment epithelial detachment was complicated by rupture of the pigment epithelium.

Woman, 67, was seen with photopsia in both eyes. Central acuity was 0.8 on the right and 1.0 on the left. Fundus examination with the Goldmann contact lens showed central pigment epithelial detachment in the macula in both eyes (Fig 10–3). Fluorescein angiography showed no evidence of subretinal neovascularization. The right eye was treated with the argon laser. Vision in the left eye was worse 6 weeks later, when central acuity was 0.5 and a large rupture of the pigment epithelial detachment along its temporal margin was observed. The pigment epithelium was folded up toward the nose and under the fovea, and the overlying neuroretina was highly elevated. The acuity 10 months later was 0.4. Cystoid changes were observed in the fovea, and areas of depigmentation were seen in the pigment epithelial fold.

Large, highly elevated central pigment epithelial detachments of 2 to 3 disk diameters were present in these eyes. Rupture of the pigment epithelium occurred 2 weeks to 2 months after detachment. In all cases the detachment tore along the temporal margin, in the area where the degenerative changes were mildest but the detachment was highest. The frequency of large ruptures of the detached pigment epithelium is unknown. Tearing of the pigment epithelium may not alter the visual prognosis, but recognition of the complication helps in interpretation of the clinical and angiographic findings in senile macular disease.

Tearing of the pigment epithelium might be prevented if the detachment can be flattened by photocoagulation, but flattening may be difficult in large, highly elevated detachments. The Moorfields Mac-

(10–11) Acta Ophthalmol. (Copenh.) 61:1–8, February 1983.

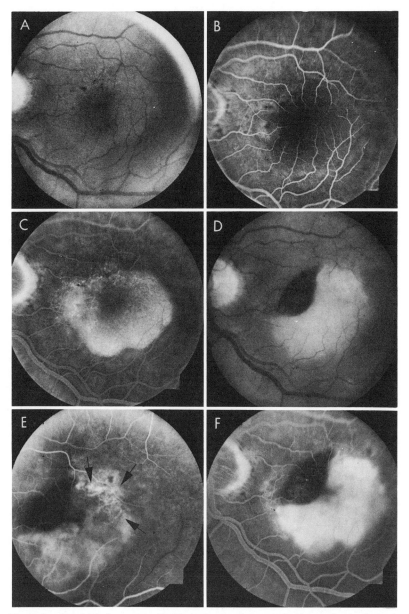

Fig 10–3.—**A,** initial photograph of left macula, showing central paleness due to pigment epithelial detachment. **B and C,** fluorescein angiograms on same day show accumulation of fluorescein under detached pigment epithelium. Small hyperfluorescent spots toward nose and above fovea correspond to drusen and pigment disturbance. **D-F,** corresponding views 2 months later show large pigment epithelial fold (*dark area*) under fovea. **E,** unobscured view of choroidal vessels temporally in area of pigment epithelial rupture (*arrows*). **F,** intense hyperfluorescence of denuded area under neuroretina; no definite new vessels are visible. (Courtesy of Laatikainen, L.: Acta Ophthalmol (Copenh.) 61:1–8, February 1983.)

ular Study Group has found that the incidence of tearing is not altered by argon laser photocoagulation.

▶ [Detachment of the retinal pigment epithelium is a fascinating and serious complication of senile macular degeneration. The author is justifiably concerned that photocoagulation may turn out not to be helpful in these cases, although there is not yet definitive data.] ◀

▶ ↓ The following 3 articles describe the ocular findings in patients with acquired immune deficiency syndrome (AIDS) seen in New York and Los Angeles hospitals. Since these articles were published the causative virus has been identified, but it could still be years before definitive treatment is available. ◀

10–12 **Acquired Immune Deficiency Syndrome: Ocular Manifestations.** Acquired immune deficiency syndrome (AIDS) is an immunologic disorder possibly caused by a transmissible infectious agent that alters lymphocyte function. Ocular disease is a frequent feature. Gary N. Holland, Jay S. Pepose, Thomas H. Pettit, Michael S. Gottlieb, Robert D. Yee, and Robert Y. Foos (Univ. of California, Los Angeles) reviewed the findings in 27 patients with AIDS who were evaluated clinically between 1981 and 1982; 10 of these and 3 additional patients had autopsies. All 30 patients fulfilled Centers for Disease Control criteria for AIDS. All but 5 had opportunistic infections; these 5 had Kaposi's sarcoma only. Only 3 patients with opportunistic infections did not have cytomegalovirus infection. All but 2 patients had a history of homosexual activity, with or without intravenous drug abuse. Profound cellular immunodeficiency was demonstrated in all patients.

Ocular abnormalities were present in 63% of the patients (table). None of those with Kaposi's sarcoma alone had ocular involvement. More than 50% of the patients had cotton-wool spots, and all had

OCULAR DISORDERS IN PATIENTS GROUPED BY ACQUIRED IMMUNODEFICIENCY
SYNDROME CLASSIFICATION

Classification	Number of Patients	Cotton-Wool Spots	Retinal Hemorrhages, Roth Spots	CMV Retinitis	Kaposi's Sarcoma (conjunctiva)	Other	No Ocular Lesions
Patients with PCP* no KS†, ±OOI‡	9	7	3	4	—	M. avium choroidal granulomas (1)	2
Patients with KS, no PCP, +OOI§	7	4	3	1	1	Conjunctivitis (1)	2
Patients with KS, no PCP, −OOI§	5	0	0	—	0	—	5
Patients with both PCP and KS, ±OOI	5	3	2	3	2	Conjunctivitis (1) and keratoconjunctivitis (1)	1
Patients with OOI only	4	2	0	0	—	Retinal periphlebitis (1) and conjunctivitis (1)	1
Total	30	16	8	8	3		11

*Pneumocystis carinii pneumonia.
†Kaposi's sarcoma.
‡Other opportunistic infections.
§Patients classified as having Kaposi's sarcoma with *Pneumocystis carinii* pneumonia have been further divided into those with and those without other opportunistic infections.
(Courtesy of Holland, G.N., et al.: Ophthalmology (Rochester) 90:859–873, August 1983.)

(10–12) Ophthalmology (Rochester) 90:859–873, August 1983.

evidence of cytomegalovirus infection. Several of these patients had areas of retinal microvascular abnormality seen on fluorescein angiography. Eight patients had retinal hemorrhages. Cytomegalovirus retinitis was present in 32% of the patients with opportunistic infections. One patient had choroidal granulomas and another had monocular retinal periphlebitis. Conjunctival Kaposi's sarcoma was present in 3 patients. Three others had mild, transient conjunctivitis. The overall case fatality rate was 57%; in patients with opportunistic infections it was 68%. Patients with cotton-wool spots had a case fatality rate of 81%, compared with a rate of 44% for the others with opportunistic infection.

The presence of cotton-wool spots, the most common ocular abnormality in this series of patients with AIDS, was strongly correlated with multiple opportunistic infections. A third of the patients with opportunistic infections had cytomegalovirus retinitis. The prognosis for these eyes is particularly poor. Kaposi's sarcoma itself can involve ocular and adnexal structures.

10–13 **Acquired Immunodeficiency Syndrome: Ophthalmic Manifestations in Ambulatory Patients.** Paul R. Rosenberg, Alan E. Uliss, Gerald H. Friedland, Carol A. Harris, Catherine Butkus Small, and Robert S. Klein (Albert Einstein College of Medicine, New York) reviewed the ocular findings in 25 ambulatory, previously healthy patients seen between 1982 and 1983 with acquired immune deficiency syndrome (AIDS). The disorder was characterized by cutaneous anergy, lymphopenia, depressed lymphocyte responses to mitogens, and opportunistic infections. The 19 men and 6 women had a median age of 32 years. Eleven patients were bisexual or homosexual, and 17 were intravenous drug abusers. Eleven patients had *Pneumocystis carinii* pneumonia as the major opportunistic infection. The ocular abnormalities are listed in the table. Ten of 18 patients with AIDS proper had ocular manifestations, but none of the 7 with AIDS prodrome were affected. Only 1 patient had decreased visual acuity in association with necrotizing retinitis consistent with cytomegalovirus infection. All but 1 of the patients with ocular abnormalities had cotton-wool spots.

Cotton-wool spots are the most common ophthalmic lesion associated with AIDS. Several of the present patients had fluorescein angiographic findings of retinal capillary nonperfusion. Other abnormalities described in AIDS include cytomegalovirus retinitis, Kaposis's sarcoma of the conjunctiva, and retinal periphlebitis. The low incidence of cytomegalovirus retinitis in the present series may be related to the fact that the group consisted chiefly of ambulatory, heterosexual drug abusers rather than promiscuous homosexual men. Three of 4 patients who died within a month of ocular examination had normal ocular findings, suggesting that ocular changes may be absent even late in the course of AIDS.

(10–13) Ophthalmology (Rochester) 90:874–878, August 1983.

CLINICAL FINDINGS IN 25 AMBULATORY PATIENTS WITH ACQUIRED IMMUNODEFICIENCY SYNDROME

Clinical Presentation	Age	Sex	Risk Factors	Acquired Opportunistic Infections	Ocular Manifestations
Prodrome					
1	26	F	IV drug abuser (IV DA)* Bisexual	Oral candidiasis (OC)	—
2	38	M	Homosexual	OC†	—
3	28	M	IV DA Homosexual	—	—
4	32	M	IV DA Heterosexual	OC	—
5	40	M	IV DA Bisexual	OC	—
6	32	M	Homosexual	OC	—
7	31	M	IV DA Heterosexual	OC	—
AIDS					
8	31	F	IV DA Heterosexual	OC; *Pneumocystis carinii* pneumonia (PCP)‡	—
9	34	M	IV DA Heterosexual	PCP; OC	—
10	22	M	IV DA Bisexual	Cryptococcal meningitis & pneumonia	—
11	34	M	Homosexual	OC; PCP	Cotton-wool spots OU§ (C-W S)
12	33	M	IV DA Heterosexual	PCP; OC	—
13	37	F	Heterosexual Wife of IV DA with AIDS	OC; PCP	C-W S OU
14	37	M	IV DA Heterosexual	OC; Esophageal cytomegalovirus ulcer	C-W S OU
15	42	F	IV DA Heterosexual	Central nervous system toxoplasmosis (CNS toxo)	—
16	32	M	IV DA Heterosexual	PCP; OC	—
17	33	F	Heterosexual Wife of IV DA	CNS Toxo	—
18	38	M	Homosexual	Kaposi's sarcoma	C-W S OU
19	44	F	Heterosexual	OC; PCP	—
20	25	M	IV DA Homosexual	OC; PCP	C-W S OU
21	25	M	Bisexual	OC; PCP; Kaposi's sarcoma	Cytomegalovirus retinitis OS
22	41	M	IV DA Heterosexual	OC; PCP	C-W S OU; Nerve fiber layer hemorrhage
23	30	M	IV DA Heterosexual	OC; PCP	C-W S OU
24	52	M	IV DA Heterosexual	OC & Esophageal candidiasis	C-W S OU; Lamellar macular hole OS
25	28	M	IV DA Bisexual	Kaposi's sarcoma	C-W S OS

*Intravenous drug abuser = IV DA.
†Oral candidiasis = OC.
‡*Pneumocystis carinii* pneumonia = PCP.
§Both eyes = OU.
(Courtesy of Rosenberg, P.R., et al.: Ophthalmology (Rochester) 90:874–878, August, 1983.)

The eye is frequently involved in AIDS, and the diagnosis should be considered in patients having cotton-wool spots in the absence of known predisposing illness. The earlier diagnosis of AIDS could reduce the number of deaths associated with opportunistic infections through early institution of specific treatment.

10–14 **Ocular Effects in Acquired Immune Deficiency Syndrome.** Acquired immune deficiency syndrome (AIDS) is an immunologic disorder prevalent in male homosexuals that is associated with various types of opportunistic infections. Joel S. Schuman and Alan H. Friedman (Mt. Sinai School of Medicine, New York) reviewed the findings in 33 patients seen in the past 2½ years with AIDS and the retinal lesions associated with the opportunistic agents affecting AIDS patients. Eighteen patients had lesions of cytomegalovirus, 11 had *Pneumocystis carinii* pneumonia, 2 had changes of toxoplasmosis, and 2 had fungal retinitis. The clinical features are summarized in the table.

The retinal lesions of cytomegalovirus infection are white and granular, and are nearly always associated with hemorrhage. These lesions progress slowly, leaving large zones of atrophy; optic atrophy often is observed. Vitreous involvement increases as the focus of retinal necrosis enlarges. The retinitis is unresponsive to all forms of

OCULAR FINDINGS IN ACQUIRED IMMUNE DEFICIENCY SYNDROME

Clinical Characteristics	Cytomegalovirus retinitis (N = 18)	*Pneumocystis carinii* pneumonia (N = 11)	Toxoplasmosis (N = 2)	Fungal retinitis (N = 2) *Candida albicans, Cryptococcus sp,*
AIDS-Susceptible group				
Homosexual	16/18	8/11	1/2	0/2
Intravenous drug user	2/18	2/11	0/2	2/2
Hemophiliac	0/18	1/11	1/2	0/2
Median Age	28.2 years	27.8 years	20.5 years	23.4 years
Sex				
Male	18/18	10/11	2/2	2/2
Female	0/18	1/11	0/2	0/2
Race				
Black	12	3	0	0
White	2	8	2	0
Hispanic	4	0	0	2
Retinitis or Retinochoroiditis	18/18 (all bilateral)	not present	2/2 (unilateral)	2/2 (unilateral)
Vitritis	12/18	not present	2/2	2/2
Optic neuritis	7/18	not present	not present	not present
Anterior uveitis	3/18	not present	not present	not present
Cotton-wool spots	not present	11/11 (bilateral in 8)	not present	not present
Response to treatment	nil	resolved spontaneously	1/2	2/2
PCP	14/18	11/11	2/2	1/2
KS	3/18	2/11	0/2	0/2
Final outcome	14/18 died	—	1/2 died	1/2 died

(Courtesy of Schuman, J.S., and Friedman, A.H.: Mt. Sinai J. Med. (NY) 50:443–446, Sept.-Oct. 1983.)

(10–14) Mt. Sinai J. Med. (NY) 50:443–446, Sept.–Oct. 1983.

antiviral therapy. The cotton-wool spots seen in patients with *P. carinii* pneumonia resemble those seen in disorders associated with circulating immune complexes or microvascular occlusive disease. Hemorrhage is infrequent. The lesions are scattered in the superficial retina of the posterior pole and tend to resolve in 6 to 8 weeks. No organisms have been observed. Toxoplasmosis can cause significant permanent visual loss, depending on the site of the lesions. The retinal lesions seen in patients with *Candida* and *Cryptococcus* infections resembled those seen in immunosuppressed patients. These lesions, if not treated, can produce vitreous abscesses and lead to retinal detachment.

The opportunistic infections associated with AIDS can involve the eyes, and ophthalmoscopy can contribute to the diagnosis. Patients with AIDS should be routinely examined for ophthalmologic involvement.

10–15 **Light-Induced Maculopathy From Operating Microscope in Extracapsular Cataract Extraction and Intraocular Lens Implantation.** H. Richard McDonald and A. Rodman Irvine (Univ. of California, San Francisco) observed a characteristic macular lesion in 6 patients having extracapsular cataract extraction and posterior chamber lens implantation. The lesion resembled that described in monkeys as a response to the coaxial illumination of the operating microscope. They are the first known patients with clinical light toxicity caused by the operating microscope. A standard operating microscope with a 30-watt bulb was used in all cases. Operating times

Fig 10–4.—A, fundus photography shows area of pigment mottling just temporal to fovea, and pale swelling of optic nerve. B, fluorescein angiography highlights area of pigment change temporal to fovea. Also observed is leakage from the ischemic disk. (Courtesy of McDonald, H.R., and Irvine, A.R.: Ophthalmology 90:945–951, August 1983.).

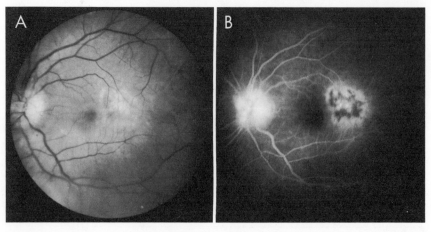

ranged from 75 to 90 minutes. All surgeons had previously performed at least 15 lens implantations. An oval area of mild yellow-white discoloration of the retina appeared 1 to 2 days postoperatively, and mottled pigmentation (Fig 10–4) developed over the next few weeks. Most lesions were near the foveola and produced a paracentral scotoma, but no compromise of central vision.

Findings in animal studies suggest that shorter wavelengths would seem to be more hazardous to the retina than longer ones. Only recently have a significant number of extracapsular extractions been done using the closed irrigation-aspiration method and lens implantation at the authors' center. The presence of the pseudophakos may be an important factor, acting to focus the illuminating light on the retina during wound closure. A long time spent in carefully removing cortical material from the posterior capsule before implanting the intraocular lens also may be important. Only a few patients have been affected; however, the lesion is easily missed and it may not be rare. Affected patients have not always shown symptoms but it may be fortunate that their lesions have been perifoveolar rather than foveolar in location. No association with aphakic or pseudophakic cystoid macular edema is apparent. Reevaluation of surgical methods and the development of more effective filters for ophthalmic instruments are indicated.

▶ [The authors of this article present compelling evidence implicating the light source of the operating microscope in retinal damage. We can not help but be concerned about all of our diagnostic instruments. Perhaps we should change to low-light levels and use image intensifiers for visualization of the eye.] ◀

▶ ↓ The authors of the following 2 articles discuss retinal detachment occurring after cataract surgery. It is evident that extracapsular surgery decreases the risk of retinal detachment. It is not clear what the effect of posterior capsulotomy on retinal detachment is, but a study of the results of YAG laser capsulotomies would be important. There is a tiny shock wave with each discharge, but certainly much less trauma to the eye occurs than that with standard posterior capsulotomy. ◀

10–16 **Prevalence of Aphakic Retinal Detachment.** S. P. B. Percival, V. Anand, and S. K. Das (Scarborough, England) in a retrospective analysis of 1,324 eyes show that the extracapsular approach has a statistically significant influence in preventing aphakic retinal detachment (ARD) and that high myopes and eyes containing iris clip lenses have a significant propensity for developing ARD.

Eyes were categorized according to postoperative refraction: Ra signified more than +8.0 diopters (D) spherical equivalent in the aphakic eye and RB signified +8.0 D or less (high myopia); a third category comprised primary intraocular lens implantation (IOL). Surgical approach was indicated as planned intracapsular extraction (IC) involving zonulysis with α-chymotrypsin followed by cryoextraction or as planned extracapsular extraction (EC) involving nucleus extraction after clean removal of a disk of anterior capsule with nontoothed

(10–16) Br. J. Ophthalmol. 67:43–45, January 1983.

INCIDENCE OF RETINAL DETACHMENT AMONG 1,324 EYES
FROM TEN YEARS OF CATARACT SURGERY

	Ra	Rb	IOL	Total
Planned IC	12/485	8/72	10/279	30/836 (3·6%)
Planned EC	2/46	1/46	1/396	4/488 (0·8%)

(Courtesy of Percival, S.P.B., et al.: Br. J. Ophthalmol. 67:43–45, January 1983.)

Kelman McPhearson forceps followed by manual aspiration of residual cortex.

The table shows the incidence of retinal detachment for each of the 6 categories. It was more than 4 times more frequent after planned IC than planned EC surgery, although 6 eyes should be excluded because retinal detachment was due to vitreous loss at surgery, a preventable complication. Vitreous hemorrhage complicated cataract surgery in 14 of the 836 IC eyes, including 3 in high myopes. After excluding the association with vitreous loss, ARD occurred in 1.9% of 482 control intracapsular eyes, 4.8% of 185 eyes containing iris clip lenses, 11.1% of 72 highly myopic intracapsular eyes, 1 of 46 highly myopic extracapsular eyes, and none of 439 nonmyopic extracapsular eyes.

The protection afforded by the extracapsular approach is encouraging, especially for myopic patients; with careful execution it obviates operative and postoperative problems with vitreous, including hemorrhage. Although ARD is known to be a bilateral disease, it is interesting to note that it occurred in 4 patients who had undergone bilateral surgery, IC in 1 eye and EC in the other, but detachment occurred only in the IC eye. This leads to the conclusion that extracapsular techniques for cataract extraction are both safe and effective.

10–17 **Retinal Detachment Following Late Posterior Capsulotomy.** The incidence of retinal detachment occurring after extracapsular cataract surgery and late posterior capsulotomy was compared with the incidence of general aphakic retinal detachment by Alice R. McPherson, Ronan E. O'Malley and Jaime Bravo (Baylor College of Medicine, Houston). Among 1,984 patients with retinal detachments, 752 had aphakic retinal detachments. Only 27 patients also underwent late posterior capsulotomy. The latter group was divided into group 1, 4 patients who underwent discission less than 1 year after cataract extraction, and group 2, composed of 23 patients undergoing discission 1 year or more after cataract surgery. Each group was further subdivided as follows: group 1A, 3 patients, and group 2A, 12 patients, whose retinal detachment occurred less than 1 year af-

(10–17) Am. J. Ophthalmol. 95:593–597, May 1983.

ter discission, and group 1B, 1 patient, and group 2B, 11 patients, whose retinal detachment occurred 1 year or more after discission. Seven eyes had implanted intraocular lenses. No significant differences with regard to extent of the retinal detachment or types or locations of the breaks between these eyes and the other 20 eyes were observed.

A steady decrease of retinal detachment in aphakic eyes occurred between 1975 (53%) and 1981 (21%). The 27 eyes contained 54 breaks, of which 24 were of the horseshoe type. No breaks were posterior to the equator, 1 was at the equator, and 29 were in the inferior quadrant. The mean interval between cataract extraction and discission was 29.1 ± 5.5 months. Of the 27 retinal detachments, 4 occurred in group 1 and 23 in group 2; 13 occurred in eyes that underwent discission from 1 to 2 years after cataract surgery and 10 in eyes that underwent discission more than 2 years later. Discission may be a definite factor in predisposing the eye to detachment, but the timing of the discission in relation to cataract surgery does not significantly affect the number of detachments. The mean interval between discission and retinal detachment was 15.3 months. Retinas became detached within 1 year of discission in 15 of the 27 eyes (groups 1A and 2A), suggesting that the detachments were directly related to the discissions. There were twice as many detachments involving all 4 quadrants in groups 1A and 2A than in groups 1B and 2B. Six eyes had detachments involving all 4 quadrants (4 in groups 1A and 2A). Of the 1,984 patients with retinal detachments, 42% had involvement of all 4 quadrants; of the 752 with aphakic retinal detachments, 53% had all 4 quadrants affected. Consequently, the 22% incidence (6 of 27 eyes) after late discission was low.

The interval between cataract surgery and discission, and between discission and retinal detachment, seemed to have a direct effect on the final functional result. Final visual acuities of 20/400 or better were attained in 22 of 23 eyes in which discission followed cataract extraction by 1 year or more, but in only 1 of 4 eyes in which the procedures were separated by less than 1 year. Delaying discission for more than 12 months may reduce the extent of retinal detachment and produce the best functional results, especially when retinal detachment is diagnosed and treated within a year after discission.

10–18 **Peripheral Circumferential Retinal Scatter Photocoagulation for Treatment of Proliferative Sickle Retinopathy.** Alan F. Cruess, Robert F. Stephens, Larry E. Magargal, and Gary C. Brown (Thomas Jefferson Univ., Philadelphia) reviewed the results of circumferential argon laser scatter photocoagulation delivered to zones of peripheral retinal capillary nonperfusion in 40 eyes of 29 patients with proliferative sickle retinopathy (PSR) in 1977 to 1982.

(10–18) *Ophthalmology* (Rochester) 90:272–278, March 1983.

Eight patients had previously received focal feeder-frond photocoagulation to 10 eyes. The mean patient age was 33 years. Most patients had hemoglobin-SC disease. The treatment technique is illustrated in Figure 10–5. If possible the entire zone of nonperfused peripheral retina was treated from just posterior to the border of capillary nonperfusion to the ora serrata. Treatment usually was with a 200-µ or 500-µ spot size, a duration of 0.1 second, and power of 100 to 400 mW. About 1,000 burns were delivered in 1 or 2 sessions.

The mean follow-up was 1.4 years. Twenty-six percent of preexisting sea fans regressed completely and 57% partially, while the remaining 17% remained stable; none progressed. Neovascularization developed de novo in only 1 eye. A good response was observed both in previously treated and in untreated eyes. Acuity responded well to treatment, especially in previously untreated eyes. Seven eyes received supplemental photocoagulation, 6 for persistent sea fan activity and 1 for new neovascularization. No complications resulted in severe permanent visual impairment. Three patients had symptomatic vitreous hemorrhage, which in 2 cases resolved with no final reduction in acuity. Only 1 eye had a symptomatic peripheral visual field defect after treatment. No retinal detachments occurred, and there was no evidence of choroidal-retinal-vitreal neovascularization in any of the treated eyes.

Peripheral circumferential retinal scatter photocoagulation is an

Fig 10–5.—Fundus drawing illustrating peripheral circumferential retinal scatter photocoagulation technique. Argon laser burns are placed approximately 1 burn-width apart throughout the entire zone of 360 degrees of peripheral retinal capillary nonperfusion. Sea fans are surrounded by laser burns but not treated directly. (Courtesy of Cruess, A.F., et al.: Ophthalmology (Rochester) 90:272–278, March 1983.)

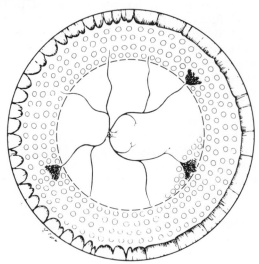

effective means of producing regression of sea fans in patients with PSR. It may also help prevent the development of de novo sea fans. The treatment appears to be safe, and less likely to cause serious complications than previously proposed laser treatment methods.

▶ [The authors of this article have described the use of extensive peripheral panretinal photocoagulation; the question that arises is whether or not all the burns were needed. The results were good but there was no control group; therefore, we will have to wait for further studies to be certain of how best to use the scatter technique.] ◀

10–19 **Further Observations Concerning Diffuse Unilateral Subacute Neuroretinitis Syndrome.** In 1978 Gass and Scelfo described a uniocular syndrome in children and young adults characterized by loss of central vision with vitreous inflammation, papillitis, and recurrent crops of evanescent gray-white lesions of the outer retina and pigment epithelium. Eventually, optic atrophy developed. J. Donald M. Gass and Robert A. Braunstein (Univ. of Miami) present evidence that diffuse unilateral subacute neuroretinitis (DUSN) is caused by at least 2 nematodes other than *Toxocara canis*. Findings in 18 patients with a mean age of 24 years were reviewed. Most patients were seen initially within a month of onset of symptoms.

At least 12 patients had multiple variably sized patches of gray-white outer retinal inflammation, and at least 4 had papillitis. A motile, tapered, unsegmented nematode was seen moving beneath the retina in 11 patients, within the retina in 5, and in the anterior vitreous in 1; in 1 patient it was either within or beneath the retina. The nematode usually was first detected in the macular region. It ranged in length from 400 to 2,000 μm. The optic nerve head was sometimes swollen, and at least 4 patients had mild optic atrophy at the outset. Eight patients were treated with oral thiabendazole. Five nematodes were photocoagulated with the argon laser or xenon light. Follow-up data are shown in the table. Only 1 patient had a definite loss of visual acuity, but at least 7 had progressive fundoscopic changes, usually with progressive field loss. Only 1 patient had a significant titer for *T. canis* on enzyme-linked immunosorbent assay. Two had mild eosinophilia.

Shorter nematodes were present in patients in this series who lived in the southeastern United States or Puerto Rico, and longer ones in those living in the northern midwestern United States. The nematodes apparently can migrate within the eye for 3 years or more, causing chronic, progressive changes in both ocular structure and function. Diffuse unilateral subacute neuroretinitis appears to represent the result of a local toxic effect of worm byproducts on the outer retina and a more diffuse toxic reaction involving both the inner and outer retinal tissues. Identification of the cause

(10–19) Arch. Ophthalmol. 101:1689–1697, November 1983.

SIGNS OF LATE STAGES OF DIFFUSE UNILATERAL SUBACUTE NEURORETINITIS DEVELOPING IN 18 PATIENTS WITH INTRAOCULAR NEMATODE*

Case	Length of Follow-up	Final Visual Acuity	Post-inflammatory Vitreous Changes	Optic Atrophy	Narrowing Retinal Arteries	Pigment Epithelial Atrophy	Subnormal Electroretinographic Findings	Other
1	29 yr	CF at 1 ft	Not stated	4+	4+	4+	Extinguished	Focal area geographic atrophy of pigment epithelium and choroid in macula
2	12 yr	20/300	Not stated	1+	1+	1+	B wave low normal in affected eye	Had typical peripheral peripapillary and macular scars of presumed ocular histoplasmosis OD; histoplasmin skin test, negative; tuberculin skin test, positive; apical lesions, lungs; sputum test, negative
3	9 yr	20/60	Not stated	0	0	1+ in macula	...	...
4	Unavailable	...	...	...	...	...	...	...
5	5 yr	CF	Yes	2+	1+	3+	Markedly abnormal, B wave < A wave	...
6	9 yr	13/200	Not stated	1+	1+	1+	Normal	...
7	2 mo	20/80	Not stated	Not stated	Not stated	Not stated	"Lower amplitudes consistent with pseudo-retinitis pigmentosa"	...
8	2 yr	20/20	Not stated	Not stated	Not stated	Not stated	...	...
9	4 yr	CF inferiorly only	Not stated	Not stated	Not stated	Not stated	...	...

No.	Duration	Visual acuity	Vitreous cells			RPE changes	EOG/ERG	
10	6 mo	20/200	Yes	0	0	Had widespread 2+ focal and diffuse changes RPE	Normal	...
11	1 yr	20/60	Not stated	3+	2+	2+	Normal (EOG normal)	...
12	4 mo	20/400	Yes	1+	1+	3+ without coarse clumps and ? tracks	Normal, not repeated	...
13	2 mo	20/50	Not stated	Yes	0	Yes	EOG subnormal before treatment; normal after treatment	...
14	4 yr	20/20	Yes	1+	1+	1+ diffuse changes with multiple peripheral focal scars	Not done	...
15	11 mo	20/25	1+ vitreous cells	0	0	Many focal atrophic RPE changes in periphery	Not done	...
16	Unavailable	...	...	...	...	...	...	...
17	37 mo since onset visual loss	1/200	2+ vitreous cells	2+	2+	2+	Markedly abnormal B wave > A wave	...
18	2 mo	CF at 3 ft	Occasional cell	2+	1+	1+	Both within normal limits, but B wave OS reduced compared with OD	...

*CF = counting fingers; RPE = retinal pigment epithelium; EOG = electro-oculogram.
(Courtesy of Gass, J.D.M., and Braunstein, R.A.: Arch. Ophthalmol. 101:1689–1697, November 1983; copyright 1983, American Medical Association.)

of the disorder is necessary to find effective preventive and therapeutic measures.

▶ [This nematode disease is not limited to the southeastern United States and must be carefully considered in a differential diagnosis of retinitis. It is encouraging that photocoagulation can be used to destroy the parasite, but the difficult diagnosis must first be made.] ◀

10–20 **Acute Retinal Necrosis (Kirisawa's Uveitis)** consists of unilateral acute uveitis with retinal periarteritis and detachment. Many of the 36 previously reported cases have been bilateral. The visual prognosis is poor. Utako Saga, Hiroko Ozawa, Sumi Soshi, Kunihiro Nagahara, Kiyoshi Akeo, Chojiro Kimura, and Yasuo Uemura (Keio Univ., Tokyo) report data on 4 cases of Kirasawa's uveitis. One is described below.

Man, 57, had blurred vision in the right eye and generalized weakness for

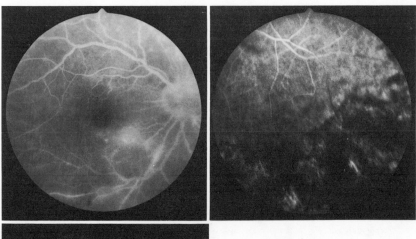

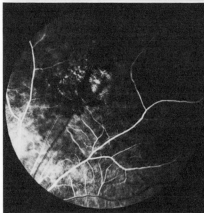

Fig 10–6 (above left).—Man aged 57 years. Fluorescein angiogram shows leakage of dye from retinal vessels but no obliteration at this time (acute stage).

Fig 10–7 (above).—Fluorescein angiogram of same patient as in Figure 10–6 shows obliteration of retinal vessels and pigment epithelial atrophy in lesions (regression stage).

Fig 10–8 (left).—Woman aged 55 years. Fluorescein angiogram shows hyperfluorescence, indicating neovascularization from choroid (cicatricial stage).

(Courtesy of Saga, U., et al.: Jpn. J. Ophthalmol. 27:353–361, 1983.)

1 week. He was found to have 2+ cells in the anterior chamber, mutton fat-like keratic precipitates, and vitreous reaction in this eye. Acuity declined progressively despite systemic and topical steroid therapy, and small white exudates appeared diffusely over the retina. The retinal arteries were extensively sheathed and narrowed. The exudates began to be absorbed, but new lesions appeared in the left eye despite large doses of intravenous and topical steroids and antibiotics. Sudden loss of vision in the right eye occurred from a retinal detachment that was considered inoperable. Fluorescein leakage from retinal vessels in the left eye (Fig 10–6) was followed by pigment epithelial atrophy and obliteration of retinal vessels (Fig 10–7). Posterior vitreous detachment developed in the left eye, followed by progressive vitreous fibrosis and retinal detachment. The retina failed to reattach despite operation. Acuity decreased to ability of finger counting in the left eye; the right eye had no light perception.

Findings of neovascularization of the choroid in another case are shown in Figure 10–8. The disease progressed rapidly from the acute to the terminal stage without remission, although some patients remain in the cicatricial stage. Treatment has not altered the course of the disorder. Posterior vitreous detachment and retinal detachment occur in the final stage. Surgery for retinal detachment was not successful in the present cases. Urayama et al. (1971) described marked perivascular infiltration of lymphocytes in the retina, choroid, and optic nerve; severe atrophy of the detached retina; and fibrous layer formation in Bruch's membrane in the periphery. Kirisawa's uveitis appears to be the same disease as acute retinal necrosis.

▶ [Acute retinal necrosis has been observed in patients in the United States and Great Britain as well as in Japan. The retina is so friable that detachment surgery inevitably fails and a search for the cause must be given high priority.] ◀

10–21 Computed Tomography in Diagnosis of Retinoblastoma. Paul G. Arrigg, Thomas R. Hedges III, and Devron H. Char evaluated the role of computer-assisted tomography (CT) in 21 children seen in the Ocular Oncology Unit at the University of California in San Francisco. All 21 underwent high-resolution, thin-section CT scan study before treatment from 1977 to 1981. Three patients with Coats' syndrome also were involved in the study. Coronal and oblique reformations were routinely obtained. Eight children with retinoblastoma had bilateral tumors. The mean age was 19 months. All children with unilateral retinoblastoma had their eyes enucleated, and all but 1 of the 8 with bilateral tumors had 1 eye enucleated.

Calcification was demonstrated by CT in at least 1 eye of all children with retinoblastoma, and all but 5 of 29 affected eyes had calcification within the tumor. All tumors without apparent calcification seen on CT were small. Calcification could not be related to age at diagnosis. A nonhomogeneous pattern of calcification was observed in eyes with large tumors (Fig 10–9) and a homogeneous

(10–21) Br. J. Ophthalmol. 67:588–591, September 1983.

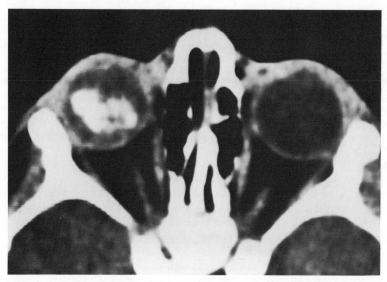

Fig 10–9.—Nonhomogeneous pattern of calcification was observed in eyes with large tumors. (Courtesy of Arrigg, P.G., et al.: Br. J. Ophthalmol. 67:588–591, September 1983.)

pattern in smaller tumors. The amount and distribution of calcium apparent on CT and at enucleation were closely correlated. Microscopic tumor spread past the lamina cribrosa of the optic nerve in 2 children was not detected by CT. There was no evidence of gross extraocular or intracranial tumor. None of the patients with Coats' syndrome had calcification on axial CT or with computer reformation.

Calcification within retinoblastomas is accurately detected by high-resolution, thin-section CT. This approach may help distinguish retinoblastomas from other lesions that can simulate them, and it may be useful in identifying retrobulbar spread, intracranial metastases, and second tumors. However, subtle retrobulbar optic nerve involvement is not reliably detected by CT. The authors currently obtain CT scans in all patients suspected of having retinoblastoma.

▶ [Computed tomography is obviously extremely helpful, especially in visualizing large tumors. We all await, however, the results of magnetic resonance imaging since it will not expose children to any X-radiation. One wonders if the eyes containing "retinocytomas" described in the following article might have been saved if magnetic resonance spectroscopy had been available.] ◀

10–22 **Retinocytoma: Benign Variant of Retinoblastoma.** A rare type of retinoblastoma consists of untreated tumors composed entirely of benign-appearing cells having photoreceptor differentiation with no

(10–22) Arch. Ophthalmol. 101:1519–1531, October 1983.

evidence of mitotic activity or necrosis. Curtis Margo, Ahmed Hidayat, Joel Kopelman, and Lorenz E. Zimmerman reviewed the findings in 5 children identified in the Registry of Ophthalmic Pathology at the Armed Forces Institute of Pathology in Washington, D.C. All 5 had 6 benign retinal tumors managed by enucleation only. The average age at enucleation was 37 months. One child had a tumor in the other eye successfully treated by irradiation and photocoagulation. Two children had a family history of retinoblastoma. One tumor was observed for 6 months before enucleation. Four children had signs of eye disease for a substantial time before evaluation; 2 were esotropic and 1 was exotropic. Four eyes contained a single small tumor, and 1 contained 2 separate tumors with similar benign histopathologic features.

Each tumor was confined to nondetached retina and obliterated the normal retinal architecture. The tumors consisted of a uniform population of cells with photoreceptor differentiation. No necrosis or mitotic activity was observed. The tumors did not invade the choroid, optic nerve, or vitreous. No areas of totally undifferentiated neuroblastotic cells were present, and there were no Flexner-Wintersteiner rosettes. The 2 tumors studied by electron microscopy consisted chiefly of neuronal cells, many of which exhibited photoreceptor differentiation. Glial cells with cytoplasmic filaments resembling astrocytes were seen occasionally. No necrosis was evident, even in areas adjacent to cells exhibiting calcific degeneration.

The term "retinocytoma" is proposed for this benign variant of retinoblastoma. Although clinically and morphologically distinct, this lesion should carry the same genetic implications associated with its malignant counterpart. It is unclear whether these tumors are benign from the outset, or whether they result from maturation of an initially malignant retinoblastoma, in analogy with the transformation of a neuroblastoma to a ganglioneuroma.

10–23 **Intraocular Lymphomas: Natural History Based on Clinico-pathologic Study of Eight Cases and Review of the Literature.** Intraocular lymphoma is rare, only about 25 such tumors having been confirmed histologically. Stephen J. Qualman, Geoffrey Mendelsohn, Risa B. Mann, and William R. Green (Johns Hopkins Univ.) reviewed the findings in 8 patients with intraocular lymphoma seen between 1965 and 1981; 6 of the tumors were associated with primary CNS lymphoma. Five of the 7 patients who died of lymphoma had autopsies. Women predominated in the series, and the average age was 61.5 years.

The sites of lymphoma in the present series and in 20 previously reported patients are shown in Figure 10–10. Most patients had unilateral reduction in visual acuity. All but 1 of those with visual symptoms had bilateral uveitis, or it rapidly developed, despite the usual

(10–23) Cancer 52:878–886, Sept. 1, 1983.

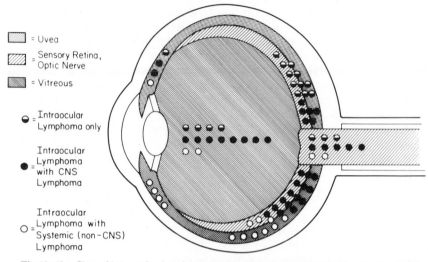

Fig 10–10.—Sites of intraocular lymphoma in 28 patients reported in the literature and in the present series. Intraocular lymphomas with no evidence of extraocular tumor (6 cases) or with CNS parenchymal involvement (14) showed preponderant involvement of vitreous, sensory retina, and subretinal pigment epithelial space (interface sensory retina and uvea). Systemic lymphomas (8, no CNS tumor) were limited mainly to uveal tract. The optic nerve head was involved in 10 instances. (Courtesy of Qualman, S.J., et al.: Cancer 52:878–886, Sept. 1, 1983.)

unilateral decrease in acuity. In 6 patients, CNS symptoms developed within 11 months to 10 years later. Two patients had early symptoms of systemic lymphoma, which was found at autopsy to involve most viscera but spared the CNS. In 6 patients lymphoma was limited to the eyes and the CNS. Only 1 patient had CNS symptoms; ocular involvement was least distinct in this patient. All CNS lymphomas exhibited dense perivascular cuffing of tumor cells and centrifugal invasion of the surrounding brain parenchyma. A similar perivascular pattern was seen in ocular tumors within the retina, but tumor infiltrates in the choroid consisted of densely packed cells without a perivascular orientation. Tumor cells were closely associated with reticulin fibers in all cases studied. All intraocular tumors were associated with inflammatory infiltrates involving both tumorous and other parts of the eyes. Intracellular immunoglobulin was demonstrated in only 1 case.

Intraocular lymphoma is often associated with isolated CNS lymphoma and is a harbinger of extraocular lymphoma. The CNS tumors tend to develop ipsilateral to the most heavily involved eye. Prompt recognition of intraocular lymphoma may permit effective management by irradiation.

▶ [Intraocular lymphomas are extremely rare, but they have 2 important features: first, they can involve all of the intraocular structures and are difficult to diagnose and second, they indicate the presence of lymphomas elsewhere in the body.] ◀

10–24 Rod and Cone Activity in Patients With Dominantly Inherited Retinitis Pigmentosa: Comparisons Between Psychophysical and Electroretinographic Measurements. Some patients with autosomal dominant retinitis pigmentosa (RP) have a profound loss of rod function and a less marked increase in the cone threshold (class I), whereas others have about equal rod and cone threshold elevations (class II). G. B. Arden, R. M. Carter, C. R. Hogg, D. J. Powell, W. J. K. Ernst, G. M. Clover, A. L. Lyness, and M. P. Quinlan (Moorsfield Eye Hosp., London) attempted to relate the electroretinographic (ERG) findings with psychophysical measurements in 57 patients with autosomal dominant RP.

The ERG findings are shown in the table. In group A patients, no ERG response was evoked by dim blue-light flashes; however, with more intense light, most patients exhibited a b wave exceeding 5 μV that was small, rising to and falling rapidly from the peak and resembling a cone response. Only group B patients had typical rod re-

Subdivision of Patients by Electroretinographic Results	Group A		Group B	
	Mean	SD	Mean	SD
Number of cases*	36		21	
Age	40		40	
	13–79		22–71	
Blue light				
V_{max} μV	11·5	±8·6	183	±116
peak time, ms*	61·5	±17·3	64	±8·5
within normal limit	0		7	
Red light				
V_{max} μV	12·5	±12·5	91	±62
peak time, ms*	55	±9·3	50	±6
within normal limit	0		4	
White light				
V_{max} μV	17·5	±17·4	230	±155
peak time, ms*	56	±10	50	±6
within normal limit	0		10	
Flicker				
% of single flash	46	±16	20	±17
ERG peak time, ms	39	±4·6	32	±4·9
within normal limit	0		10	
Goldmann field size				
(mean outer margin, degrees)	18	±13	33	±15
within normal limits	0		3	

*Note those cases where absent response has been neglected in calculations.

(Courtesy of Arden, G.B., et al.: Br. J. Ophthalmol. 67:405–418, July 1983.)

(10–24) Br. J. Ophthalmol. 67:405–418, July 1983.

sponses. The cone ERGs in group A were smaller and more delayed than in group B patients. Young and old patients were found in both groups. Twenty of the group A patients had psychophysical thresholds exclusively determined by cones (A_1), and 16 had evidence of rod function (A_2). The range of amplitudes of the cone ERGs was similar in these subgroups. When a computer model was developed to relate the psychophysical threshold measurements to the ERG data, one subgroup of patients was found to have a scotopic ERG smaller than expected from visual field losses, whereas in the other group the psychophysical elevation of rod visual threshold was greater than expected from the ERG findings.

Some patients with autosomal dominant RP have rod photoreceptors that absorb the same proportion of incident light as in normal persons and have rod signals of normal size. It is possible that the rods become noisy so that the signals that adapt bipolar cells develop in darkness, without affecting the mechanism generating the b wave. Alternately, the b wave current generators could be reduced in magnitude, or the current pathways modified. In these cases the effect of the disease on the ERG would be due to damage to cells that are not photoreceptors. Loss of perceptual sensitivity that is not reflected in the ERG also could be explained by a functional disturbance at some stage subsequent to the neuronal activity that generates the b wave.

11. Neuro-Ophthalmology

Optic Neuritis—Current Status

MARCEL FRENKEL, M.D.

Eye and Ear Infirmary
University of Illinois, Chicago

Acute unilateral optic neuritis is a perplexing problem for the clinician. In the typical situation the patient is a young person past puberty and younger than age 45. The major symptom is acute loss of vision in one eye for 12 to 72 hours with vision ranging from 20/40–20/60 to no light perception. In many instances there is pain on motion of the globe during the first few days. A history of an upper respiratory infection some days to weeks previously may be elicited. The physical findings include pupillary escape and color perception desaturation which may best be elicited by an alternate cover test. If the involvement of the optic nerve is close to the papilla, blurring of the disk margins, dilation of veins, exudation, and hemorrhages may occur that are usually of a mild degree but rarely may be so extensive as to mimic a central vein obstruction. If the papillary portion of the optic nerve is spared, the examination of the optic fundus may be entirely normal. In some 10% of patients it is reported that a peripheral vasculitis may be observed. Pain on motion of the globe reflects an inflammatory reaction involving the sheath of the optic nerve at the orbital apex where its sheath is contiguous or merges with the sheaths of the ocular muscles at the annulus of Zinn; pain is elicited on motion.

Visual field testing usually discloses central, paracentral, or cecocentral scotomas. Occasionally an arcuate defect may be detected, which identifies the vascular inflammatory mediation in this disorder. If a small central scotoma may not be detectable on central field or Goldmann perimetry using white light, a small red target presented centrally may disclose the defect. The Amsler grid is extremely useful in detecting such central aberrations. This method of detection is best performed with the red grid where the central defect will be demonstrable in most cases or may be enhanced on alternate cover testing.

The question of etiologic diagnosis is always difficult. In most cases such optic neuritides fall into the category of what we must at this point call idiopathic, lacking any discrete positive factor. However, among differential diagnostic factors, one must consider whether the optic neuropathy is isolated or whether it is part of a more generalized demyelinizing process (in most cases multiple sclerosis) or whether it represents a vasculopathy such as lupus erythematosus, an infiltrating neoplastic process, or leukemic infiltration of the optic nerve. Optic neuritis may be the first involvement in viral and bacterial processes such as infectious mononucleosis, Guillain-Barré syndrome, cytomegalic virus, and a host of other inflammatory reactions including the granulomas of tuberculosis, sarcoid, and syphilis. Infrequently, compressive neuropathies may manifest acutely and one must always be cautious in interpreting the patient's report of a sudden onset of visual loss. Often the defect is noticed after an injury, while sighting a gun, or while closing an eye to apply makeup. Among the important compressive lesions to be considered are pituitary adenomas, meningiomas of the tuberculum sella, parachiasmal area, or the optic nerve sheath itself, or cysts and neoplasms of the nasal or paranasal sinuses. Aneurysms of the anterior cerebral anterior communicating arterial system occasionally may be directed downward. Notochordal remnants and craniopharyngiomas may manifest in the second to fifth decades and mimic optic neuritis. In the age group at risk, arteriosclerotic occlusive vascular disease is unusual, but retinal or ophthalmic migraine may be present with acute unilateral visual loss which may persist with residual central, arcuate, or sectorial field defects. Headache may not necessarily be a symptom.

The medical history may be as important as the physical examination in determining if the optic neuropathy is a component of a more disseminated affliction. Transient episodes such as Bell's palsy, trigeminal neuralgia, or labyrinthitis, which rarely occur in the age group in question may point to a generalized demyelinizing process. More commonly, one may elicit a history of transient diplopia, weakness, paresthesia, or bladder dysfunction. Uthoff's sign, an increase in visual loss characteristic of demyelinization, reflects a delayed conduction due to an increase in body temperature after exercise or bathing.

While many authorities believe that a typical picture compatible with optic neuritis requires no investigation, the author's experience does not confirm this view. Therefore, a usual workup mayy include the testing of visually evoked responses to determine the possible involvement of the fellow optic nerve. Brain stem and auditory-evoked responses may indicate other conduction defects, as may somatosensory-evoked responses along the limbs. Subclinical conduction delays are seen in multiple sclerosis.

Computerized axial tomography and, in the future, nuclear magnetic resonance testing are valid for several reasons. The first is to demonstrate the presence of the frequently swollen optic nerve in an idiopathic optic neuritis. They may also disclose the presence of compressive lesions and, in some instances, with infusion, may also demonstrate an aneurysm. It is important to indicate to the radiologist that the main concern relates to the prechiasmal and perichiasmal portions of the optic system. Secondly, the radiologic studies may show cerebral or brain stem plaques of demyelinization which would indicate a more generalized syndrome. Finally, and more controversial, is the applicability of lumbar puncture. Should every patient with optic neuritis have a spinal puncture? In those circumstances when a spinal puncture is at all feasible, it is relevant. It is useful in confirming the diagnosis of an idiopathic disturbance and ruling out associated disease.

In approximately 40% of instances, isolated optic neuritis is associated with oligoclonal banding on immune electrophoresis with an increase in the immunoglobulin G fraction (IgG) to approximately 150% of its normal level. This finding may occur in the presence of normal spinal fluid protein levels and in the absence of any pleocytosis. According to Scandinavian investigators, when oligoclonal banding occurs, the risk of a patient with an isolated optic neuritis developing multiple sclerosis within 5 years appears to rise to the vicinity of 80%. When such banding is absent, the risk of dissemination is considered to be in the range of 5%. A less specific index of demyelinization is the isolation of myelin basic protein in the cerebrospinal fluid which tends to indicate a widespread process. Elevated protein levels with polyclonal grouping may be indicative of a collagen vascular disturbance. A nonspecific elevation in protein may reflect a neoplasm at the base of the skull. More generally, a complete blood count and peripheral blood smear as well as a determination of the sedimentation rate are reasonable diagnostic approaches.

The neurologic examination may be brief but should include a check of olfaction and a test of the integrity of the ocular motor system. Frequently overlooked by ophthalmologists is the integrity of the corneal reflex and sensation along the trigeminal distribution. Suck and snout reflexes as well as an increase in the jaw jerk reflex indicate bilateral corticobulbar disturbances. Limb weakness, asymmetry in the deep tendon reflexes, and loss of superficial abdominal reflexes with abnormal plantar reflexes confirm disseminated lesions. Of particular relevance to the ophthalmologist is the possibility of uncovering nystagmus and a current or previous internuclear ophthalmoplegia. There may be no apparent defect on pursuit but repetitive saccadic movements may reveal a lag in adduction which reflects some prior insult.

The etiology of optic neuritis in its idiopathic form is still a mystery. Etiology may be linked to geographic distribution of demyelinizing syndromes in general, these being more prevalent in cold and temperate latitudes such as Northern Europe, the Great Lakes region of the United States, and tending to be less frequent in Mediterranean and tropical climates. When considering multiple sclerosis, many studies have shown that the incidence of multiple sclerosis following a unilateral acute optic neuritis may range anywhere from 17% to 50%. It is likely that the true incidence is in the range of 25% to 35%. Possibly, the remaining instances of idiopathic optic neuritis may represent a forme fruste of multiple sclerosis.

Although one must not equate optic neuritis with multiple sclerosis, the etiologies may be similar. One should consider the theories which have been invoked to explain the latter. The most prevalent current theory is that this syndrome represents an immune disturbance following a viral infection with repeated episodes of demyelinization on stimulation of immune complex formation. An alternative theory is that of a slow virus, the prototype being subacute sclerosing panencephalitis, a progressively fatal disorder seen in children and young adults. Although nucleocapsids have been found in neural tissue from patients with multiple sclerosis, a viral etiology has not been defined. Demyelinization may represent the concurrence of genetic predisposition with an external insult such as a virus. Human lymphocyte antigens (HLA-Dw2, HLA-3 and HLA-B7) seem to be associated with a higher susceptibility to multiple sclerosis and may represent the background on which additional factors will play a role.

Treatment

The treatment of idiopathic optic neuritis is currently in flux. The spontaneous recovery rate has not been determined. Most patients will recover vision to a level close to that existing before inflammation regardless of the peak visual loss. Indeed, patients with no light perception may recover to 20/20 or 20/25 levels. Because of the remitting nature of the neuritis the validity of corticosteroid therapy is not established. It appears to shorten the exacerbation without improving the ultimate visual prognosis beyond its natural course.

In practical terms, we use a short course of steroids in the range of 60 to 80 mg of prednisone orally per day for 7 to 10 days or a 5- to 7-day course of ACTH intravenously when vision in the presenting eye is 20/200 or less. If there has been no recovery in the first eye, steroids are used when there is any degree of visual loss in the fellow eye. One must consider that a therapeutic response does not necessarily substantiate a diagnosis of idiopathic optic neuritis since steroids may shrink edematous compressive tumors.

There has been recent interest in the use of more potent cytotoxic and immunosuppressive agents in the treatment of optic neuritis and generalized multiple sclerosis. Intrathecal injections of interferon-B have yielded an initial improvement in clinical status in a short follow-up period. Plasmapheresis has been suggested but the results are uncertain. Because of the remitting nature of demyelinizing syndromes, it is extremely difficult to arrive at easy conclusions regarding therapeutic benefit.

One of the important questions which confronts the ophthalmologist is whether to apprise the patient of the possible link of idiopathic optic neuritis with generalized demyelinization. The statistical incidence of multiple sclerosis ranges from 50% in earlier studies to levels of 17% in more recent surveys. In the past, it had generally been inadvisable to discuss the possible evolution into multiple sclerosis because of the connotation of severe disability. While the prognosis has not changed, the patient is now believed to have a "right to know." It may be crucial for a young patient to be aware of the potential for disability since he or she may be making life decisions regarding family formation, or educational or business commitments. Aware of the statistical possibilities, the patient, rather than the physician, can assume the responsibility for important choices.

By defining prognostic factors such as oligoclonal banding, HLA analysis, and the results of visually evoked and brain stem auditory responses, it may be possible for the clinician to arrive at a realistic and ethically sound basis for selecting those patients who should be informed of the possible implications45of acute optic neuritis.

▶ ↓ There is debate concerning the treatment of carotid artery obstructive disease, however, its diagnosis is still necessary. In the following 2 articles, the authors discuss the effectiveness of invasive and noninvasive tests in the detection of carotid artery disease. Ophthalmodynamometry is still a valuable test, but the question is, should all patients with amaurosis fugax have arteriography? If a third have treatable lesions and digital intravenous subtraction arteriography may miss symptomatic shallow ulcers, then the answer must be yes. Let us hope that magnetic resonance flow studies will some day eliminate the need for invasive studies. ◀

11–1 **Ophthalmodynamometry Revisited.** To determine the accuracy of ophthalmodynamometry in detecting significant carotid stenosis, as verified by angiography, Marc A. Mullie and Trevor H. Kirkham (McGill Univ., Montreal) used ophthalmodynamometry to evaluate data on 100 patients with symptoms of amaurosis fugax or transient cerebral ischemic attacks who were scheduled to undergo bilateral carotid angiography. The criteria for a positive, or abnormal, test result included a corrected systolic pressure of 70 mm Hg or less, a corrected diastolic pressure of 25 mm Hg or less, and a difference of 20% or more between the systolic or diastolic readings from the 2 sides. The criterion for a positive or abnormal angiogram result was demonstration of significant (50% or more) stenosis of the internal carotid artery between its origin and that of the ophthalmic artery. The sensitivity, specificity, and overall accuracy of ophthalmodynamometry in detecting significant stenosis of the internal carotid artery were determined for each of the 3 criteria.

Of the 3 criteria for a positive result, a corrected systolic pressure of 70 mm Hg or less had the highest sensitivity (95%) and overall

(11–1) Can. J. Ophthalmol. 18:165–168, May 1983.

accuracy (88%). With the use of all 3 criteria, only 1 of which had to be met in an individual case, ophthalmodynamometry identified significant carotid obstruction with 80% sensitivity, 78% accuracy, and a false positive rate of 25%. The purpose of all noninvasive tests of carotid function is to identify those patients who have significant disease that is curable by surgery and, consequently, those who should undergo angiography. Angiography remains the standard of comparison for the noninvasive tests despite its shortcomings in detecting atheromatous plaques and ulceration.

Ophthalmodynamometry is used on the assumption that central retinal artery pressure reflects internal carotid artery pressure, because the ophthalmic artery is the first major branch of the internal carotid artery and the central retinal artery is an end artery. Ophthalmodynamometry measures pressure, not blood flow, through the central retinal artery system. The reasons for false positive results of ophthalmodynamometry include the following: the end points are subject to measurement error; cardiac arrhythmias may cause inaccurate readings; generalized atherosclerosis in the aortic arch and its branches may alter pressure-flow relationships in the internal carotid artery; and a stenosed or occluded ophthalmic artery lowers the pressure on that side, whereas a carotid obstruction distal to the origin of the ophthalmic artery may raise the pressure and elevate the ophthalmodynamometry reading.

Ophthalmodynamometry is a simple tool, valuable in detecting carotid artery obstruction, and can play a role in stroke prevention. All patients with amaurosis fugax or transient cerebral ischemia attacks should undergo angiography if they are potential candidates for surgery, whatever the ophthalmodynamometry result.

11–2 **Amaurosis Fugax: Results of Arteriography in 59 Patients.** Amaurosis fugax is a recognized warning symptom of impending cerebral or retinal infarction. Several workers have reported abnormal angiographic findings in more than 90% of patients (table). Harold P. Adams, Jr., Steven F. Putman, James J. Corbett, Brian P. Sires, and H. Stanley Thompson (Univ. of Iowa, Iowa City) reviewed the cerebral angiographic findings in 59 patients with transient monocular blindness who were examined between 1975 and 1982. Patients with central retinal artery occlusion and no previous amaurosis fugax, and those with established migraine, were excluded. Three patients with branch retinal arterial occlusion were included. The 34 men and 25 women were aged 24 to 80 years; most were older than age 55. All had recent symptoms, but some sustained attacks for more than a year.

Five patients had strokes, and 2 of them had residual neurologic abnormalities. Eleven patients were thought to have episodes representing hemispheric transient ischemic attacks and 8, vertebrobasilar

(11–2) Stroke 14:742–744, Sept.–Oct. 1983.

SUMMARY OF REPORTED RESULTS OF ARTERIOGRAPHY IN PATIENTS WITH AMAUROSIS FUGAX

| | Total number patients | Number of patients with | | | |
		Carotid artery stenosis	Carotid artery ulcer	Carotid artery occlusion	Normal
Marshall and Meadows	27	11 (41%)	—	5 (18%)	11 (41%)
Kollartis et al. (81 vessels)	45	38 (47%)	18 (22%)	12 (15%)	13 (16%)
Ramirez-Lassepas et al.	27	20 (74%)	—	6 (22%)	1 (4%)
Hooshmand et al.	34	12 (35%)	18 (53%)	2 (6%)	2 (6%)
Lemak and Fields	234	151 (65%)	—	32 (13%)	51 (22%)
Mungas and Baker	107	80 (75%)	—	—	12 (11%)
Pessin et al.	43	20 (47%)	4 (9%)	7 (16%)	9 (21%)
Wilson et al.	43	16 (37%)	8 (19%)	3 (7%)	16 (37%)
Thiele et al.	94	49* (52%)	37 (39%)	—	8 (9%)
Parkin et al.	38	21 (55%)	12 (31%)	4 (11%)	1 (3%)
Present report (60 vessels)	59	15 (25%)	8 (14%)	10 (17%)	20 (33%)

*Ten patients with only stenosis; 39 with stenotic and ulcerated lesions.
(Courtesy of Adams, H.P., Jr., et al.: Stroke 14:742–744, Sept.-Oct. 1983; by permission of American Heart Association, Inc.)

attacks. Angiographic findings were normal in 19 patients. Fifteen patients had stenosis of the origin of the internal carotid artery, and 8 others had prominent plaques without significant stenosis or ulceration. Two patients had stenosis of the external carotid artery, and 1 had isolated stenosis of the ophthalmic artery. Complete occlusion of the internal or common carotid was seen in 10 patients. One patient had kinking of the internal carotid artery, and 2 had fibromuscular dysplasia. The angiographic findings could not be related to the clinical history or various demographic factors. All patients with a stroke, however, had abnormal findings on angiography. Neither Doppler flow study nor oculoplethysmography was a reliable indicator of the angiographic findings.

About 34% of the patients in this series with amaurosis fugax had no carotid abnormalities observed on angiography, and fewer than 34% had carotid stenosis. Angiography remains the single best means of diagnosis, although it may fail to demonstrate small lesions and is not without complications. All patients with transient monocular blindness must be assumed to have carotid artery disease until this is ruled out, but emboli can arise from several other sites in these patients.

11–3 **Eye Signs in 611 Cases of Posterior Fossa Aneurysms: Their Diagnostic and Prognostic Value.** A. J. McKinna (Univ. of Western Ontario, London, Ont.) reviews the ophthalmologic aspects of 611 posterior fossa aneurysms seen between 1965 and 1980; the neurosurgical aspects were previously reported (Drake, 1982).

(11–3) Can. J. Ophthalmol. 18:3–6, February 1983.

The 390 females and 221 males in the study were aged 10 to 71 years (average, 41 years). The saccular or "berry," congenital type of aneurysm was by far the most common. Most lesions were located in the basilar artery and bifurcation (70%) or in the vertebral artery (10%). One factor that may have led to rupture of the aneurysm or enlargement to a size sufficient to cause symptoms was hypertension, which was present in 26% of the patients. Presenting signs and symptoms included severe headache, loss of consciousness (often transient and recurrent), and diplopia (table). Eye signs of a serious intracranial disorder were present in 50% of the patients. Only computed tomography and four-vessel angiography were able to demonstrate small aneurysms in the posterior fossa; routine skull films and incomplete angiography were not useful.

Of the 611 patients, 598 underwent surgery. Many patients had postoperative neurologic deficits that usually cleared quickly. Many also had eye signs, including third cranial nerve plasy in 375 patients (63%) which cleared in 83%, usually quickly.

Results of surgery were good in 78% of the patients, fair in 10%, and poor (patient totally dependent) in 4%; 46 patients (8%) died within a few weeks after surgery, usually (39 cases) of causes related to the aneurysm or operation. Average age was similar among patients with poor or fatal outcomes and those with better results. Hypertension was present in 50% of patients who died and 25% of those with poor results, suggesting that it is an unfavorable sign, but not a contraindication to surgery when controlled. Aneurysms larger than 2.5 cm in diameter were found in 55% of patients with poor or fatal outcomes but in only 17% of the entire series of 611 patients. Omi-

INITIAL SIGNS AND SYMPTOMS IN 611 CASES

Sign or symptom	No. (and %) of cases
Severe headache	503 (82)
Loss of consciousness	258 (42)
Diplopia	215 (35)
Third cranial nerve palsy	130
Sixth cranial nerve palsy	40
Defective upward gaze	30
Skew deviation	9
Fourth cranial nerve palsy	3
Bilateral external ophthalmoplegia	3
Mental confusion (including amnesia, drowsiness and dysphasia)	124 (20)
Hemiplegia	119 (19)
Neck pain	102 (17)
Major visual field defects	42 (7)
Ataxia	35 (6)
Retinal and/or vitreous hemorrhages	29 (5)
Papilledema	23 (4)

(Courtesy of McKinna, A.J.: Can. J. Ophthalmol. 18:3–6, February 1983.)

nous preoperative eye signs included major defects in ocular motility or the visual field, which were found in 89% of patients with poor or fatal outcome.

▶ [The author of this article reviewed the eye data from the patients in a neurosurgical series. A third had diplopia, usually with third nerve involvement, but the author's point is that 50% had at least one eye sign. This is obviously a very serious disease in which the patients may initially be seen by an ophthalmologist because of diplopia.] ◀

11–4 **Analysis of Characteristic Eye Movement Abnormalities in Internuclear Ophthalmoplegia.** The syndrome of internuclear ophthalmoplegia (INO) is characterized by impaired adduction of the eye on the side of the medial longitudinal fasciculus lesion and dissociated nystagmus of the contralateral abducting eye.

Timothy B. Crane, Robert D. Yee, Robert W. Baloh, and Robert S. Hepler (Univ. of California, Los Angeles) used quantitative electro-oculographic recording techniques to analyze the frequency of the 4 characteristic eye movement abnormalities in 13 men and 8 women, aged 25 to 73 years, with INO. Thirteen patients had bilateral medial longitudinal fasciculus lesions, making a total of 34 lesions for analysis.

Slowing of the adducting saccade was present in all 34 eyes. The other characteristic eye movement disorders were found less frequently: dissociated nystagmus at 30 degrees of eccentric gaze (31 of 34), dysmetria of the abducting eye (28 of 34), and limitation of adduction (20 of 34).

The most sensitive pattern for detecting INO seems to be slowing of the adducting saccade combined wtih either dissociated nystagmus or dysmetria of the abducting eye. These features should be closely evaluated clinically and by eye movement recordings when looking for subtle signs of an INO.

▶ [Quantitative electro-oculography is not universally available, but it is impressive that 100% of the patients had measurable slowing of adduction.] ◀

11–5 **Pupil Sparing in Oculomotor Palsy: Brief Overview.** The clinical tenet that sparing of the pupil in patients with oculomotor nerve palsy is predictive of an extraaxial ischemic lesion, whereas pupil involvement is predictive of an extraaxial compressive lesion, has some important exceptions. Stephen E. Nadeau and Jonathan D. Trobe (Univ. of Florida, Gainesville) describe 2 patients with pupil-sparing oculomotor nerve palsy caused by midbrain infarction and glioma. A brief review of the literature is provided.

CASE 1.—Man, 62, was admitted to the hospital with the acute onset of dizziness, confusion, and headache. He was lethargic and had atrial fibrillation with a rapid ventricular response. Goldmann perimetry disclosed a left homonymous hemianopia and a right homonymous superior quadrantanopia. Paresis of the left gaze was observed. Supraduction was absent in the righ-

(11–4)   Arch. Ophthalmol. 101:206–210, February 1983.
(11–5)   Ann. Neurol. 13:143–148, February 1983.

eye. With the left eye fixing, a 30-degree right hypotropia was observed. There was minimal levator function and a 5-mm ptosis of the right upper lid. The pupils measured 3 mm in dim illumination and showed a normal reaction to light and near stimulus. A dense supranuclear facial paresis on the left side was observed, and the uvula deviated slightly to the right. The patient had a moderate hemiparesis of the left side that was more pronounced in the arm than in the leg, left-sided hyperreflexia, and a left-sided Babinski sign. A computed tomographic (CT) scan revealed areas of diminished attenuation consistent with the presence of infarction in the right cerebral peduncle and midbrain tegmentum, the left inferior temporal lobe, and both occipital lobes, leading to the clinical diagnosis of embolic infarction.

CASE 2.—Man, 27, was admitted to the hospital with progressive drooping of the right upper lid, diplopia, and left-sided weakness of 3 weeks' duration. He was mildly lethargic and displayed a pseudobulbar affect. Bilateral horizontal gaze paresis, which was more pronounced to the left, was present. The oculocephalic maneuver elicited excursions of greater amplitude than did saccades or pursuit. Upgaze impersistence with nystagmus was observed. Supraduction and infraduction were reduced in the right eye, and right upper lid ptosis of 4 mm was present. The pupils measured 4 mm in dim illumination and showed a normal reaction to direct light and near stimulus. The left corneal reflex was slightly diminished. A supranuclear facial paresis was seen, and a dense hemiparesis of the right side, which was most pronounced in the arm, was present. The finger-to-nose test indicated slight ataxia on the right side. The reflexes on the left side were hyperactive and an extensor plantar response was observed on the same side. Sensation was normal. A CT scan demonstrated a 2-cm contrast-enhancing mass in the right cerebral peduncle. A biopsy specimen taken from this area showed a grade 3 astrocytoma.

Preservation of pupillary function neither specifically localizes nor defines the cause of palsy. A review of the literature indicates that pupil-sparing oculomotor palsy may occur in intraaxial lesions, in a small proportion of subarachnoid compressive lesions, and in a high proportion of cavernous sinus compressive lesions. It is likely that the phenomenon of pupillary sparing depends on the nature of the causative lesion, its clinical course, and the portion of the nerve that has been damaged.

▶ [In spite of these exceptions to the rule, if a patient has diabetes with pupil-sparing and oculomotor palsy, further studies would not seem to be necessary.] ◀

11–6 **Tolosa-Hunt Syndrome (THS)** is discussed by R. Sandyk (Johannesburg). Only about 50 patients with THS have been described. The syndrome is characterized by steady ocular pain, involvement of the cranial nerves passing through the cavernous sinus, and spontaneous remissions and exacerbations. Extreme sensitivity to steroid therapy also is characteristic. The third, fourth, and sixth cranial nerves, the first division of the fifth nerve, and the pericarotid oculosympathetic fibers may be affected. Partial or complete ptosis is a constant clinical sign of THS, and residual neurologic deficit is frequent. Recurrences

(11–6) S. Afr. Med. J. 63:577–578, Apr. 9, 1983.

usually affect the same side. High-dose steroid therapy leads to significant neurologic improvement and may prevent residual damage. Systemic manifestations of THS are rare. A granulomatous process is found at the level of the anterior cavernous sinus, superior orbital fissure, and orbital apex. The inflammation is nonspecific.

Patients suspected of having THS should be examined by arteriography and possibly by orbital venography. Sellar and orbital radiography and CT also may be helpful. The cerebrospinal fluid is normal in most patients. Surgical exploration is not necessary if there is a good response to steroid therapy. The differential diagnosis includes temporal arteritis, orbital myositis, diabetic ophthalmoplegia, intracavernous carotid aneurysm, nasopharyngeal and orbital tumor, and ophthalmic migraine. High-dose steroid therapy should produce a good response in 24 to 48 hours. Treatment can be repeated if there are recurrences, but long-term steroid therapy does not seem to be beneficial.

11–7 **High-Resolution CT of Lesions of the Optic Nerve** is discussed by Robert G. Peyster, Eric D. Hoover, Beverly L. Hershey, and Marvin E. Haskin (Hahnemann Med. College, Philadelphia). High-resolution computed tomographic (CT) scanning makes it possible to evaluate optic nerve lesions accurately in both axial and coronal planes. Both neoplastic and nonneoplastic conditions can be studied in this way. A GE/8800 scanner was used in this study, with iodinated contrast injection if not contraindicated. Routine studies consisted of 5-mm axial and coronal sections; 1.5-mm sections were obtained when indicated. The combination of CT findings, clinical data, and associated abnormalities will lead to a correct diagnosis in most instances.

Smaller optic nerve gliomas are characterized by fusiform enlargement of the nerve silhouette, while larger masses may be eccentric or multilobulated and may have higher density values. Enhancement generally is less intense than in meningiomas. Computed tomography is useful in showing intracranial extension of an orbital glioma. Optic nerve-sheath meningiomas generally lead to thickening of the nerve sheath. The normal optic nerve running through the tumor produces a "tram-track" appearance (Fig 11–1). Enhancement is less intense than in intracranial meningiomas. Neuromas of the optic nerve sheath and other tumors can produce optic nerve enlargement seen on CT.

Bilateral enlargement of the optic nerve and sheath has been observed in patients with increased intracranial pressure and papilledema and in patients with chronic pseudotumor cerebri. Optic neuritis may be manifested by enlargement and contrast enhancement of the nerve. Enlargement of the optic nerve and sheath may be seen in the advanced stages of Graves' disease. Other causes include toxoplasmosis, tuberculosis, sarcoidosis, and traumatic hematoma. Dru-

(11–7) AJR 140:869–874, May 1983.

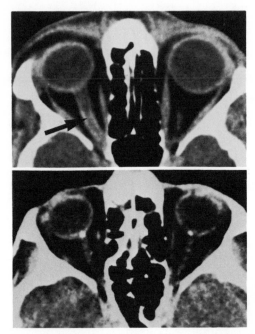

Fig 11–1 (top).—Optic nerve sheath meningioma with tram-track sign. Axial computed tomogram shows enlargement of optic nerve and sheath with lower-absorption nerve *(arrow)* encased by thickened sheath.

Fig 11–2 (bottom).—Axial scan of optic nerve drusen shows bilateral calcifications at insertion of optic nerves on globes.

(Courtesy of Peyster, R.G., et al.: AJR 140:869–874, May 1983; copyright 1983, reproduced by permission of American Journal of Roentgenology.)

sen often calcify and are readily recognized on CT as punctate high densities at the junction of the optic nerve and globe (Fig 11–2).

▶ [The high-resolution CT imaging is spectacular but the radiation dose is as high as it was with standard, less effective x-ray studies. Perhaps new technology will make it possible to reduce the radiation but, of course, magnetic resonance imaging eliminates it entirely.] ◀

11–8 **Suprasellar and Olfactory Meningiomas: Report on a Series of 153 Personal Cases.** C. L. Solero, S. Giombini, and G. Morello (Milan) report the results of surgery in 153 patients with anterior fossa midline meningioma treated between 1947 and 1977. There were 55 suprasellar and 98 olfactory meningiomas in the series. Females predominated. Ages at operation ranged from 18 to 72 years. Presenting symptoms are shown in Table 1, and the findings in Table 2. Pneumoencephalography, though currently not often used, yielded useful findings in 81% of the patients, as did brain scanning in 88% and angiography in 98%. A right frontal craniotomy usually was per-

(11–8) Acta Neurochir. (Wien) 67:181–194, 1983.

TABLE 1.—SYMPTOMS ON ADMISSION

Symptom	Suprasellar		Olfactory	
	Number of cases	%	Number of cases	%
Headache	14	(25.5)	47	(48)
Visual loss	54	(98)	53	(54)
Mental changes	6	(11.9)	33	(33.6)
Epilepsy	2	(3.6)	22	(22.4)
Anosmia	1	(1.8)	39	(39.7)
Motor deficits	1	(1.8)	4	(4)

(Courtesy of Solero, C.L., et al.: Acta Neurochir. (Wien) 67:181–194, 1983; Berlin-Heidelberg-New York; Springer.)

TABLE 2.—SIGNS ON ADMISSION

Signs	Suprasellar		Olfactory	
	Number of cases	%	Number of cases	%
State of consciousness:				
normal	47	(85.4)	33	(33.6)
euphoria	7	(12.7)	58	(59.1)
drowsiness	1	(1.8)	7	(7.1)
Visual loss	54	(98.1)	57	(58.1)
Visual field impairment	39	(70 9)	47	(47.9)
Fundus examination:				
optic atrophy	43	(78.1)	31	(31.6)
papilloedema	1	(1.8)	30	(30.6)
Foster-Kennedy syndrome	3	(5.4)	4	(4.1)
Anosmia	6	(10.9)	66	(67.3)
Hemiparesis	8	(14.5)	32	(32.6)

(Courtesy of Solero, C.L., et al.: Acta Neurochir. (Wien) 67:181–194, 1983; Berlin-Heidelberg-New York; Springer.)

formed. Small tumors were removed piecemeal, and larger ones were electrocoagulated before being scalloped out by diathermy. The optic nerve was severed in 9 patients who were already blind in 1 eye. A flap of pericranium or fascia lata was used to prevent dural leakage of cerebrospinal fluid (CSF) in about 25% of the patients. Tumor removal was complete in 88% overall, including 78% of the suprasellar meningiomas and 94% of the olfactory meningiomas.

The overall operative mortality was 20%. Both patient age and tumor volume were important factors in outcome. Fifteen patients had postoperative complications. Four had meningitis, caused in 3 instances by CSF rhinorrhea. Permanent sequelae included motor deficits in 4 patients, mental deterioration in 4, and diabetes insipidus in 1. Four of 93 patients followed up for a mean of 10½ years after operation had recurrences after presumably radical surgery. Thirteen patients were seriously or totally disabled from sequelae of surgery or the regrowth of incompletely removed tumor. Vision in none of 25 patients with normal vision preoperatively was compromised, and 7 of 68 with visual impairment regained normal vision; 28 others were considerably improved after operation.

Early removal of olfactory and suprasellar meningiomas, with improved diagnostic methods, can be expected to improve the immediate and long-term outcome. The present results were obtained by traditional surgical methods rather than by microsurgical techniques.

▶ [Visual loss was the most frequent symptom, however, it might be that many of the patients in this series did not seek help until late in the course of their disease. On the other hand, ocular signs dominate the clinical picture, with a high incidence of visual field defects and optic disk pathology.] ◀

11–9   **Complications of Herpes Zoster Ophthalmicus.** Larry W. Womack and Thomas J. Liesegang (Mayo Clinic) reviewed the findings in 53 women and 33 men, aged 20 to 88 years (average, 65 years), who were seen at Mayo Clinic between 1975 and 1980 with acute (64 patients) or subacute or chronic (22 patients) herpes zoster ophthalmicus. The right eye was involved in 38 patients and the left in 48. No patient had bilateral involvement of previous episodes of herpes zoster ophthalmicus.

Many patients had preeruptive pain in the eye or trigeminal nerve pain, but the diagnosis rarely was made before the eruption. The most common pattern of skin distribution was concomitant eruption along the frontal, lacrimal, and nasociliary branches of the ophthalmic division of the trigeminal nerve. Of the 64 patients with severe disease, 18 (28%) had only eyelid vesicles without development of ocular or adnexal disease. Of the total study series of 86 patients, 61 (71%) had ocular involvement (table), but no case of optic nerve or retinal involvement was found. Of serious concern were 4 patients with neurologic complications, including 2 with contralateral hemiplegia and 2 with segmental cerebral arteritis. Because the neurologic complications occur several months after the episode of herpes zoster ophthalmicus, the association is often overlooked and the opportunity to treat systemically with corticosteroids is missed.

The ocular complications necessitated 11 ocular operations in 8 patients, including tarsorrhaphy for neurotrophic keratitis in 6 patients. Substantial visual loss was associated with herpes zoster ophthalmicus in 24 patients (28%); this was severe (with visual acuity worse than 20/200) in 10 patients. Associated conditions seen in 21 of the 86 patients included malignancies in 13 and forms of vasculitis in 4; there were no lymphomas.

Only 36 of the 64 patients (56%) with acute disease required ther-

(11–9) Arch. Ophthalmol. 101:42–45, January 1983.

apy. Four of 11 treated with prednisone had moderate postherpetic neuralgia. Topically applied 1% prednisolone acetate was used in 26 patients, and 23 received topical cycloplegic agents.

Topically applied 1% prednisolone acetate is often useful in the treatment of corneal, scleral, or uveal inflammation and in the ocular

---

OCULAR COMPLICATIONS IN 86 PATIENTS WITH HERPES ZOSTER
OPHTHALMICUS

Complication	No. of Patients
Lid involvement	
Entropion with trichiasis of upper lid	5
Ptosis	1
Cicatricial ectropion with exposure of cornea	2
Scarring of both upper and lower lids	3
Total	**11**
Corneal involvement	
Acute epithelial keratitis	
Pseudodendritic keratitis	7
Punctate epithelial keratitis	12
Mucous plaques	2
Total	**19 ***
Acute anterior stromal infiltrates	7
Disciform keratitis	17
Sclerokeratitis	2
Neurotrophic keratitis	10
Late dendritic keratitis	1
Perforation	1
Total	**47 ***
Scleral involvement	
Episcleritis (recurrent)	1
Scleritis	3
Total	**4**
Canalicular scarring	2
Uveitis	
Diffuse	33
Localized	2
Sectorial iris atrophy	15
Total	**37 ***
Glaucoma (secondary)	10
Persistent	2
Cataract	7
Neuro-ophthalmic involvement	
Cranial nerve palsy	3
Contralateral hemiplegia	2
Segmental cerebral arteritis	2
Total	**7**
Postherpetic neuralgia	15

*Some patients had more than one manifestation of involvement.
(Courtesy of Womack, L.W., and Liesegang, T.J.: Arch. Ophthalmol. 101:42–45, January 1983; copyright 1983, American Medical Association; by permission of Mayo Foundation.)

hypertensive response, but it must often be used in large doses, monitored closely, administered for long periods, and carefully tapered. Recognition of superimposed bacterial, fungal, or herpes simplex disease is important, as is recognition of conditions that will not respond to topically applied prednisolone, such as neurotrophic keratitis. The role of prednisoone in the treatment of herpes zoster ophthalmicus cannot be determined from this study.

▶ [One does not usually think of visual loss in cases of herpes zoster but 25% of patients in this Mayo Clinic series had a significant decrease in acuity. There still is no definitive data for the effectiveness of topical corticosteroid, although in some clinics it has been used for many years with apparently good results and few complications.] ◀

▶ ↓ The following 2 articles demonstrate the extremes of pupil changes with subtle defects measured by pupillography on the one hand and marked irregularity of significance to the neurosurgeon, on the other. The ophthalmologist is not likely to encounter the latter, but headache is a common symptom. ◀

11-10   **The Pupil and Headaches.** Horner's syndrome is the most common ocular abnormality described in patients with vascular headache. Peter Herman (Mt. Sinai School of Medicine, New York) performed pupillography before and after the instillation of cocaine eyedrops in 17 females and 3 males, mean age 39 years, with chronic vascular headaches. Sixteen patients had classic or common migraine and 4 had cluster headaches. Six patients had headache during the examination. Pupillography was repeated 30 to 35 minutes after instillation of 5% cocaine into each eye.

Pupillography showed anisocoria in 65% of the patients initially and in 90% after cocaine instillation. The smaller pupil was ipsilateral or contralateral to the headache in similar numbers of patients. The findings are shown in the table. Three patients had normal responses and 3 had a complete lack of response to cocaine instillation. The pupillary response to light decreased after cocaine instillation in 15 of 20 patients and increased in 4. Pupillary constriction was especially reduced in the cluster headache group.

Patients with cluster headache and migraine may have a subtle

RESULTS OF COCAINE INSTILLATION IN INTERMEDIATE-RESPONSE PATIENTS

	Intermediate* Cocaine Response	Pupil Size (mm) Right	Left	Ptosis	Reverse Ptosis	Constriction to Light % Before Cocaine Right	Left	Constriction to Light % After Cocaine Right	Left
ALL VASCULAR HEADACHE	15	6.1	6.0	In 9 out of 11 cases seen	None in 11	25.0	25.5	20.0	20.0
MIGRAINE (Classic and common)	11	6.0	5.9	6	—	26.0	25.0	24.0	24.0
CLUSTER	4	6.2	6.1	3	—	24.3	24.7	16.7	16.5

*Intermediate response is dilation of less than 30%.
(Courtesy of Herman, P.: Headache 23:102–105, May 1983.)

(11–10) Headache 23:102–105, May 1983.

chronic sympathetic deficiency affecting both the pupil and the eyelid. At times, the deficiency may worsen, leading to a prominent Horner's syndrome. Pupillography with sympathomimetic eyedrops is a convenient and objective means of diagnosing clinically difficult cases of vascular headache. Eyedrops probably should not be used in patients with headaches and pupillary dilatation.

11–11 **Oval Pupil: Clinical Significance and Relationship to Intracranial Hypertension.** Lawrence F. Marshall, David Barba, Belinda M. Toole, and Sharon A. Bowers (San Diego) observed the oval, or "football," pupil in 15 neurosurgical patients. They were among 141 patients older than age 15 seen in a 2-year period in whom the intracranial pressure (ICP) was continuously monitored. In 13 patients the ICP was 22 to 38 mm Hg when the oval pupil was first observed. In another patient from whom an epidural hematoma was removed, the bone flap could not be replaced because of brain swelling. Fourteen patients had intracranial hypertension at the time that the pupillary abnormality was first noted; in 9 of these the pupil returned to normal shape and size after reduction of the ICP. In the 4 whose ICP was not satisfactorily controlled, the pupil became progressively larger, round, fixed, and unreactive. One patient with control of ICP had persistent pupillary abnormality 3 months after injury, suggesting irreversible injury to the third nerve or to the midbrain.

The oval pupil was associated with moderate intracranial hypertension in nearly all of the present patients. Control of ICP usually was associated with return to a normal pupil, whereas failure of ICP control was associated with development of a fixed, dilated, unreactive pupil. Monitoring the ICP is essential for the proper management of patients with severe brain injury, but the oval pupil is indicative of clinically significant intracranial hypertension in most instances. If an oval pupil is observed in a patient with head injury, subarachnoid hemorrhage, or other intracranial catastrophe, prompt treatment is indicated even if the clinical status appears to be good.

11–12 **The 20/20 Eye in Multiple Sclerosis.** Mark J. Kupersmith, J. I. Nelson, William H. Seiple, Ronald E. Carr, and Penny A. Weiss (New York Univ.) evaluated the visual pathways of 24 patients, mean age 32, with definite or probable multiple sclerosis (MS), 20/20 Snellen visual acuity, and no history of optic neuritis. Twenty-five controls with normal neuro-ophthalmologic findings also were assessed. Psychophysical studies of contrast thresholds were done in 18 patients. Both transient and steady-state contrast visual-evoked potentials (VEPs) were recorded.

Delayed latencies were identified in transient VEP recordings in 38% of the patients with MS, and interocular latency differences were abnormal in 67% of them. All patients with abnormal latencies in

(11–11) J. Neurosurg. 58:566–568, April 1983.
(11–12) Neurology (Cleve.) 33:1015–1020, August 1983.

either eye had abnormal interocular latency differences. The results of contrast VEPs were abnormal in 46% of the MS patients. Psychophysical studies of contrast sensitivity showed abnormal results in 78% of the patients in the study. Color vision abnormalities were found in 4 of the 24 patients evaluated. The findings correlated poorly with cerebrospinal fluid abnormalities. Eight of 22 MS patients had relative afferent pupillary defects. Funduscopy showed abnormalities of the optic nerve or nerve fiber layer in 11 of 22 patients. Also, 75% of the eyes with abnormal fundi had abnormal findings on contrast VEPs, and 80% of these patients also had abnormal psychophysically determined contrast thresholds.

Psychophysical contrast and VEP studies are helpful in demonstrating subtle visual impairment in patients with MS. However, psychophysical testing requires good patient cooperation and is a subjective approach. Although they are objective, VEP studies should be extended to measure the full modulation transer function. It may prove helpful to assess the horizontal, vertical, and oblique orientations separately with respect to both latency and contrast sensitivity.

▶ [This is a sophisticated study but the Arden grating set is not a very scientific test. It is now clear that visual-evoked response testing with grating targets that can be varied in orientation as well as spatial frequency and contrast is the most sensitive.] ◀

11–13 **Prospective Examinations of Benign Paroxysmal Positional Nystagmus** are discussed by A. Rast and K. Hess (Univ. of Zurich, Switzerland). Benign paroxysmal positional nystagmus (BPN) is the most frequently seen cause of vestibular vertigo. Precise reports about the usual course of the disease do not exist. In a prospective study, 47 out of 55 patients with BPN were examined after 3 to 4½ years. In 44% of the patients, nystagmus disappeared in an average of 8.6 months. During follow-up, 25% of the patients (28%) still suffered regularly from positional nystagmus. In another 25% of the patients (28%) episodic nystagmus had occurred for years and averaged 3.6 episodes per patient. In 25% of the patients no causative factors were found. In 33% of these patients, head injury was found to be the cause of BPN. In a few patients BPN was found to be directly connected with nontraumatic labyrinth affection, intermittent vertebrobasilar insufficiency, or anesthesia.

The course of BPN is more resistant and less predictable than was previously believed. It is noteworthy that no patient showed up after the first examination and that patients with a resistant course of the disease never requested therapy on their own. The benign nature of the disease may account for this attitude and most patients learn to adjust to the symptom and are only mildly handicapped by BPN. No patient in this study was threatened with severe damage caused by nystagmus and an indication for neurectomy was not discussed. In

(11–13) Schweiz. Med. Wochenschr. 113:504–507, Apr. 9, 1983.

any case such a decision should wait at least 2 years. Physiotherapy, recommended by some clinicians, seems to suppress BPN. However, its effectiveness for the chronic condition still needs to be studied.

About 50% of the patients had a history or results of examination that showed acute unilateral vestibular deficiency, such as an acute peripheral vestibular pathologic condition whose cause also was unknown. In addition it can be expected that vestibulopathy with late BPN is a matter of the labyrinth and not the vestibular nerve or ganglion. The reason why some patients do not become symptom-free may be a degenerative labyrinth process with chronic or periodic liberation of pathogenic cell detritus.

▶ ↓ In the following 2 articles the authors discuss functional visual loss. There seems to be 2 extremes: the sophisticated malingerer who wishes to profit from his or her visual problems and the patient with hysteria. Unfortunately most patients fall on the continuum between the 2 extremes. These articles help us understand more about these patients. ◀

11–14 **Functional Visual Loss.**—*I. A true psychiatric disorder?*—Roger G. Kathol, Terry A. Cox, James J. Corbett, H. Stanley Thompson, and John Clancy point out that 1% to 5% of patients seen by ophthalmologists have functional visual loss (acuity below 20/30 with the best correction) not related to an apparent physical cause. The entity has been referred to as hysterical amblyopia, functional amblyopia, and ocular malingering. Patients may be seen with constricted or spiral visual fields or focal field defects. The acuity usually is worse than 20/40, but it is normal on retesting or when the patient is encouraged, or when a subterfuge is used.

There is little evidence that functional visual loss is always a manifestation of conversion hysteria or that CNS dysequilibrium is responsible, but Babinski's suggestion that the patient is suggestible seems to be valid. Some patients undoubtedly are malingerers, and it may not be possible to distinguish conscious from unconscious behavior by signs and symptoms alone. Few studies have been done on psychiatric disorders in patients with functional visual loss, but psychiatric disease is far from uniformly present in these patients, and no particular type of disorder is especially prevalent.

Nearly 50% of the patients continue to exhibit or complain of visual difficulty. No treatment has been found to be particularly helpful. Hypnosis-narcosis, behavior modification, and psychotherapy have all been tried. The lack of efficacy of a variety of measures supports the view that some patients with functional visual loss are merely suggestible. Visual field testing lends itself to variation in response in suggestible persons. Suggestion has succeeded in the treatment of as many as 90% of patients with visual acuity abnormalities and also in some patients with visual field abnormalities. A psychiatric diagnosis should not be made in patients with functional visual loss but no evi-

(11–14) Psychol. Med. 13:307–314, May 1983; 315–324, May 1983.

dence of psychiatric disorder. This could help avoid unnecessary and ineffective treatment.

II. Psychiatric Aspects in 42 Patients Followed Up for Four Years.— Kathol, Cox, Corbett, Thompson, and Clancy followed up 42 of 80 patients seen in 1973 to 1979 at the University of Iowa Hospitals with functional visual loss. They had initially been seen with constricted or spiral visual fields, focal visual field defects that resolved on retesting or with subterfuge or that did not follow expected laws of physiology, or visual acuity abnormalities that fluctuated over time or were corrected with subterfuge. Organic pathology explaining the abnormalities was lacking. Mean follow-up was 53 months.

The most common presenting complaints were blurred or reduced visual acuity, headache, and loss of side vision. Nine patients had no visual symptoms. Twenty-three of the 42 patients continued to meet criteria for functional visual loss at follow-up. All had spiral or constricted visual fields, and 6 had field defects as well. Two had loss of acuity. Only 8 patients reported incapacity resulting from their visual difficulties. Recovery was associated with symptoms present for less than 2 years, absence of a psychiatric diagnosis, and lack of treatment. Twenty-two patients in all had a psychiatric diagnosis other than conversion disorder or factitious disorder at follow-up. Somatization disorder was most frequent. Ten patients had findings consistent with a diagnosis of conversion disorder. Organic pathology was found at presentation in 10 cases. Reassurance alone was more likely to be followed by recovery than nonspecific measures such as glasses and nonmedicinal eyedrops.

Twenty of the original 42 patients with functional visual loss had no evident psychiatric disorder. The findings support Babinski's view that this disorder sometimes represents merely increased suggestibility. Daily life may not be disrupted even if the condition persists, and psychiatric intervention appears unnecessary. Patients with concurrent psychiatric disease are more likely to have persistent findings of functional visual loss, but they have not been shown to respond even to psychiatric treatment. The psychiatric disorder itself should be the focus of treatment in these patients.

12. Medical Ophthalmology and Drug Therapy

Treatment of Ocular Inflammatory Disease With Nonsteroidal Antiinflammatory Drugs

LEE M. JAMPOL, M.D.

Northwestern University, Chicago

Prostaglandins, unsaturated fatty acid derivatives, are important mediators of inflammation in the eye[1] and elsewhere in the body. In recent years, an array of nonsteroidal antiinflammatory drugs (NSAIDs) has been developed (table). These drugs inhibit cyclo-oxygenase, an enzyme important in the synthesis of prostaglandins from their precursors. These drugs are widely utilized in therapy for arthritis and other acquired diseases of the connective tissue. It has recently been recognized that NSAIDs may be helpful in therapy for ocular inflammation as well. This discussion will briefly review use of NSAIDs for ocular disease.

NONSTEROIDAL ANTIINFLAMMATORY DRUGS CURRENTLY IN USE

1. Pyrazolones
   phenylbutazone (Butazolidin)
   oxyphenbutazone (Tandearil)
2. Indolacetic acids
   indomethacin (Indocin)
   sulindac (Clinoril)
3. Pyrrolacetic acids
   tolmetin (Tolectin)
4. Proprionic acids
   ibuprofen (Motrin, Rufen)
   fenoprofen (Nalfon)
   naproxen (Naprosyn)
5. Anthranilic acids
   mefanamic acid (Ponstel)
   meclofenamate (Meclomen)
6. Others
   aspirin
   diflunisal (Dolobid)
   acetaminophen
   piroxicam (Feldene)

Aphakic Cystoid Macular Edema

Collection of fluid in the macula with the formation of cystic spaces is a common complication in the eye.[2] It is seen in patients with uveitis, diabetes mellitus, retinal vascular occlusions, and in many other situations. Cystoid macular edema in the aphakic or pseudophakic eye, the Irvine-Gass syndrome, is a significant cause of visual loss after cataract surgery. Miyake et al.[3] have presented evidence that prostaglandins are synthesized and released in the eye following cataract surgery. It has thus been suggested that prostaglandin synthesis, presumably by tissues in the anterior segment, is responsible for the occurrence of cystoid macula edema following cataract surgery. Inhibitors of prostaglandin synthesis have been utilized for the prophylaxis (prevention) or therapy of cystoid macular edema.[4]

Topical indomethacin preparations have been shown to be effective in the prophylaxis of angiographic aphakic cystoid macular edema.[5, 6, 7] It should be noted, however, that the incidence of the visually significant cystoid macular edema is much lower that that of angiographic cystoid macular edema; it is unclear if topical indomethacin is also effective in preventing clincally significant aphakic cystoid macular edema.

Once cystoid macular edema is established, it seems logical that therapeutic use of topical NSAIDs may be useful. However, to date no therapeutic trials have demonstrated a significant benefit.[8] At present, no topical commercial preparation of NSAIDs has been approved for release in the United States.

One study has also shown that systemic use of indomethacin is valuable in the prophylaxis of aphakic cystoid macular edema.[9] However, in this trial, side effects of the drug were common. As is true for topical agents, so far no trial has demonstrated a therapeutic effect of systemic NSAIDs. However, anecdotal cases have suggested a possible role for this therapy.

We utilize systemic indomethacin, 25–50 mg t.i.d. orally in patients with aphakic cystoid macular edema which does not clear spontaneously. We have also used topical 1% indomethacin in similar situations. Further clinical trials should prove or disprove the long-term benefit of this therapy.

Scleritis

Oral oxyphenbutazone (Tandearil), 100 mg q.i.d. or indomethacin (Indocin) 25–50 mg t.i.d. are of benefit in the therapy of scleritis.[10] These agents are much more potent than topical corticosteroids but probably are less potent than systemic corticosteroids. In desperate situations, cytotoxic drugs also are more effective. The duration of therapy necessary for scleritis varies greatly from case to case.

Uveitis

Corticosteroids, either topical, periocular, or systemic, are frequently used in therapy for uveitis. Side effects of the corticosteroids however, are significant in terms of cataract formation, inhibition of wound healing, predisposition to infection, and elevated intraocular pressure. A topical or systemic NSAID that would be effective for uveitis is desirable. In experimental situations, topical or systemic antiinflammatory agents such as oxyphenbutazone and indomethacin have been shown to be effective in animal models of uveitis. They have also been used for some cases of human anterior nongranulomatous uveitis.[11] However, in our experience they appear to be weaker than potent topical or systemic corticosteroids. At present, NSAIDs are rarely utilized in the United States in therapy for uveitis.

Dilation of the Pupil During Surgery

During surgical or laser manipulations in the anterior segment, miosis may develop. In surgical procedures when access to the posterior segment is a necessity, miosis can greatly hinder technique. Atropine-like drugs and sympathomimetic drugs will cause dilation of the pupil but with trauma to the iris, the pupil may still constrict. Clinical trials have suggested that topical applications of NSAIDs may prolong pupillary dilation.[12, 13]

Glaucomatocyclitic Crisis

Patients with this syndrome demonstrate unilateral attacks of elevated intraocular pressure associated with very mild anterior chamber reaction and an open filtration angle. It has been suggested that prostaglandins mediate this response and Japanese studies have shown elevated prostaglandins in the aqueous humor.[14] As a result, oral indomethacin has been used and has been reported to return the elevated intraocular pressure to normal faster than standard therapies, including acetazolamide, epinephrine, and dexamathasone.[14]

Postcataract Hypertension

With tight cataract wound closure, elevation of intraocular pressure in the first 48 hours after the operation is common. This elevation is probably related to a breakdown of the blood-aqueous barrier with increased aqueous formation. Administration of aspirin and perhaps other NSAIDs may be valuable in preventing this pressure rise.[15]

Treatment of Postcataract Inflammation

Topical indomethacin has been reported to be effective in preventing postcataract flare, miosis, and corneal edema.[16] However, it is possible that topical NSAIDs inhibit wound healing. Further studies are necessary in this area (see below).

Ocular Side Effects of Systemic NSAIDs

Indomethacin, one of the most widely used NSAIDs, has been reported to cause corneal deposits and retinal dysfunction.[17] However, subsequent studies have not confirmed the side effects of retinal abnormalities.[18] Considering the widespread use of this drug, if significant ocular toxicity occurs, it must be rare.

Ibuprofen, another commonly prescribed drug for arthritis, has been reported to cause central visual loss.[19, 20] This "toxic amblyopia" with a central scotoma, color visual loss, and normal fundus examination is often seen 1 to 3 weeks after beginning administration of the drug. The visual loss appears to be reversible in almost all cases. A similar side effect has been seen in one patient treated with benoxaprofen, a new NSAID that has been removed from the market because of hepatic and renal toxicity.

Ocular Side Effects of Topical NSAIDs

Topical indomethacin appears to cause minimal side effects. There may be stinging at the time of administration and punctate keratitis. One concern about the use of these drugs is their possible effect on wound healing. To date, conflicting conclusions have been reached in this area. It has also been suggested that the topical NSAIDs may worsen the course of herpes simplex keratitis. In this respect they may be similar to corticosteroids. Significant systemic side effects from topical NSAIDs have not been reported.

Systemic Side Effects of Systemic NSAIDs

The NSAIDs are potent drugs that may have significant systemic side effects of which ophthalmologists using these drugs must be aware. Gastrointestinal symptoms may occur. All of these agents to a greater or lesser degree can interfere with platelet function and thereby cause bleeding. This is an important consideration in patients who have bleeding into the eye following trauma or are undergoing surgery in which bleeding is a potential complication. The effect on platelets from a NSAID lasts several days. The NSAIDs may also cause skin rash, bone marrow suppression, hepatic toxicity, depressed renal function, and central nervous system symptoms including headaches, dizziness, and confusion. Aspirin and some of the other drugs may cause tinnitus and hearing loss with the use of high doses. Asthmatic attacks may be precipitated in susceptible patients. Aspirin has been linked to Reyes' syndrome in children with viral illness. Recently benoxaprofen has been removed from the market because of reported hepatic and renal complications.

Summary

Nonsteroidal antiinflammatory drugs are potent medications that are already widely utilized in therapy for many ocular conditions. Side effects are a serious problem with the use of these drugs systemically. In the future effective topical NSAIDs will probably be used in therapy for many ocular diseases.

References

1. Stjernschantz, J.: Autacoids and Neuropeptides. In Sears, M. (ed.): *Pharmacology of the Eye*. Springer-Verlag Berlin, 1983, pp. 312–329.
2. Laatikainen, L.: Cystoid macular edema. Clinical course and characteristics. In Sears, M. (ed.): *Surgical Pharmacology of the Eye*. Raven Press, New York (In press).
3. Miyake, K., Sugiyama, S., Norimatsu, I., et al.: Prevention of cystoid macular edema after lens extraction by topical indomethacin III. Radioimmunoassay measurement of prostaglandins in the aqueous during and after lens extraction procedure. *Graefes Arch. Clin. Exp. Ophthalmol.* 209:83–88, 1978.
4. Jampol, L.M.: Pharmacologic therapy of aphakic cystoid macular edema: A review. *Ophthalmology* 89:891–897, 1982.
5. Miyake, K., Sakamura, S., and Miura H.: Long-term follow-up study on prevention of aphakic cystoid macular edema by topical indomethacin. *Br. J. Ophthalmol.* 64:324–328, 1980.
6. Kraff, M.C., Sanders, D.R., Jampol, L.M., et al.: Prophylaxis of pseudophakic cystoid macular edema with topical indomethacin. *Ophthalmology* 89:885–890, 1982.
7. Yannuzzi, L.A., Landau, A.N., and Turtz, A.I.: Incidence of aphakic cystoid macular edema with the use of topical indomethacin. *Ophthalmology* 88:947–954, 1981.
8. Burnett, J., Tessler, H., Isenberg, S., et al.: Double-masked trial of fenoprofen sodium treatment of chronic aphakic cystoid macular edema. *Ophthalmic Surg.* 14:150–152, 1983.
9. Klein, R.M., Katzin, H.M., and Yannuzzi, L.A.: The effect of indomethacin pretreatment on aphakic cystoid macular edema. *Am. J. Ophthalmol.* 87:487–489, 1979.
10. Watson, P.G., and Hazleman, B.L.: *The Sclera and Systemic Disorders.* W.B. Saunders, London, 1976, pp. 384–390.
11. Hunter, P.J.L., Fowler, P.D., and Wilkinson, P.: Treatment of anterior uveitis. Comparison of oral oxyphenbutazone and topical steroids. *Br. J. Ophthalmol.* 57:892–896, 1973.
12. Sawa, M., and Masuda, K.: Topical indomethacin in soft cataract aspiration. *Jpn. J. Ophthalmol.* 20:514–519, 1976.
13. Keulen de Vos II, C.J., van Rij, G., Renardel de Lavalette, J.C.G., et al.:

Effect of indomethacin in preventing surgically induced miosis. *Br. J. Ophthalmol.* 67:94–96, 1983.

14. Misada, K., Izawa, Y., and Mishima S.: Prostaglandins and glaucomatocyclitic crisis. *Jpn. J. Ophthalmol.* 19:368–375, 1975.
15. Rich, W.J.C.C.: Prevention of postoperative ocular hypertension by prostaglandin inhibitors. *Trans. Ophthalmol. Soc. UK* 97:268–271, 1977.
16. Mochizuki, M., Sawa, M., and Masuda, K.: Topical indomethacin in intracapsular extraction of senile cataract. *Jpn. J. Ophthalmol.* 21:215–226, 1977.
17. Burns, C.A.: Indomethacin, reduced retinal sensitivity, and corneal deposits. *Am. J. Ophthalmol.* 66:825–835, 1968.
18. Carr, R.E., and Siegel, I.M.: Retinal function in patients treated with indomethacin. *Am. J. Ophthalmol.* 75:302–306, 1973.
19. Collum, L.M.T., and Bowen, D.I.: Ocular side effects of ibuprofen. *Br. J. Ophthalmol.* 55:472–477, 1971.
20. Palmer, C.A.L.: Toxic amblyopia from ibuprofen. *Br. Med. J.* 3:765, 1972.

12–1 **Cyclosporin A Therapy in Treatment of Intraocular Inflammatory Disease Resistant To Systemic Corticosteroids and Cytotoxic Agents.** Side effects are frequent with both corticosteroid and cytotoxic drug therapy for noninfectious intraocular inflammatory disorders. Robert B. Nussenblatt, Alan G. Palestine, and Chi-Chao Chan (Natl. Inst. of Health) successfully treated 15 of 16 patients who had severe posterior uveitis of presumed noninfectious origin with cyclosporin A. The patients had bilateral, sight-threatening, chiefly intermediate or posterior uveitis that had failed to respond fully to either daily systemic corticosteroid therapy or cytotoxic agents. The patients were aged 20 to 67 years. All had active inflammatory disease at the outset of study and had recently had a decrease in acuity of at least 2 lines on the Snellen chart. All eyes but 2 had acuities worse than 20/40. Cyclosporin A was initially given in an oral dosage of 10 mg/kg daily, and the dosage was subsequently adjusted to the inflammatory response. Follow-up ranged from 2 to 18 months.

All but 1 of the 16 patients had long-term improvement in visual acuity, intraocular inflammation, or both. Twelve had improvement in acuity of 2 lines or more. Some patients had further improvement in vision after several months of treatment. Vitreal inflammation responded more slowly than anterior chamber involvement. Four patients received topical corticosteroid therapy besides cyclosporin A. Five patients had renal toxicity and 2 had evidence of hepatic toxicity.

Cyclosporin A has effectively reduced inflammation in patients with severe intraocular noninfectious inflammatory disorders unresponsive to conventional immunosuppressive therapy. Visual acuity has improved in most cases. Renal and liver toxic effects are a consideration, but cyclosporin A nevertheless is expected to have an important role in the management of severe, blinding inflammatory intraocular disorders.

(12–1) Am. J. Ophthalmol. 96:275–282, September 1983.

▶ [Cyclosporin A is a promising new treatment for uveitis and, although its side effects are potentially serious, they can be controlled. It may be that local application will be possible and effective. (See Dr. Tessler's introduction to Chapter 8.)] ◀

12–2 **Systemic Effects of Topical Ophthalmic Medications.** Topically applied ophthalmic drugs have the potential for significant systemic absorption, which may result in widespread adverse side effects. Beatrice L. Selvin (Univ. of Maryland Hosp., Baltimore) discusses in a review of the literature, the potential side effects of topically applied autonomic drugs used in ophthalmic practice.

Systemic absorption can occur through the nasal mucosa, gastrointestinal (GI) tract, or the circulation. Topically applied autonomic drugs that produce mydriasis, miosis, and cycloplegia are commonly used for examination of the eye, control of glaucoma, and relief of minor symptoms. As the systemic effects caused by ocular instillation of the sympathomimetic drugs epinephrine and phenylephrine are primarily cardiovascular, the ophthalmologist should be aware of the cardiac status of the patient. The anticholinergic drugs atropine, scopolamine, and homatropine, as well as cyclopentolate and tropicamide, are readily absorbed transconjunctivally and through the nasal mucosa and GI tract. The side effects of these drugs primarily involve the CNS. Physostigmine, the traditional antidote to central anticholinergic poisoning, also reverses many of the peripheral effects of anticholinergic drugs.

Among the parasympathomimetic drugs, pilocarpine is the most commonly used agent for the treatment of primary glaucoma and neutralization of dilating drops. The adverse side effects of this drug are characterized primarily by exaggeration of the parasympathomimetic effects. Carbachol has a longer duration of action than pilocarpine and similar, but more toxic side effects. Conjunctival instillation of physostigmine, a "reversible" anticholinesterase agent, may produce the already-known adverse systemic effects of the drug. The systemic effects of echothiophate iodide, an "irreversible" anticholinesterase drug, are due to the accumulation of acetylcholine at neuromuscular junctions and synapses throughout the central and peripheral nervous systems. Thus the side effects of echothiophate, which include GI disturbances, depressed cardiac function, respiratory symptoms, CNS effects, and neuromuscular disorders, generally do not appear for weeks or months after initiation of therapy, and the association between toxicosis symptoms and ocular therapy is often unrecognized. The oximes provide a specific antidote to echothiophate toxicosis. Timolol, a β-adrenergic antagonist that lowers intraocular pressure, should be prescribed with caution.

All physicians involved in the care of patients should be familiar with the actions, interactions, and toxic effects of ocularly instilled medications. In many cases, the prevention of systemic side effects

(12–2) South. Med. J. 76:349–358, March 1983.

requires the discreet use of these drugs. If surgery is required, consultation between the ophthalmologist and anesthesiologist regarding long-term and perioperative use of ocular medication is imperative.

▶ [This article is a fine review of systemic problems associated with topical ophthalmic medications. Systemic absorption occurs by means of several routes; however, it is important to remember that the nasolacrimal duct, if not occluded, provides immediate access to the nasal mucosa. Absorption across the nasal mucosa is as rapid as intravenous injection. Ophthalmologists rely on blinking to remove excess medication after its instillation by eyedrops, but blinking also provides the pumping action for nasolacrimal fluid movement.] ◄

12–3 **Effects of Sodium Hyaluronate, Chondroitin Sulfate, and Methylcellulose on the Corneal Endothelium and Intraocular Pressure.** One approach to minimizing endothelial cell damage from an intraocular lens is coating of the implant with high-viscosity substances. Scott M. Mac Rae, Henry F. Edelhauser, Robert A. Hyndiuk, Eileen M. Burd, and Richard O. Schultz (Med. College of Wisconsin, Milwaukee) examined the efficacy and toxicity of 3 such substances—sodium hyaluronate (Healon), chondroitin sulfate, and methylcellulose. In vitro corneal perfusion studies were performed on rabbit eyes. The substances were also injected into the anterior chamber of rabbit and cynomolgus monkey eyes, and sequential intraocular pressure measurements were recorded. The degree of endothelial protection af-

Fig 12–1.—Average intraocular pressure in monkeys after injection of each test substance; *BSS*, balanced salt solution. (Courtesy of Mac Rae, S.M., et al.: Am. J. Ophthalmol. 95:332–341, March 1983.)

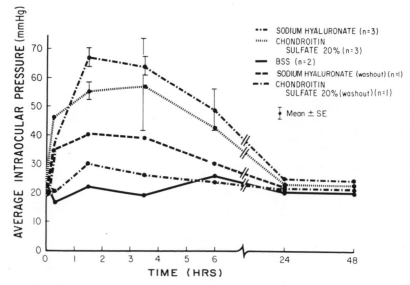

(12–3) Am. J. Ophthalmol. 95:332–341, March 1983.

forded by the substances was determined when the endothelium of rabbit corneas was abraded in vitro.

Corneal thickness was not significantly altered by 1:2 diluted 1% sodium hyaluronate, 0.4% methylcellulose, or 10% chondroitin sulfate. Endothelial cell patterns were maintained during perfusion on specular microscopy, and no ultrastructural abnormalities occurred. Corneal thickness decreased when 20% chondroitin sulfate was perfused, especially when it was mixed with balanced salt solution, and endothelial cell edema was observed. Intraocular pressures increased when the substances were injected into the anterior chamber of rabbit eyes. A substantial rise in pressure also was seen in monkey eyes (Fig 12–1). In both groups, pressures returned to baseline within 48 hours. Endothelial abrasion tests showed that both 1% sodium hyaluronate and 20% chondroitin sulfate provided excellent endothelial protection from polymethylmethacrylate lens surfaces. Less protection was provided by 10% chondroitin sulfate and 0.4% methylcellulose.

Both sodium hyaluronate and 20% chondroitin sulfate protect the corneal endothelium from damage by intraocular lenses and are nontoxic, although the latter is hyperosmolar and causes corneal thinning. A sharp rise in intraocular pressure can occur with both substances, and anterior chamber washout is indicated when a significant volume of either substance is used.

▶ [The high-viscosity substances protect the corneal endothelium and are a great boon to lens-implant surgeons, especially in teaching hospitals. The problem of the induced ocular hypertension, however, has not been solved. The authors of this article conclude that the material should be irrigated from the eye. However, this is an extra manipulation and no doubt hard on the eye as well as on the surgeon since the material looks like vitreous. More pharmacologic work needs to be done.] ◀

▶ ↓Acyclovir (acycloguanosine) is an effective antiherpesvirus agent. In the following 2 articles, the authors have shown that the drug is more effective when used in combination with either interferon or with the corticosteroid betamethasone. Both the Holland group (acyclovir plus interferon) and the Ireland (acyclovir plus betamethasone) believe they have demonstrated the best combined therapy. It is evident that more work needs to be done and perhaps a combination of 3 drugs would be most effective. The use of corticosteroids in herpetic disease does make one a little uneasy, however. ◀

12–4 **Combination Therapy for Dendritic Keratitis With Acyclovir and α-Interferon.** Erik W. J. de Koning, O. Paul van Bijsterveld (Utrecht, Holland) and Kari Cantell (Helsinki) compared the effect of treatment with acyclovir combined with α-interferon or albumin-placebo in 59 patients with superficial herpetic keratitis. Eleven patients had a geographic ulcer, 28 had large dendrites, and 20 had small dendrites. Nine of the latter patients had stellate keratitis. All patients received 3% acyclovir ophthalmic ointment 5 times a day, with simultaneous administration of eyedrops containing 30 million international units per ml of α-interferon (human leukocyte interferon) or placebo. The 2 treatment groups were well matched demographically

(12–4) Arch. Ophthalmol. 101:1866–1868, December 1983.

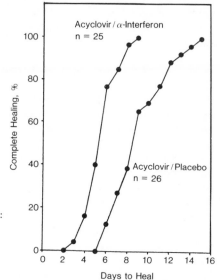

Fig 12–2.—Time to complete healing of dendritic keratitis in patients treated with acyclovir plus α-interferon or acyclovir plus placebo. (Courtesy of de Koning, E.W.J., et al.: Arch. Ophthalmol. 101:1866–1868, December 1983; copyright 1983, American Medical Association.)

and clinically. Twenty-five of the 51 evaluable patients received combined treatment with interferon.

The average time to partial healing was 2.8 days with combined active treatment and 5.0 days with acyclovir plus placebo. Times to complete healing are compared in Figure 12–2. The average time to complete healing was 5.8 days with combined active treatment and 9.3 days with acyclovir plus placebo. The average time required for complete healing of geographic ulcers was 6.8 days with combined active treatment and 10.7 days with acyclovir plus placebo.

Dendritic keratitis was healed more rapidly with combined acyclovir and α-interferon therapy than with acyclovir plus placebo in this trial. The results were better than those obtained in a previously reported study using trifluridine as an antiviral agent. Toxic side effects were infrequent and fewer than in trifluridine-treated patients. In 2 patients treated with acyclovir plus placebo, mild punctate keratopathy developed. The best current treatment of dendritic keratitis appears to be acyclovir or trifluridine in combination with a potent interferon.

12–5 **Acyclovir (Zovirax) in Herpetic Disciform Keratitis.** Viral antigen is present in white blood cells in the anterior chamber in patients with disciform keratitis and iritis. Acyclovir is an antiviral agent that can penetrate the intact corneal epithelium and stroma and achieve therapeutic levels in the aqueous humor. L. M. T. Col-

(12–5) Br. J. Ophthalmol. 67:115–118, February 1983.

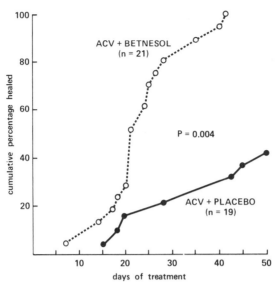

Fig 12–3.—Time to healing in patients with disciform keratitis given acyclovir and Betnesol (betamethasone) or acyclovir and placebo. (Courtesy of Collum, L.M.T., et al.: Br. J. Ophthalmol. 67:115–118, February 1983.)

lum, P. Logan (Dublin) and T. Ravenscroft (Kent, England) evaluated the effect of topical acyclovir, alone and combined with dilute steroid drops, in 40 patients with a clinical diagnosis of disciform keratitis. All patients were treated with 3% acyclovir ophthalmic ointment and then were assigned to treatment with 0.01% betamethasone drops or a placebo in a double-blind design. Treatment was given to the infected eye 5 times daily. Drops of 1% homatropine also were used; the eye was not padded.

The 19 patients treated with acyclovir alone and the 21 also given steroid drops were comparable in most clinical respects. The latter patients healed in a median of 21 days, but 11 of the patients treated with acyclovir alone were withdrawn from the study because of deterioration or a failure to improve within 2 weeks (Fig 12–3). Similar results were obtained when patients receiving steroids at the outset were excluded from analysis. Healing occurred significantly more rapidly in the patients given both acyclovir and steroids. Both uveitis and corneal thickness tended to respond more to combined treatment. Changes in visual acuity were similar in the 2 treatment groups, but 4 patients given acyclovir alone and 1 given combined treatment had worsening acuity. The only adverse event was mild, transient unctate keratopathy reported in 3 patients.

Combined antiviral and steroid therapy appears indicated in the management of disciform keratitis. A rapid clinical response is consistently obtained with virtually no adverse effects using acyclovir in combination with diluted steroid drops.

▶ ↓ We are still learning about the side effects of timolol. In the first of the following 2 articles, the more common contraindication of bronchospastic pulmonary disease is discussed. In the second article, however, a new problem is described. Timolol not only dangerously masks hypoglycemic symptoms in diabetic patients, but appears to inhibit their response to the administration of glucose. This is only the second such report, but timolol should be prescribed with considerable caution for patients with fragile diabetes. ◀

12–6   **Respiratory Arrest Following First Dose of Timolol Ophthalmic Solution.** Timolol maleate is a nonselective β blocker used as an ophthalmic solution to treat glaucoma. However, therapeutic doses can cause a significant reduction in airflow in patients with bronchospastic pulmonary disease. David S. Prince and Nathan H. Carliner (Univ. of Maryland, Baltimore) report findings in a patient who had a potentially fatal respiratory arrest within 30 minutes of receiving the first dose of timolol ophthalmic solution.

Man, 67, was receiving treatment for chronic obstructive lung disease, noncritical calcific aortic stenosis, essential hypertension, and glaucoma. He was taking hydrochlorothiazide, theophylline, and metaproterenol. Moderate obstructive lung disease, reported 7 months earlier, did not respond to bronchodilator therapy. Timolol in a 0.5% solution was prescribed because of progression of glaucoma despite pilocarpine treatment. Shortness of breath began within 5 minutes of instillation of a drop of solution in each eye and was not relieved by inhalation of metaproterenol. Dyspnea progressed rapidly, marked cyanosis developed, and the patient became unresponsive and apneic. Ventilatory assistance was instituted before admission to the hospital, where an endotracheal tube was inserted for mechanical ventilation. Intravenous aminophylline, steroids, and aerosolized isoetharine were administered. Wheezing was observed bilaterally when the patient began to recover. The arterial blood pH was 7.07; the Pco_2, 93 mm Hg; and the Po_2, 197 mm Hg during 50% oxygen inhalation. The patient was extubated after 17 hours despite intermittent wheezing.

Timolol probably provoked bronchospasm in this patient. Patients with bronchospastic lung disease who are candidates for timolol treatment should receive the first dose under supervision and should continue to be closely followed up for as long as timolol therapy is administered. Spirometry is useful before and after topical administration of the drug. Patients with obstructive airway disease may be critically dependent on β-adrenergic stimulation for the maintenance of airway patency, and timolol should be used only as a last resort when other methods have failed to control glaucoma.

12–7   **Ophthalmic Timolol Treatment Causing Altered Hypoglycemic Response in a Diabetic Patient.** Only one previous report has appeared of a dangerous change in the pattern of hypoglycemic episodes in a diabetic patient due to timolol maleate therapy. Tryg

---

(12–6) Chest 84:640–641, November 1983.
(12–7) Arch. Intern. Med. 143:1627, August 1983.

M. Velde and Fran E. Kaiser (Univ. of Minnesota, Minneapolis) report data on a similar case.

Man, 65, with type II diabetes, had received 1 to 4 units of Semilente and 25 units of lente insulin each morning for 25 years and had about 1 hypoglycemic episode a month. Open-angle glaucoma had been treated with ophthalmic solutions of pilocarpine and epinephrine. Timolol was substituted for epinephrine because of conjunctival irritation. One drop of 0.25% solution was used in each eye twice daily. A 0.5% solution was substituted within 2 months. The patient began to have 2 to 3 hypoglycemic episodes a month. Changes in mental status, rather than sweating or uneasiness, were first noticed. Far more glucose was needed than previously to reverse the episodes. Two reactions associated with grand mal seizures occurred, and timolol therapy was discontinued. The patient continued to have several hypoglycemic reactions a month with sweating and uneasiness, which were rapidly reversed by ingestion of a candy bar or a few packets of sugar. No further seizures or changes in mental status occurred.

Hypoglycemic episodes progressed to the point of dysfunction of the CNS before being detected when this patient was receiving timolol therapy for glaucoma. Relative resistance to glucose administration also was observed. There is considerable evidence that nonselective β-blockade can influence recovery from hypoglycemia. Systemic β-blockade blunts catecholamine-mediated hypoglycemic symptoms and metabolic compensatory mechanisms, both of which are important in prompt recovery from hypoglycemia.

Caution is needed in even using topical β-adrenergic blockers in diabetic patients who are prone to hypoglycemia.

12–8 **Aminocaproic Acid Decreases Secondary Hemorrhage After Traumatic Hyphema.** To determine whether administration of aminocaproic acid can reduce the incidence of secondary hemorrhage after nonperforating ocular trauma, and whether it can do so in the currently recommended dosage, John J. McGetrick, Lee M. Jampol, Morton F. Goldberg, Marcel Frenkel, and Richard G. Fiscella (Univ. of Illinois, Chicago) prospectively studied data on 48 consecutive patients (49 eyes) aged 6 to 40 years during a 6-month period. Excluded were those with sickle hemoglobin or a history of intravascular coagulopathy, pregnant patients, and those requiring immediate surgery. Males comprised 81% of the study group.

Assignment to treatment with aminocaproic acid or placebo was done in a double-blind fashion by computerized randomization. Twenty-eight (57%) patients received aminocaproic acid, 100 mg/kg orally every 4 hours up to a maximal dose of 5 g every 4 hours (30 gm/day) for 5 days; oral placebo was given to 20 (43%) patients every 4 hours for 5 days. Admission orders included no reading, patch and shield to the involved eye, 1% atropine sulfate 4 times a day to the affected eye, and oral acetaminophen up to 650 mg as needed for pain; no aspirin was given.

(12–8) Arch. Ophthalmol. 101:1031–1033, July 1983.

One (3.6%) of 28 eyes in patients given aminocaproic acid rebled, whereas 7 (33.3%) of 21 eyes in patients given placebo rebled; this difference was statistically significant ($P < .01$). In the aminocaproic acid-treated group 19 (68%) patients received the maximal dose (5 gm every 4 hours, 30 gm/24 hours); the other patients received lower doses according to their weight. Comparison of the incidence of secondary hemorrhage in the group receiving the maximal dose of aminocaproic acid (5%) with that in the placebo-treated group (33%) was statistically significantly different ($P < .05$). Nausea or vomiting occurred in 6 (21%) patients given aminocaproic acid; when treatment was stopped in 2 of these patients, 1 rebled subsequently. Visual acuity on admission and final visual acuity showed no significant difference between the 2 groups (table). All hyphemas in the aminocaproic acid-treated group initially filled less than 25% of the anterior chamber; in the placebo group, 86% of the hyphemas filled less than 25%. Clotted blood was visibly present in the anterior chamber for a mean of 4.5 days in the aminocaproic acid-treated group, and for a mean of 6.3 days in the placebo group.

Secondary hemorrhage usually occurs between the second and sixth days after initial trauma and is probably related to clot lysis and retraction from the previously traumatized blood vessels. Aminocaproic

INITIAL AND FINAL VISUAL ACUITIES

	No. (%) of Eyes	
Acuity	Aminocaproic Acid	Placebo
Initial Values		
≥6/12 or better	11 (39.3)	6 (28.6)
6/15-6/30	7 (25.0)	4 (19.0)
6/60-6/120	1 (3.6)	3 (14.0)
Counting fingers	3 (10.7)	2 (9.5)
Hand motion	2 (7.1)	1 (4.8)
Light perception	3 (10.7)	5 (23.8)
No light perception	0	0
Central steady fixation	1 (3.6)	0
Final Values		
≥6/12	22 (78.6)	14 (66.6)
6/15-6/30	1 (3.6)	3 (14.0)
6/60-6/120	2 (7.1)	3 (14.0)
Counting fingers	1 (3.6)	0
Hand motion	0	0
Light perception	1 (3.6)	0
No light perception	0	1 (4.8)
Central steady fixation	1 (3.6)	0

(Courtesy of McGetrick, J.J., et al.: Arch. Ophthalmol. 101:1031–1033, July 1983; copyright 1983, American Medical Association.)

acid, an antifibrinolytic agent, prevents the conversion of plasmino-
gen to plasmin, preventing or delaying clot dissolution. Aminocaproic
acid therapy is contraindicated when an intravascular clotting process is present and during pregnancy. Caution should be observed
with its use in patients who have cardiac, hepatic, renal, or sickle cell
disease. Also, care must be taken not to discontinue aminocaproic
acid therapy owing to nausea or other mild adverse reactions, because
there is an increased risk of secondary hemorrhage when therapy is
discontinued prematurely. If prochlorperazine does not stop nausea
and vomiting, the dosage of aminocaproic acid should be decreased
rather than discontinued completely.

▶ [Aminocaproic acid is an antifibrinolytic agent which should slow clot dissolution
and theoretically give more time for traumatized vessels to heal. Its efficacy in traumatic
hyphema has been debated, but this study suggests it may reduce secondary bleeding
in those patients in whom there are no systemic diseases contraindicating its use.] ◀

12-9 **Incidence of Serious or Fatal Accidents During Fluorescein
Angiography.** L. Zografos (Lausanne, France) conducted a survey involving 260 clinics in 30 different countries, comprising 594,687 angiographies. However, these figures should not be viewed as indicative of
the total number of angiographies practiced in these countries or the
world, since questionnaires were sent only to the principal ophthalmologic centers, and responses were received from only 60% of these.

There were 12 fatal accidents (1 in 49,577 angiographies) and 33
serious incidents (1 in 18,020 angiographies); the latter included only
accidents that occurred during the course of or immediately following
fluorescein angiography and necessitating reanimation.

The total number of angiographies affected in a particular clinic
reflects the experience of its personnel and their ability to respond to
the various problems which may arise in the course of this procedure.
Among 123 clinics in which less than 1,000 angiographies were performed, 7 accidents were reported, which represents 1 accident in
5,666 angiographies, reflecting a risk factor clearly elevated from the
global figure of 1 accident in 13,215 procedures. It may be assumed
that the inexperience of the examiners also increases the patient's
anxiety during an exceptional examination linked to a menacing ocular pathologic condition—a situation undoubtedly contributive to a
cardiovascular accident.

Although the age of the patient would not seem to play a role in frequency of accidents, it certainly influences its severity. Moreover, a history of arterial hypertension, diabetes, coronary pathology, or vascular
sclerosis clearly represents a predisposing factor. On the other hand,
neither time elapsed after injection nor concentration of fluorescein
would seem to play a role in the frequency of accidents. Still, the total
number of accidents is noteworthy for an examination considered inof-
fensive. One should insist on qualified personnel and avoid the practice

(12–9) J. Fr. Ophtalmol. 6:495–506, 1983.

of this procedure in elderly patients whose general health is poor.

▶ [It is obvious that fluorescein angiography is not an entirely benign diagnostic procedure. Nonetheless, all would not agree with the author's opinion that elderly patients with poor health be excluded. It is this elderly population that have the treatable neovascular membranes and proliferative retinopathies amenable to laser therapy. Perhaps the best approach is a carefully acquired history and qualified personnel.] ◀

13. Surgery

Yag Laser Photodisruption

MORTON F. GOLDBERG, M.D.

Eye and Ear Infirmary
University of Illinois, Chicago

The availability of YAG (yttrium-aluminum-garnet) lasers in North America for the past 1 to 2 years has enabled ophthalmologists to assess personally the indications, techniques, and complications of this important new therapeutic modality. The overwhelming European enthusiasm for this technique has been reaffirmed for some clinical indications, and characteristic complications have also been discovered. Pathogenesis of the complications and long-term results have yet to be documented in detail in this country, but our preliminary conclusions clearly indicate that YAG laser photodisruption has a definite place in modern ophthalmic surgery. At the time of this writing, however, the Food and Drug Administration continues to categorize YAG lasers as investigative devices, and distribution of instruments by their manufacturers has been greatly curtailed. Nonetheless, it is obvious to those ophthalmologists using the initially distributed instruments that a new era of "noninvasive" surgery has dawned with substantial benefits to patients, physicians, and to society at large. In many cases, complicated diseases are now amenable to outpatient, noninvasive therapy, and costs that previously would have been imposed by operating room usage and inpatient care have disappeared. The following summary discusses indications, techniques, and complications of YAG laser therapy for some common ophthalmic diseases.

I. Indications

REALISTIC INDICATIONS

Pupillary Membranes

Pupillary membranes constitute the most common and most appropriate indication for YAG laser therapy. After conventional intracapsular or extracapsular cataract extraction, a variety of pupillary membranes may form, including opacified portions of retained anterior capsule, posterior capsule, both capsules (with or without cortical debris), and others. These capsules may become opacified in either aphakic or pseudophakic eyes. In the case of pseudophakic eyes, opacified capsular material may occur in the presence of intraocular lenses placed in the anterior chamber, in the pupillary plane, or in the posterior chamber. All of these capsules are amenable to YAG laser photodisruption, and preliminary results obtained in our and in many other centers indicate clearly an extremely high (more than 95%) anatomical success rate is opening such capsules to create optically clear spaces.

Postuveitic pupillary membranes can be more difficult to open than pupillary membranes after cataract extraction. Postuveitic membranes are often thicker and denser than the thin membranes that characterize the postoperative aphakic or pseudophakic eye. They also tend to be found in eyes that have had various other complications, including loss of transparency of the cornea (due to chronic inflammation or secondary glaucoma) and vascularized posterior synechiae, which may bleed during photodisruption or which may cover most of the postuveitic membrane. Such eyes frequently require invasive surgery such as pars plana membranectomy or translimbal membranectomy with scissors, punches, or automated vitrectomy machines.

Complications of YAG laser membranotomies in the pupillary space are more common than one would have believed from the initial European literature. Most of them, if detected early and if treated properly, leave no permanent sequelae and are easily managed. These complications include secondary glaucoma, which often occurs during the first 24 hours after treatment and which is most efficiently detected within several hours after treatment; transient iritis; and, rarely, microhyphemas, which are almost invariably self-limited. Although some ophthalmologists have recommended routine administration of antiglaucomatous agents (for example, Timoptic) and corticosteroids following YAG laser capsulotomy or membranotomy, we have used these preparations only when the diagnosis of laser-induced glaucoma or iritis has been made. In virtually all cases, topical administration of these drugs has controlled the complications within a matter of hours or days. Nevertheless, because the pressure peaks following YAG laser membranotomy can be substantial, occasionally exceeding 50 mm Hg, this complication should not be considered lightly. Preliminary investigations using tonographic techniques suggest that the transient glaucoma is related to a decrease in outflow facility, possibly due to liberated lenticular or proteinaceous debris that occludes the trabecular meshwork.

Additional complications, which have been reported in only a handful of cases relative to the large number of patients treated, include corneal edema and retinal detachment. In the case of corneal edema, it is not known whether the corneas were already predisposed to decompensate from previous intraocular lens or other forms of surgery or whether the corneal disease is a direct consequence of YAG laser treatment. If the laser itself is responsible, it is possible that the shock waves themselves or scattered debris liberated by them result in physical damage to the corneal endothelium. It is also possible that the infrared irradiation itself has exceeded the threshold for direct damage to the corneal endothelium during the initial treatment sessions. This is particularly true if optical breakdown occurs in or near the corneal endothelium.

In the case of retinal detachment, it is presently unknown if these aphakic eyes would have developed retinal detachments even without YAG laser therapy. Aphakic eyes are obviously more susceptible to retinal detachment than they would have been in their phakic state. As yet, the cause-and-effect relationship between YAG laser membranotomy and subsequent retinal detachment has not been proved, but the chronologic association of retinal detachment with preceding YAG laser membranotomy in a few cases is important enough that all patients should have this and other potential complications explained to them in the process of obtaining informed consent. Furthermore, all patients having undergone YAG laser membranotomy should have their peripheral fundi inspected thereafter to detect retinal breaks that may have occurred. Prophylactic photocoagulation of the retinal breaks utilizing, for example, an argon laser, may be extremely beneficial.

Iridotomy and Coreplasty

Cutting peripheral holes in the iris to relieve pupillary block is a relatively straightforward indication for YAG laser therapy. To date, experience with the argon laser far exceeds that with the YAG laser, but it is apparent that the success rate is higher with the YAG laser. Far fewer laser shots are necessary, and the opening tends to be substantially larger than with the argon laser. The shape and size of the iris opening are somewhat unpredictable, however, and long ovoid tears may occur. The rate of immediate bleeding from the torn iris is also substantially higher with the YAG laser than with the argon laser, but, for the most part, these microhyphemas are cleared from the anterior chamber quickly and without permanent complications. Occasionally, iris perforation will not be possible if the cornea is translucent from high intraocular pressure or some other corneal disease. In most circumstances, however, the YAG laser is an efficient means of cutting a hole in the peripheral iris. Some measure of control over the size and shape of the opening and also the ease of perforation can be obtained by pretreating the peripheral iris with a thermal laser burn, such as that from an argon laser or from a YAG laser operating in the thermal mode. Immediate treatment in the co-agulated, stretched iris is followed in most cases by a round opening confined to the pretreated area. Similar techniques can be employed for making a linear opening in an updrawn pupil (optical iridotomy). To date, the possible long-term effects of YAG laser iridotomy on the crystalline lens have not been described. Short-term studies, however, report no induced cataracts thus far.

Incarcerated Vitreous

Many eyes withstand vitreous incarcerated in limbal wounds with-out complication. If complications such as updrawn pupil, corneal edema, or cystoid macular edema supervene, however, an attempt at surgical correction is worth considering. It is technically possible in most cases to cut vitreous strands by YAG laser photodisruption near their areas of insertion at the limbus. As a result, updrawn or notched pupils and iris crowded into the anterior chamber angle can be returned to their normal anatomical configurations. There is no doubt, therefore, that the anatomical state of the anterior segment of the eye can be restored to a more nearly normal appearance. Whether or not visual acuity will be beneficially affected due to dehydration of the cornea or to relief of macular edema has not yet been unequivo-cally established.

It is technically easiest to cut the incarcerated vitreous where the gelatinous sheets come to their narrowest dimensions. This area is usually found immediately adjacent to the points of incarceration. Thus, explosions from the YAG laser must occur close to the corneal endothelium, trabecular meshwork, and face of the ciliary body in the anterior chamber angle. Common complications, therefore, include di-rect explosions at the level of the corneal endothelium and local hem-orrhages emanating from the face of the ciliary body into the anterior chamber. To date, these complications have been self-limited in our experience, but, as in all cases of YAG laser therapy, precise focus and awareness of the proximity of adjacent intraocular structures are essential if the complication rate is to be minimized.

Synechiolysis

Both anterior and posterior synechiolysis are also technically fea-sible by YAG laser photodisruption. Anterior synechiolysis is most easily accomplished after pretreatment with pilocarpine (to help re-store a central, circular pupil). If there is a sheet of vitreous between the anterior surface of the iris and the corneal endothelium, optical breakdown should occur within this vitreous material. Otherwise, di-rect explosions in the cornea are inevitable.

Posterior synechiolysis is most safely achieved when the eye is aphakic or pseudophakic. Pretreatment with a sympathomimetic agent is beneficial both in an attempt to reduce laser-induced hemorrhage and to help tear the posterior synechiae free once some initial cutting from laser explosions occurs. It has been claimed that the YAG laser is gentle enough to cut posterior synechiae off a crystalline lens. This would appear to be excessively hazardous in most circumstances, and is therefore presently contraindicated in our practice because disruption of the anterior lens capsule could easily occur and traumatic cataract thereby be induced.

Anterior and Midvitreous Bands

Cutting an anterior or midvitreous band can be attempted if there are optical indications or if the retina is being detached by a discrete vitreous band. It is safest to cut vitreous bands in an aphakic eye. If the crystalline lens is in situ, extreme caution should be observed because intravitreal explosions within approximately 3 to 4 mm of the posterior lens capsule can inadvertently rupture it and produce a traumatic cataract. Cutting of vitreous bands can also be attempted if a circumscribed band is causing clinically important traction on the retina, even if visual acuity is not currently compromised. In many cases, the vitreous band, upon careful inspection by contact lens biomicroscopy, proves to be not a single discrete structure, but rather a set of interdigitating membranous and meshlike tissues. Complete transection of these almost invisible structures is often difficult, and traction therefore may not be relieved despite partial vitreolysis.

Breakage of Residual Cortical Material

Breakage of residual cortical material is sometimes desirable to enhance spontaneous absorption of cataractous debris left in an eye following incomplete cataract extraction. Clarification of the visual axis can be achieved quicker in certain circumstances and the rate of absorption of the lens material can also be accelerated. Complications include low-grade iritis and trabecular blockade with secondary glaucoma. These are usually easily managed by topical administration of appropriate medications.

POTENTIAL INDICATIONS

Posterior Vitreous Bands

Deep or posterior vitreous bands interfering with the visual axis or causing sufficient traction to detach the macula or cause recurrent vitreous hemorrhage may be cut by YAG laser photodisruption. Substantial hazards exist, including hemorrhage from blood within intravitreal bands, failure to appreciate the full extent of a vitreous membrane (which superficially looks like a discrete band, but which in reality represents just one sheet of extensive interlacing vitreous membranes), and explosions near enough to the surface of the retina that shock-induced chorioretinal trauma or hemorrhages occur. Extreme care should be taken when optical breakdown occurs at about 3 to 4 mm from the retina, since the shock wave can be powerful enough to rupture the retinal tissue, a retinal blood vessel, the macula, or optic nerve head tissue. It is therefore best to avoid treating immediately anterior to the optic nerve head, the macula, and major retinal vessels. Relatively safe places to treat include intravitreal areas anterior to previously photocoagulated fundus (photocoagulation scars that have been created in the past). Small chorioretinal hemorrhages are not uncommon when treating close to the wall of the eye, but somewhat surprisingly rhegmatogenous retinal detachments appear to be infrequent after such complications. Since the hemorrhages may be initiated at the level of the choroid, with subsequent passage of blood through ruptured Bruch's membrane and sensory retina into the vitreous, it is possible that longer follow-up will disclose the presence of choriovitreal or chorioretinal neovascularization. Only time will tell. Treating in the deep vitreous is often complicated by the presence of murky fluid caused by previous hemorrhage, such as that associated with proliferative diabetic retinopathy or by laser-induced bleeding. In these circumstances, rather high energy levels must be achieved to create optical breakdown, and the risk to the retina from large shock waves is substantial. It is best to terminate the procedure and try again on another day. To date, convincing evidence that deep vitreolysis with the YAG laser is sufficiently safe and effective to warrant widespread use has not been provided.

Opening a Sealed Filtration Bleb

Using appropriate gonioprisms, explosions can be made with a YAG laser in the region of the trabecular meshwork. Such explosions, on occasion, may open a sealed bleb. Large series of cases with appropriate follow-up have not been reported, and the role of the YAG laser in this clinical situation has not yet been established. Similarly, the use of the YAG laser as a primary therapeutic modality for creation of a filtering bleb or as an adjunct to surgical creation of a filtering bleb has not been established, despite its advocacy in the literature.

Thermal Usage of the YAG Laser

Certain commercial instruments, such as the Lasag Microruptor II, have the capacity of creating relatively long discharges (milliseconds) so that linear absorption and thermal coagulation can occur, analogous to that achieved with argon and krypton laser photocoagulators.

Advocates of this form of experimental therapy have suggested that the YAG laser, used in the thermal mode, may be useful for laser trabeculoplasty, coagulation of the iris prior to iridotomy or coreplasty, coagulation of vascularized vitreous bands prior to photodisruption, for fundus coagulation of proliferative retinopathies or of disciform macular degeneration, and for transscleral cyclophotocoagulation. Compelling evidence with long-term follow-up has not yet been presented.

Techniques

Obtain Informed Consent

As in all operative interventions, appropriately informed consent must be obtained from the patient before inception of therapy. The patient should be made aware of the investigative nature of YAG lasers and of the limited follow-up data currently available. Alternative forms of therapy should be explained and questions answered. Loss of vision can occur from YAG laser therapy through a variety of means, including corneal decompensation, glaucoma, iritis and its complications, retinal detachment, cystoid macular edema, and so on. Whether all of these complications are a direct result of the YAG laser has not yet been established, but patients should be made fully aware of the potential for loss of vision. As in all cases of surgical therapy, the risk-to-benefit ratio must be assessed by the ophthalmologist and explained to the patient. In most cases, the therapeutic options for the patient include invasive surgery (such as surgical discission, pars plana or translimbal vitrectomy, or membranectomy, and so on). In some circumstances, an individual patient may elect to maintain the status quo and trust to the natural course of the disease. In other circumstances, the patient may elect invasive surgery. In most cases, however, the YAG laser provides a preferable option, and most patients, when confronted with a serious intraocular disease affecting vision, prefer the noninvasive nature of the YAG laser despite its experimental nature and the lack of long-term follow-up data.

Capsulotomy and Membranotomy

It is important to be aware of the pupillary axis so that the opening in the opacified tissue will coincide with it. It is thus desirable to begin the YAG laser procedure with the pupil in its normal configuration. If it becomes technically difficult to make a sufficiently large opening, the pupil can be dilated once a central opening has been made. If the pupil is dilated prior to beginning therapy, it is frequently difficult to know the exact location of the pupillary axis. Thus, an opening larger than that required for visual improvement must be made to insure that the pupillary axis falls within the opened membrane.

The ophthalmologist should be aware of the location and type of any intraocular lens. The initial shot of the laser should, in general, be made just off the visual axis in the event pitting of the lens occurs. Once the appropriate dosage parameters are developed (number of millijoules, number of pulses per burst, etc.), the visual axis can then be treated directly. Patients with glass intraocular lenses should not be treated because shattering of the glass can occur. It is relatively safe to treat pupillary membranes adjacent to polymethylmethacry-late intraocular lenses because, even if pitting occurs, it is rare for visual acuity to be degraded. Some glare, however, may be created, but this has not proved to be disabling in our experience. Intraocular lenses with their convex surface placed posteriorly may be difficult to treat effectively if the posterior capsule is adherent to the posterior curve. It is extremely difficult in such circumstances to cut the membrane without pitting the intraocular llens, because the posterior surface of the intraocular lens is not in a single plane of focus, but is continuously changing from one point to the next.

It is essential to know if a patient iridectomy is present at the time of creating a laser-induced capsulotomy. If not, it is possible for vitreous material to herniate through the opening in the membrane and cause pupillary block. This is particularly likely to occur if the eye is aphakic. Although it is less apt to occur if the eye is pseudophakic, vitreous material can herniate through the opening and around the implant into the anterior chamber, and blockage of the pupil or of the trabecular meshwork can occur in this fashion. Accordingly, the surgeon may wish to create a laser-induced iridotomy at the time of capsulotomy. In many circumstances, this is not absolutely necessary, but the patient should be followed up carefully for the occurrence of glaucoma, and, if it develops because of these considerations, YAG laser iridotomy is then definitely indicated.

Whether or not a large or a small opening should be made depends on the status of the eye and the ophthalmologist's prediction for future complications and the need for additional therapy. If the eye is aphakic, a small opening may minimize vitreous prolapse, thereby protecting against the development of pupillary block or of vitreocorneal touch. If the eye has substantial guttata, a small opening again may minimize vitreous prolapse and the possibility of vitreocorneal touch and eventual corneal decompensation. On the other hand, if the patient is known to have a retinal pathologic condition requiring careful ophthalmoscopic inspection, laser photocoagulation of the fundus, or eventual retinal surgery, a large opening should be made.

With respect to the technique of opening a posterior capsule, it is desirable, as in the case of surgical discission, to cut at right angles to tension lines so that the opening naturally enlarges as the first cuts are made. Making a central cruciate cut with the YAG laser is also often sufficient, and successive explosions should be placed at the extremities of the initial cuts in the membranes. With this technique, the openings tend to "unzip" themselves. If a particularly good view of the fundus is desired, a circular opening can be made and a trephination of the membrane can be accomplished. After which, the membrane can be cut into small fragments or simply allowed to fall gravitationally into the inferior vitreous.

At the start of the membranotomy, a deliberate attempt to place the explosions just posterior to the membrane in the anterior vitreous, rather than within the membrane, is desirable to protect the intraocular lens. With the Lasag Microruptor II, this is achieved automatically with a dial setting on the console. In other commercial instruments, this technique can be accomplished by deliberate defocusing, utilizing the dioptric scale on the slit-lamp oculars.

Use of specially made contact lenses is highly desirable, since the eye is mechanically stabilized, the image is magnified, and the cone angle of the laser beam is increased. This enables optical breakdown to occur at lower energy settings. Lenses now commercially available include the Lasag series, the Abraham lens, and the Peyman 12.5-mm lens manufactured by Ocular Instruments. Sample initial settings with the Lasag instrument are 1 to 2 millijoules in fundamental mode at 1 pulse per discharge. After the focusing and the dosage parameters are established, the pulse rate can be increased to 4 pulses per burst even in the presence of an intraocular lens. However, if pitting of the lens is occurring at 1 pulse per burst, the rate of firing should not be increased for fear of making the pitting even worse. Fankhauser has recommended that a pulse energy of 4 to 5 millijoule should not be exceeded for fear of damaging the intraocular lens severely. Most of our retropseudophakic membranes have been opened with fundamental mode therapy, and the multimode capability has rarely been required to date.

Iridotomy

It is desirable to attempt iridotomies where the cornea is clearest. In addition, the iridotomy should be made in the peripheral iris so that the distance between the explosion and the crystalline lens is maximized. However, an iridotomy made too far toward the iris root can explode the greater arterial circle. Even if the greater arterial circle itself is not damaged, microhyphemas frequently occur after YAG laser iridotomy. These almost invariably stop spontaneously or can be stopped by moderate pressure on the eye with the contact lens.

Contact lenses available for iridotomy include the Lasag series, the Abraham anterior segment lens, and the Peyman anterior segment lens. Some ophthalmologists prefer to pretreat the iris with thermal mode YAG or with an argon laser. The advantages include possible coagulation of small blood vessels in the iris and possible stretching of the iris so that penetration by the YAG laser is accomplished with less tendency to bleed and at lower energy settings. In any event, the contact lens is particularly desirable, and it is helpful to keep the beam perpendicular to the surface of the iris. Sample initial settings utilizing the Lasag Microruptor II include 4 to 6 millijoule in fundamental mode at 4 pulses per burst. Fankhauser has recommended that the energy level not exceed 16 millijoule. We have rarely found it necessary to exceed 8 millijoule.

Incarcerated Vitreous, Updrawn Pupil, and Anterior Synechiae

Pretreatment with topical pilocarpine has proved beneficial in our experience because pupillary sphincter activity helps to restore the normal anterior segment configuration once restraining bands in the anterior chamber angle are cut with the YAG laser. Use of a specially designed contact lens is essential because some incarcerated vitreous bands are simply too strong to be cut without the effects of the special goniolens in place. The Lasag angle contact lenses are particularly helpful in this regard. Incarcerated vitreous strands can be exceedingly difficult to see during YAG laser photodisruption. Furthermore, if any fibrin or blood collects in the anterior chamber, the ability to achieve optical breakdown is diminished, and it is wise to discontinue treatment until another day. In any event, magnification, illumination, and visual contrast must be maximized. If a beam splitter is present in the delivery system, it should be removed. The power of the oculars should be changed so that the highest power eyepieces available are used. The room itself should be pitch black. After the incarcerated vitreous is cut by the YAG laser, the angle of the anterior chamber should be checked on the best available slit lamp. Frequently, gossamer or cobweb-like strands will still be incarcerated in the limbal wound, and angle landmarks must be memorized so that these tiny strands can be found and treated with the laser delivery system. Unfortunately, the laser delivery systems do not appear to resolve optically the finest vitreous strands as well as the best available slit lamps.

Sample initial settings are 4 to 6 millijoule in the multimode format with 4 to 9 pulses per burst. It is wise not to exceed 8 to 10 millijoule. Care must be taken to prevent optical breakdown near the corneal endothelium or the face of the ciliary body in the anterior chamber angle. Frequent hemorrhages from the face of the ciliary body occur doing this procedure but can be controlled by moderate pressure exerted via the contact lens.

This form of YAG laser photodisruption can be technically difficult and tedious, and repeated sessions separated by days or weeks are often necessary.

Deep Vitreous Bands

It is essential to have detailed knowledge of the extent of deep vitreal bands prior to beginning YAG laser photodisruption. It is desirable, therefore, to make a careful biomicroscopic drawing of the bands and associated membranes. Landmarks must include any vessels within the membranes, the location of the optic disk and macula, and the proximity, if any, to underlying major retinal blood vessels and old or fresh photocoagulation scars in the fundus. In addition, ultrasonic determination of the position of the band relative to the wall of the eye and adjacent retina should be made before beginning therapy. Photodisruption should not be attempted within 3 to 4 mm of vital retinal or optic nerve structures. Similarly, photodisruption should not be attempted within 3 to 4 mm of the posterior lens capsule if the crystalline lens remains in situ.

Specialized contact lenses (the Peyman 18- and 25-mm lenses) are important in mid- and deep vitreous photodisruption. The conventional Goldmann fundus contact lenses do not appear as useful in this respect, because they do not increase the cone angle. Sample initial settings are 6 to 7 millijoule in a multimode format with 4 to 6 pulses per burst. Fankhauser has recommended that maximal pulse energy should be approximately 5 to 10 millijoule when the laser focus is about 3 mm from the posterior capsule of the crystalline lens. He also recommends that the pulse energy should not exceed about 4 to 5 millijoule when the laser focus is about 3 mm from the retina. Our patients have frequently required substantially higher pulse energy due to murkiness of the vitreous associated with previous intravitreal hemorrhaging, and we have avoided retinal trauma in these cases with energy settings of 10 to 14 millijoule. Nevertheless, this is an extremely hazardous undertaking, and the energy setting should be initiated at a low level and increased only as necessary.

As in the case of anterior vitreolysis, deep vitreolysis often requires repeated sessions and great patience. The proper indications and techniques of deep vitreolysis are in a state of flux, and the proper role of the YAG laser in this area has not yet been defined.

Postoperative Management

The eye should be inspected several hours following treatment and again after approximately 1 day, 1 week, 1 month, and 3 months, respectively. Additional checkups may be required. Inspection for best-corrected visual acuity, iridocyclitis, glaucoma, anatomical status of the anterior chamber angle, and presence or absence of retinal breaks and detachments should be conducted. The patient should be instructed to call the ophthalmologist immediately if any new symptoms occur.

13–1 **Effect of Indomethacin in Preventing Surgically Induced Miosis.** Miosis from surgical trauma is a frequent problem in extracapsular cataract operations. It can occur despite preoperative dilation with anticholinergic and sympathomimetic agents and may impede the removal of lens material and the implantation of an intraocular lens in the posterior capsule. Prostaglandins appear to be at least partly responsible for the miosis. H. C. J. Keulen-de Vos, G. Van Rij, J. C. G. Renardel de Lavalette, and J. T. G. Jansen (Erasmus Univ., Rotterdam, Netherlands) undertook a double-blind study of preoperative treatment with 0.5% indomethacin to prevent miosis during extracapsular cataract extraction. Sixty-four patients with senile cataract, whose mean age was 71 years, participated in the study. Study patients had 0.5% aqueous indomethacin drops instilled twice the night before operation and three times on the day of operation, from 2 hours to 15 minutes before operation. Mydriasis was achieved with combined 0.5% tropicamide and 5% phenylephrine drops. The study and placebo groups were comparable.

Pupillary constriction from the start of operation through irrigation and aspiration was less in indomethacin-pretreated patients than in those given placebo drops. Mean pupillary constrictions were 2.4 and 3.1 mm, respectively. The difference in pupillary constriction was greatest after expression of the lens nucleus. No significant group differences were found in relation to the length of operation or delay in operating. Pupillary constriction did not differ in relation to iris color.

Pretreatment with topical indomethacin drops before extracapsular cataract operations with lens implantation significantly inhibited miosis in this study, presumably through inhibition of prostaglandin synthesis. Relative widening of the operative field resulted, making removal of lens material and implantation of the intraocular lens easier and thereby minimizing peroperative and postoperative complications.

▶ [There are many variables affecting pupil size during cataract surgery. The authors of this article have performed a randomized trial and found that indomethacin seems helpful, although the effect was small.] ◀

▶ ↓ In the following 3 articles, the authors describe their experience with the pulse neodymium:YAG laser. The FDA has not made a final decision about its safety and effectiveness, but so many operations are being done that it is probably irrelevant. We are, however, beginning to see a few complications; pupillary block following capsulotomy is described in the third article. There is little doubt, however, that as long as extracapsular cataract extraction remains popular, the YAG laser will be an essential part of the procedure. Technology moves very rapidly, however, and we cannot guess what will be in vogue 10 years from now. One could reasonably guess, however, that a two-stage procedure may not survive without at least some modification. ◀

13–2 **Laser Photodisruptors: Damage Mechanisms, Instrument Design, and Safety** are discussed by Martin A. Mainster, David H.

(13–1) Br. J. Ophthalmol. 67:94–96, February 1983.
(13–2) Ophthalmology (Rochester) 90:973–991, August 1983.

Sliney, C. Davis Belcher III, and Sheldon M. Buzney. The short-pulse neodymium (Nd):yttrium-aluminum-garnet (YAG) crystal laser systems permit noninvasive incision of transparent intraocular structures. Disruption occurs from the delivery of great optical power to a small focal spot, rather than by light absorption in pigmented tissues, as with conventional lasers. The Nd:YAG laser photodisruptors consist of a Q-switched or mode-locked source, a delivery system producing a typical spot 25 to 50 μm in diameter, and a helium-neon laser providing a red aiming-focusing beam. These systems are designed chiefly to disrupt the lens capsule, pupillary membranes, and anterior vitreous bands. The extent of exposure of posterior segment structures to near-infrared radiation determine the safety of an Nd:YAG laser photodisruptor system. The effects of optical breakdown on the transmission of laser radiation were assessed using a developmental clinical laser system.

The mechanisms of disruption of transparent membranes by short-pulse Nd:YAG lasers are illustrated in Figure 13–1. The optical breakdown threshold in homogeneous substances generally is reduced with an increased pulse duration, an increased focal spot area, and a higher wavelength of incident laser light. The threshold is lowered by the presence of microscopic impurities in the target

Fig 13–1.—Short-pulse laser systems can disrupt transparent membranes by 3 nonlinear mechanisms: (1) very high irradiances disintegrate tissues in the focal volume, stripping electrons from atoms ("ionizing" them) and creating a "plasma," or a gaseous state consisting of electrons and ions; (2) the plasma expands outward rapidly, causing shock and acoustic (pressure) waves that disrupt tissue around the area of disintegration; and (3) latent stress in the membrane can cause additional disruption when the laser makes an incision. (Courtesy of Mainster, M.A., et al.: Ophthalmology (Rochester) 90:973–991, August 1983.)

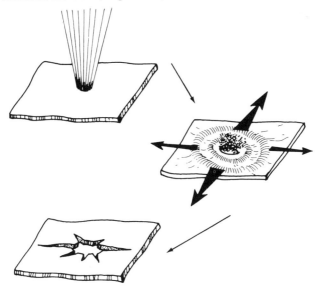

material, which act as sites for focal heating and starting electrons. The extent of the zone of mechanically disrupted tissue surrounding an area of optimal breakdown depends on the irradiance and total energy in the laser pulse, the time that the pulse sustains the plasma or other wave-producing effect, and the mechanical properties of the target tissues. The near-infrared radiation from an Nd:YAG laser is poorly absorbed by both hemoglobin and water, and therefore provides greater penetration of highly vascularized tissues than other types of laser radiation. The use of long-pulse Nd:YAG laser radiation in retinal photocoagulation has been proposed. The safety margin, however, is expected to be much lower than that with a continuous wave argon green or even a krypton red laser. The retinal damage threshold increases with the wavelength, as shown in Figure 13–2.

Short-pulse laser systems hold great promise in ophthalmic surgery, but the instrumentation is still evolving and potential hazards exist.

It is best to avoid photodisruptor use in hazy media, and to make sure that the focal plane of the beam is at least 5 mm anterior to the retina or posterior to the crystalline lens.

Fig 13–2.—Spectral transmission of human ocular media (*curve 1,* left ordinate scale) characterizes the percentage of light passing through the media at various wavelengths. The relative spectral absorption of the human retinal pigment epithelium and choroid (*curve 2,* right ordinate scale) characterizes the percentage of light absorbed in these tissues at various wavelengths. The relative spectral absorption measured in a second independent study (*curve 3,* right ordinate scale) may be more applicable to small spot sizes. Relevant laser wavelengths are indicated. The wavelength dependence of nonlinear optical breakdown (plasma formation) in ocular media cannot be predicted from the spectral transmission of the media. (Courtesy of Mainster, M.A., et al.: Ophthalmology (Rochester) 90:973–991, August 1983.)

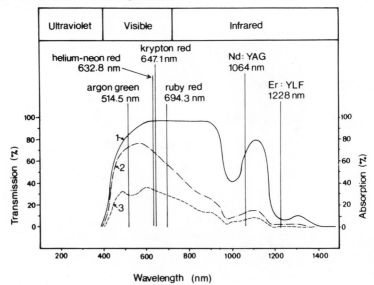

13–3 **Neodymium-YAG Laser for Posterior Capsulotomy.** The increase in extracapsular cataract extractions in the United States has spurred interest in management of the opaque posterior capsule. Arlo C. Terry, Walter J. Stark, A. Edward Maumenee, and Warren Fagadau (Johns Hopkins Hosp., Baltimore) used the neodymium-yttrium-aluminum-garnet (YAG) laser to perform posterior capsulotomy in 49 eyes undergoing extracapsular cataract extraction. Twenty-seven eyes had an implanted posterior chamber intraocular lens, 1 had an anterior chamber lens, and 2 had iris plane lenses. Capsulotomy was done an average of 21 months after cataract extraction. An average of 36 bursts was used to create an opening in the posterior capsule. A power setting of 2 millijoule was effective. All capsulotomies but 1 required only a single treatment session.

A clear pupillary space (Fig 13–3) was achieved in all eyes. Visual acuity improved by 1 or more Snellen lines in all but 4 eyes, and by 3 or more lines in 33 eyes. Acuity was 2 or more lines better than the best recorded after cataract extraction in 13 eyes. However, eyes did not return to the best acuity recorded after cataract extraction. The intraocular pressure increased by 4 mm Hg or more in 37 eyes, and was 50 mm Hg or higher in 4 eyes after capsulotomy, but only 2 eyes required treatment to control the intraocular pressure 4 months after treatment. Damage to the intraocular lens from laser treatment occurred in 12 eyes, but did not adversely affect visual acuity or produce inflammation. One eye had bleeding from iris neovascularization adjacent to the site of treatment. Specular microscopy showed no

Fig 13–3.—Clear pupillary opening is seen after discission of an opaque posterior capsule was achieved with the neodymium-yttrium/aluminum/garnet laser. (Courtesy of Terry, A.C., et al.: Am. J. Ophthalmol. 96:716–720, December 1983.)

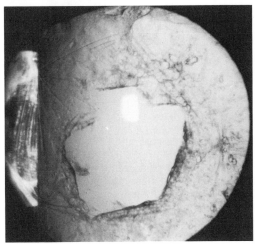

(13–3)   Am. J. Ophthalmol. 96:716–720, December 1983.

significant endothelial cell loss in the 14 eyes examined. No retinal damage was apparent.

The neodymium-YAG laser effectively cuts the opaque posterior capsule in patients having extracapsular cataract extraction, but further studies are needed to confirm the safety of the procedure before its widespread use. In 6 of 19 eyes without implants in the present series rupture of the anterior hyaloid face occurred with forward displacement of vitreous into the anterior chamber; a rhegmatogenous retinal detachment developed subsequently in 1 of these eyes.

13–4   **Pupillary Block Following Nd:YAG Laser Capsulotomy.** The use of the Nd:YAG (neodymium:yttrium-aluminum-garnet) laser for capsulotomy has been believed to be relatively free of complications. Jon M. Ruderman, Paul G. Mitchell, and Manus Kraff (Univ. of Illinois, Chicago) report a case in which pupillary block, elevated intraocular pressure, and transient loss of vision developed 5 hours after Nd:YAG laser capsulotomy.

Man, 23, was examined in July 1982 with a history of cataracts that resulted from stepping on an electric power cable in 1979. The cataracts had been treated by phacoemulsification and the patient claimed to have regained good visual acuity. During the next 3 years his vision deteriorated to a best-corrected acuity of 6/90, (20/300) and 6/120 (20/400) in the right and left eyes, respectively. The ocular examination was unremarkable except for partial opacification of the posterior capsules with Elschnig's pearls in both eyes. Laser interferometry (Rodenstock) indicated a visual potential of 6/15 (20/50) and 6/30 (20/100) in the right and left eyes, respectively. A cross-shaped Nd:YAG laser capsulotomy was performed in both eyes through 7-mm pupils previously dilated with tropicamide and phenylephrine (number of laser discharges, 300 OD and 319 OS; beam diameter, 50 μ). Immediately after the procedure the patient's best vision was 6/7.5 (20/25) in both eyes. There was minimal cell and flare in the anterior chamber, the pupillary aperture was clear, and the anterior hyaloid face was intact. Postoperative intraocular pressure was 18 mm Hg bilaterally. The patient was given a regimen of 1% prednisolone acetate, 3 times a day. Five hours after the operation he experienced pain in the right eye, along with nausea and vomiting. After 4 hours, vision in the right eye had greatly decreased and the patient was instructed to begin digital ocular massage and to report to the clinic.

Vision had improved considerably on arrival less than 1 hour later. Visual acuity was 6/30 (20/100) in the right eye and 6/7.5 (20/25) in the left eye. The conjunctiva of the right eye were hyperemic, the cornea showed microcystic edema, and the iris was in bombé configuration. Prolapse of the vitreous face into the anterior chamber was observed. The margins of the capsulotomy in the right eye could not be visualized through a nonreactive 4-mm pupil. The view of the fundus was hazy, but it seemed to be normal. Aphakic pupillary block by vitreous prolapse was diagnosed and the patient was immediately given 0.5% timolol eyedrops, 500 mg of acetazolamide, and 4 ounces of a glycerin solution orally. Immediate gonioscopy showed the angle to be closed, but the pupil dilated and the angle opened before the examination was completed. The iris fell back and the intraocular pressure dropped to 8 mm Hg.

(13–4)   Ophthalmic Surg. 14:418–419, May 1983.

Within 30 minutes the vision in the right eye had returned to 6/7.5 (20/25). It was now evident that the vitreous face had prolapsed into the anterior chamber, almost to the cornea, and that the capsulotomy was considerably wider than it had been at the conclusion of Nd:YAG laser surgery. Argon laser peripheral iridotomy was performed later the same day to prevent recurrence of the pupillary block.

This case represents a severe complication from Nd:YAG capsulotomy, which does not appear to have been previously reported. Ironically, the Nd:YAG laser could have been used to prevent or treat this complication if the surgeon had created an iridotomy or incised the anterior hyaloid face at the time of posterior capsulotomy. As a relatively high percentage of posterior capsules will eventually opacify, the surgeon who plans an extracapsular cataract extraction should consider performing a peripheral iridectomy at the time of surgery.

13–5 **Pupillary Block After Interocular Lens Implantation.** Pupillary block is a complication of cataract surgery that leads to peripheral anterior synechiae and chronic angle-closure glaucoma, a complication that may be avoided by combining cataract extraction with iridectomy. E. Michael Van Buskirk (Oregon Health Sciences Univ., Portland) reports data on 17 patients (table), aged 40 to 86 years, who had pupillary block that was detected 1 week to 3 years after intraocular lens implantation. Six types of anterior chamber lenses accounted for 16 of the incidents. One case is described below.

CLINICAL SUMMARY OF 17 CASES OF PUPILLARY BLOCK AFTER INTRAOCULAR LENS IMPLANTATION

Patient No.	Age (yrs)	Cataract Procedure*	Intraocular Lens Used	No. of Iridotomies[†]	Time Elapsed to Pupillary Block	Peripheral Anterior Synechiae (clock hrs)	Intraocular Pressure (mm Hg)
1	72	ICCE	Leiske	1	3 mos	8	20
2	75	ICCE	Choyce	1	3 yrs	8	38
3	67	ICCE	Tennant-Anchor	1	3 mos	12	36
4	72	ICCE	Leiske	1	Unknown	12	52
5	40	ECCE	Tennant-Anchor	1	1 to 2 mos	0	14
6	77	ECCE	Sinsky	0	3 wks	1	22
7	72	ICCE	Optiflex-Cilco	1	2 mos	11	26
8	72	ICCE	Leiske	1	1 mo	7	17
9	72	ICCE	Kelman	1	3 mos	4	18
10	86	ICCE	Leiske	2	3 wks	7	18
11	80	ICCE	Optiflex-Cilco	1	3 mos	8	24
12[‡]	86	ICCE	Choyce	2	7 mos	4	35
13[‡]	72	ICCE	Kelman-AC21	1	7 mos	—[§]	38
14[‡]	66	ICCE	Kelman	1	2 mos	—[§]	25
15[‡]	84	ICCE	Leiske	1	1 wk	0	24
16	71	ICCE	Choyce	1	6 wks	6	24
17	65	ICCE	Choyce	1	1 mo	1	22

*ICCE = intracapsular cataract extraction; ECCE = extracapsular cataract extraction.
†Sixteen of 17 patients underwent laser iridotomy. Patient 12 underwent surgical iridectomy.
‡Data obtained by telephone rather than by direct examination.
§Gonioscopic data unavailable.
(Courtesy of Van Buskirk, E.M.: Am. J. Ophthalmol. 99:55–59, January 1983.)

(13–5) Am. J. Ophthalmol. 95:55–59, January 1983.

Woman, 72, underwent lens extraction with peripheral iridectomy and implantation of a Choyce anterior chamber intraocular lens in the right eye. Slight blurring of vision was noticed 3 years later. Intraocular pressure was 28 mm Hg and the anterior chamber was peripherally flat with the iris bulging around the intraocular lens, which had rotated to occlude both iridectomies. Laser iridotomies performed at the 6, 1, and 11 o'clock positions restored the anterior chamber to the normal aphakic position. Antiglaucomatous therapy was required for intraocular pressure in excess of 30 mm Hg due to synechial closure of two thirds of the anterior chamber angle.

Pupillary block in an aphakic eye results from blockage of the pupillary and iridectomy apertures at their posterior surface by vitreous face, which causes entrapment of aqueous humor in the posterior chamber, iris bombé, and closure of the anterior chamber angle. Although iridotomy eliminates pupillary block, glaucoma medications or further surgery may be necessary. Pupillary block in an eye with an implanted intraocular lens should be treated as a clinical emergency to prevent angle-closure glaucoma. Prevention of pupillary block by adequate surgical iridectomies during cataract surgery is preferable to any form of postoperative treatment.

As it is the optical portion of the intraocular lens that occludes the pupil, variations in foot-plate design probably will not prevent pupillary block. Designs that prevent rotation of the lens and occlusion of the iridectomies would be helpful in reducing the incidence of this complication. Meanwhile, at least 2 peripheral iridectomies should be placed far enough apart to prevent their simultaneous occlusion by the intraocular lens.

▶ [All but one of the cases of pupillary block were in eyes with an anterior chamber lens. It may not be due to the lens but rather why this type of lens was used. Many cataract surgeons use an anterior chamber lens if something happens during surgery preventing the implantation of a posterior chamber lens. It might be better to abandon lens implantation if all does not go perfectly during surgery.] ◀

13–6   **Healon as an Emergency Aid.** H. Neubauer (Univ. of Cologne, W. Germany) used sodium hyaluronate (Healon) in follow-up surgery of the anterior segment. In complications after intraocular lens (IOL) implantation, position correction of the clip lens with introduction of Healon through a cannula and separate access is indispensable (Fig 13–4). While Healon is recommended for stabilization of the anterior chamber in risky situations, it can also be used as a viscous spatula. When a more or less complete anterior synechia exists at the incision site it can be atraumatically dissolved by inserting a cannula behind the synechia and filling the space between the angle of the chamber and the synechia with Healon. So far Healon has not caused any problems with regard to tissue compatibility, viscosity, resorption, or its optical quality in the anterior chamber.

Ten patients had massive anterior synechiae with distortion of the pupil after cataract extraction. Secondary glaucoma was prevented in

(13–6) Klin. Monatsbl. Augenheilkd. 182:269–271, April 1983.

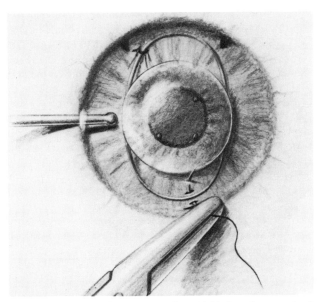

Fig 13–4.—Viscous stabilization of anterior chamber with McCannel suture after lower luxation of iris-clip lens. Central anterior chamber is filled with Healon by means of paracentesis. Button cannula remains in place during successive McCannel suture in which needle is introduced through limbus parallel corneal incision. (Courtesy of Neubauer, H.: Klin. Monatsbl. Augenheilkd. 182:269–271, April 1983.)

3 of these patients most likely by removal of the anterior synechiae and centralization of the pupil at the right time. Among 5 patients with secondary glaucoma after cataract surgery, 2 required further treatment for secondary glaucoma and 1 patient had relapse of the distorted pupil and secondary glaucoma even after the third Healon synechiolysis. In 2 chronically and unsuccessfully operated-on glaucomatous eyes a synechiolysis proved effective, but did not change the glaucoma. Previous unsuccessful synechiolyses without Healon shows the excellent benefit of Healon in extended synechiolysis treatment.

It is understandable that the use of Healon has no effect on an already severely damaged angle of the chamber. Therefore, early synechiolysis with Healon can be beneficial especially in cases of distortion of the pupil after cataract extraction with insufficient cleansing of the vitreous. In reviewing results of secondary treatment given after injuries, use of Healon in risky situations should be encouraged as a means of stabilizing the anterior chamber with a viscous fluid. However, it still will take time to determine the routine indication for this expensive medication and eventually to find less costly viscous media that produces comparable results.

▶ [Healon is superb for the maintenance of the anterior chamber in all sorts of secondary procedures. It is important to note, however, that the substance does not flow around the eye like saline solution. Thus, to fill the entire anterior chamber, the cannula must be moved throughout the area including across the eye to the opposite side.] ◄

13–7 **Methylcellulose Instead of Healon in Extracapsular Surgery With Intraocular Lens Implantation.** Danièle Aron-Rosa, Howard C. Cohn, Jean-Jacques Aron, and Charles Bouquety compared the results of extracapsular cataract extractions with posterior chamber lens implantation in which 1% methylcellulose or air was used. A total of 150 eyes in 138 patients were operated on, 75 with methylcellulose and 75 with air. Endothelial cell counts were repeated 8 to 12 weeks after operation in 70 eyes of 63 patients given implants with methylcellulose and 63 eyes of 58 patients given implants with air. The respective mean ages were 65 and 67 years. The surgical technique included an yttrium-aluminum-garnet laser anterior capsulotomy.

Preoperative central endothelial cell densities were comparable in the 2 groups. Patients given implants with methylcellulose had a mean loss of 8% determined by postoperative evaluation, compared with 25% in the group given implants with air. The difference was highly significant. The mean best-corrected acuity was 20/25 in each group. All intraocular pressure elevations resolved within 6 days of operation. There was no significant difference in postoperative inflammation in the 2 groups.

Endothelial cell loss in extracapsular cataract operations with posterior chamber lens implantation can be greatly reduced by implanting the lens with methylcellulose rather than air. The methylcellulose apparently acts as a protective cushion between the implant and the endothelium, and better visibility is provided, reducing the risk of inadvertent endothelial contact. Methylcellulose is less viscous than Healon and is easier to wash out of the anterior chamber. Healon may be preferable when vitreous pressure threatens, as in young patients. No toxicity has been observed with the use of methylcellulose. Only methylcellulose prepared without preservatives in a 0.49% salt solution should be used.

▶ [The authors of this article present useful information, although their control probably should have been Healon instead of air. There may be less of an intraocular pressure rise with methylcellulose than with Healon, and air itself may have a detrimental effect on the corneal endothelium.] ◄

13–8 **Surgical Management of Cataract Associated With Chronic Uveitis** is described by Matthew E. Dangel, Walter J. Stark, and Ronald G. Michels (Johns Hopkins Hosp., Baltimore). Cataracts associated with uveitis often are associated with extensive posterior synechiae, and obstruction of aqueous flow may result in iris bombé. Hypotony is a common feature of these eyes. The patients often are young, which makes intracapsular extraction potentially hazardous,

(13–7) Ophthalmology (Rochester) 90:1235–1238, October 1983.
(13–8) Ophthalmic Surg. 14:145–149, February 1983.

and conventional extracapsular extraction also is difficult. Vitrectomy instrumentation permits the controlled removal of opaque lens material in these cases.

TECHNIQUE.—Limbal incisions are made through clear cornea after ultrasound examination, and an infusion needle and a small-diameter vitrectomy instrument are inserted. The infusion needle or a thin spatula is used to free adhesions between the pupillary margin and the lens (Fig 13–5). If neces-

Fig 13–5 (top).—Bimanual technique for removal of complicated cataract. Spatula is used to rupture synechiae between iris margin and anterior lens capsule. Infusion needle is then used to rupture synechiae on other side of eye.

Fig 13–6 (bottom).—Partial superior iridectomy is performed with vitrectomy probe to enlarge pupil further after rupture of all posterior synechiae.

(Courtesy of Dangel, M.E., et al.: Ophthalmic Surg. 14:145–149, February 1983.)

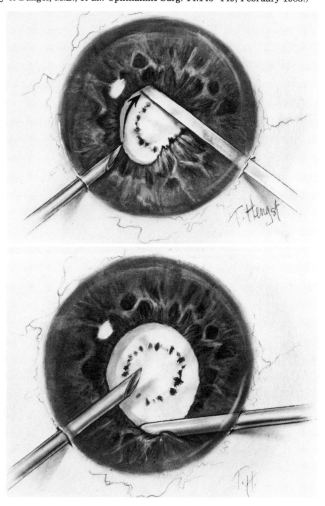

sary, a superior sector iridectomy and inferior sphincterotomy are done with the vitrectomy probe (Fig 13–6). A small opening in the anterior lens capsule then is made with the infusion needle (Fig 13–7), and the vitrectomy probe is inserted to remove both cortical and nuclear lens material if it is soft (Fig 13–8). If the lens nucleus is firm, an ultrasonic needle can be used to emulsify and remove it. In the presence of iris bombé and a shallow anterior chamber, a limbal approach can be used, and the vitrectomy instruments can be inserted through the peripheral aspect of the iris into the lens. Excision of vitreous gel often can be achieved through a limbal approach if the vitreous is diffusely opaque. Dense fibrotic tissue in the posterior lens capsule or a thick

Fig 13–7 (top).—After pupillary opening has been enlarged by rupture of posterior synechiae and iris has been partially excised with vitrectomy probe, small incision is made in anterior lens capsule with tip of infusion needle.

Fig 13–8 (bottom).—Opaque nuclear and cortical lens material is excised with vitrectomy probe introduced through small incision in anterior lens capsule.

(Courtesy of Dangel, M.E., et al.: Ophthalmic Surg. 14:145–149, February 1983.)

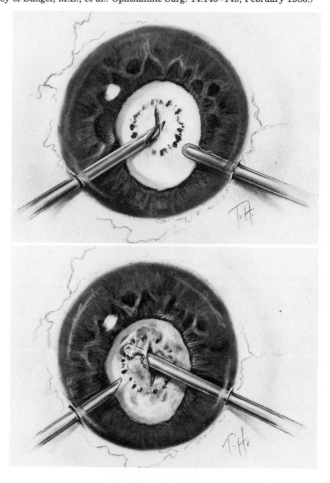

retrolenticular membrane is excised if present. The anterior chamber is filled with air before the instruments are withdrawn. The limbal incisions are closed with 10–0 monofilament nylon sutures. Gentamicin and a depot steroid are injected into the subconjunctival space at the end of the operation.

This method was used in 8 eyes of 5 patients with complicated cataracts associated with uveitis. Vision had been markedly reduced in all eyes and was improved postoperatively. There were no operative complications. Surgery did not appear to worsen the ocular inflammation, although all patients received topical steroids postoperatively. Intraocular pressures did not change significantly after surgery. There were no retinal tears or detachments,

This approach is preferable to conventional methods in the management of complicated cataracts associated with chronic uveitis.

▶ [Closed-eye anterior segment reconstruction with vitrectomy instrumentation has saved many eyes that would have been lost prior to the technology. Indeed, opening chronically inflamed eyes carried extreme risk, and breaking the posterior synechiae was difficult if not impossible. More eyes may have benefited from anterior segment surgery with infusion-suction cutters than from posterior segment operations.] ◀

▶ ↓ The authors of the following 2 articles carefully tested the effects of irrigating the eye with saline and silver protein solutions. The solutions had no effect on the ocular bacterial counts. We look forward to their continued work to provide information about what will safely reduce conjunctival bacteria preoperatively. ◀

13–9 **Chemical Preparation of the Eye in Ophthalmic Surgery.** *I. Effect of conjunctival irrigation.*—Chemical preparation of the eye just before operation represents the last chance to achieve a sterile field. Sherwin Isenberg, Leonard Apt, and Robert Yoshimuri (Univ. of California, Los Angeles) examined the effects of irrigation, as part of the preoperative chemical preparation of the eye, on the conjunctival flora in 40 consecutively seen patients undergoing ocular surgery. No antibiotics were used preoperatively. One eye was irrigated with sterile physiologic saline solution, while the other was not irrigated. Further preparation was performed with hexachlorophene solution, applied to the surrounding skin and lid margins. The inferotemporal or inferonasal conjunctival cul-de-sac was cultured. The mean number of colonies was increased by less than 1% after chemical preparation in control eyes, but by 18% in the irrigated eyes. The mean number of species isolated increased 23% in the control eyes and 46% in the irrigated eyes, a significant difference.

Irrigation of the eye with saline solution appears to increase the number of bacterial species and possibly the colony count of bacteria in the conjunctival cul-de-sac. Irrigation may wash organisms hidden within the conjunctiva to the surface, or organisms on the skin may be carried into the eye. Although irrigation may be indicated to remove debris from the eye or to wash out medication, it should not be used solely in an attempt to sterilize the ocular surface.

II. Effectiveness of mild silver protein solution.—Although many

(13–9) Arch. Ophthalmol. 101:761–763, May 1983; 764–765, May 1983.

ophthalmologists continue to use a 20% silver protein solution for antimicrobial purposes, no controlled clinical studies have proved its effectiveness when used to prepare the eye for surgery. Isenberg, Apt, and Yoshimuri investigated the usefulness of this solution as an antimicrobial measure in 32 patients undergoing ophthalmic surgery. None had received antibiotic therapy or had active infection at the time of operation. One drop of 20% mild silver protein solution was instilled in the inferior conjunctival fornix of one eye. Hexachlorophene soap was applied to the surrounding skin regions, and the eye receiving silver protein solution then was irrigated with normal saline solution. The numbers of both colonies and species were greater after preparation than before in both treated and control eyes, but in no case was the increase significant at the 5% level. Only 3 of 15 initially sterile eyes remained sterile after preparation. The organisms isolated included diphtheroids, *staphylococcus epidermidis, Propionibacterium acnes, Candida albicans,* and *Klebsiella.*

The mild silver protein solution can darkly stain mucus or debris on the conjunctiva, eyelids, or skin and thereby serves as a marker for the adequacy of preparation of the eye. It is not, however, an apparently significant bactericidal agent when used in the human conjunctiva.

13–10 **Postoperative Infections in Ophthalmology: Clinical, Pathologic and Medicolegal Considerations.** M. Taglioni, P. Besson, Ph. Sourdille, F. Hervouet, S. Liotet, and L. Guillaumet (Paris) investigated the frequency of postoperative infection in open globe ocular surgery, its various clinical aspects, and predisposing factors. Although frequency is difficult to determine given the heterogenous nature of available statistics, a considerable decrease of such occurrences is evident since 1945–1950.

Traumatic surgery clearly has the greatest risk of infection, particularly when involving a foreign body, and percentages as high as 5.57% have been reported, whereas surgery for cataract or glaucoma appears to be a relatively safe procedure. The clinical course of such infection may vary from early acute fulminating infection to low-grade inflammatory lesions that are questionably related to allergy. Both the curative and prophylactic aspects of treatment are fraught with difficulty, particularly the former because the responsible organism may not always be determined. Cultures of aqueous humor have been found to give better results than those of the vitreous humor, although current statistics show no more than a 50% rate of success in determining the infectious agent. As soon as the infection is diagnosed, lavage of the anterior chamber is followed by topical and systemic administration of the appropriate antibiotic. Steroids and atropine will enhance the results whatever the pathologic nature of the lesion, although a wait of 24 to 48 hours after institution of antibiot-

(13–10) J. Fr. Ophtalmol. 6:161–177, 1982.

ics is preferred before deciding on their administration. If pus reappears in the anterior chamber, the process of lavage and injection may have to be repeated several times.

Use of vitrectomy is disputed, and has been relegated only to desperate cases. The preventive aspects of treatment involve a variety of elements, such as the condition of the surgical theater, the sterilization of instruments, and the formation of the surgical team.

▶ [The incidence of postoperative infections is less than 0.1% but, nonetheless, infection will eventually happen in just about every ophthalmic surgeon's practice. Unfortunately, in the United States, patients are inclined to sue because of a poor result, regardless of the quality of the medical care they received.] ◀

13–11 **Regional Analgesia Combined With Intravenous Sedation in Major Eyelid Surgery: Alternative to Induced Hypotension.** R. S. Neill (Canniesburn Hosp., Glasgow, Scotland) describes the use of this alternative technique in 14 elderly patients who required excision and reconstruction for eyelid carcinoma. These 8 women and 6 men with an average age of 80 years were considered "at risk" for general anesthesia with or without induced hypotension. Twelve of the 14 had coexisting medical conditions. (Five cases are described below.)

Sensation to the orbit and surrounding area (Fig 13–9) is supplied by 4 branches from the first division of the fifth cranial nerve and 2 branches from the second division. To induce regional nerve blockade dental cartridge syringes fitted with 27G needles are used. The trochlear nerves and supraorbital nerve can normally be blocked from a single midline injection site on the nasal bridge by first directing the needle downward and laterally. The infraorbital nerve can be blocked from an intraoral approach by inserting the needle into the upper buccal sulcus. The zygomaticofacial nerve is blocked by palpating the foramen and injecting in a radial direction from it. Anesthesia of the conjunctiva is obtained by instillation of local anesthetic drops (amethocaine 1.0%). A supplementary injection of a little local anesthetic may be necessary at the lid margin or canthus.

CASE 1.—Woman, 74, had basal cell carcinoma of the right lower eyelid. Regional anesthesia was achieved with infraorbital, trochlear, supraorbital, lacrimal, and zygomaticofacial nerve blocks by using 6 ml of 2% lignocaine with epinephrine 1:80,000. Amethocaine was instilled into the conjunctiva.

CASE 2.—Woman, 73, had basal cell carcinoma at the left medial canthus. Premedication with 25 mg of pethidine and 50 mg of promethazine was supplemented by 3.5 mg of morphine intravenously. Anesthesia was achieved with infraorbital and supraorbital nerve blocks by using 4 ml of 2% lignocaine with epinephrine 1:80,000.

CASE 3.—Woman, 78, with basal cell carcinoma of the right medial canthus had no premedication but received slow intravenous injection of 9 mg of morphine and 9 mg of droperidol for sedation. Regional anesthesia was achieved as described in the previous case.

(13–11)   Br. J. Plast. Surg. 36:29–35, January 1983.

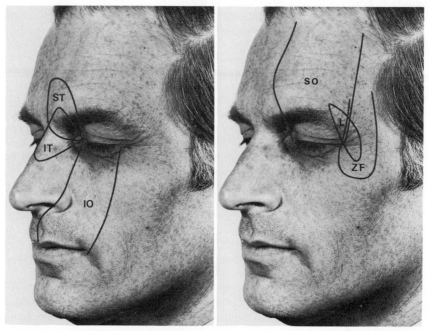

Fig 13–9.—Area of sensation supplied by fifth cranial nerve. ST = supratrochlear nerve; IT = infratrochlear nerve; IO = infraorbital nerve; SO = supraorbital nerve; L = lacrimal nerve; and ZF = zygomaticofacial nerve. (Courtesy of Neill, R.S.: Br. J. Plast. Surg. 36:29–35, January 1983.)

CASE 4.—Man, 70, with basal cell carcinoma of the left lower eyelid received no premedication, adequate sedation being achieved with 7 mg of morphine and 7 mg of droperidol. Regional anesthesia was achieved as described above. A small amount of local anesthetic was used in the lid margin.

CASE 5.—Man, 68, with full-width basal cell carcinoma of the left lower eyelid received no premedication but was sedated with 10 mg of morphine and 10 mg of droperidol. Regional anesthesia was achieved as described above. Amethocaine was instilled into the conjunctiva and the nasal septum was anesthetized with 10% cocaine applied by Q Tips.

In these 14 patients the combination of careful intravenous sedation with regional nerve block allowed extensive and prolonged procedures to be performed with minimal upset to the patient. It provides a safe alternative to profound induced hypotension in "at risk" elderly patients.

► [This is a fine article by an anesthesiologist who describes in precise detail how to block the first and second divisions of the fifth cranial nerve. The infraorbital nerve block method is of special interest since a potentially dangerous canal injection is not necessary.] ◄

13-12 **Ten Caveats in Keratorefractive Surgery.** J. James Rowsey

(13–12) Ophthalmology (Rochester) 90:148–155, February 1983.

(Univ. of Oklahoma, Oklahoma City) outlines the various ways in which the topographic corneal shifts occurring during and after cataract surgery, keratorefractive surgery, and ocular trauma are associated with refractive alterations. The normal cornea flattens over any traumatic or surgical incision in the area of the incision. A controlled flattening provides the basis for myopic correction in radial keratotomy. Traumatic incisions around the visual axis may be associated with unequal flattening in the peripheral cornea, resulting in irregular astigmatism. Radial corneal incisions flatten the adjacent cornea and also the cornea 90 degrees away, by about half the former amount. The cornea-flattening effect is more prominent as incisions approach the visual axis, and it becomes maximal as incisions traverse the visual axis.

The cornea flattens directly over any sutured incision, regardless of the suturing method used. A compressive effect of tight sutures prevents gaping of the wound, and distinct corneal flattening results. The flattening is manifested by ring separation or broadening, indicating a longer radius of corneal curvature. With loose sutures, the limbal cornea flattens in the nearby region, steepens 90 degrees away, and flattens 180 degrees away. With tight sutures the limbal cornea steepens in the immediate vicinity, flattens 90 degrees away, and steepens 180 degrees away. The cornea flattens over wedge resections or tucks, and steepens anterior to these maneuvers.

Tissue removal, whether traumatic or surgical in origin, leads to corneal flattening over the site of removal. Suture removal early after operation may be associated with release of the flattening effect and decreased astigmatism, but there is a risk of wound dehiscence and leakage. Full-thickness addition of corneal tissue produces corneal steepening over the site of the addition and flattens the adjacent cornea. Tissue addition to a traumatically flattened region of cornea may permit a return to contact lens use.

▶ [Perhaps the good that has come out of keratorefractive surgery thus far is that it has made us more careful and precise in the closure of our cataract incisions.] ◀

13–13 **Surgical Technique and Postoperative Treatment in Perforating Injuries of the Lens.** Extensive experimental research proved that the healing of lens capsule wounds can be supported effectively by application of a fibrin tissue adhesive. The result is a circumscribed scar in an otherwise clear lens. The clinical application of the method was also successful. Preliminary results have been published and a review of all cases is in preparation. W. Buschmann (Univ. of Würzburg, W. Germany) reports on the indications, techniques, and postoperative treatment.

The application of the fibrinogen tissue adhesive is indicated if spontaneous healing cannot by expected or has failed and the major parts of the lens are still clear. Even large traumatic posterior sub-

(13–13) Klin. Monatsbl. Augenheilkd. 183:241–245, October 1983.

capsular rosettes may disappear after closure of the lens-capsule wound. Therefore, they are by no means a contraindication for this lens-saving fibrinogen application.

The tissue adhesive should be applied as soon as possible after injury. Especially in larger lens-capsule lesions it is regularly applied as part of surgical care. Successful application of the tissue adhesive is still possible in the days following a perforating injury if the lens-capsule wound is small and the progress of lens opacification is slow. Up to now only the easiest application technique has been used in clinical work. Thrombin solution and fibrinogen concentrate are applied successively to the lesion area and its surroundings, using thin, blunt needles. Swollen, denatured lens fibers should be removed before application. In case of perforation of the anterior and posterior lens capsule, fibrin closure of the anterior lesion is usually sufficient. A corneoscleral incision and full exposition of the lens wound to be sealed will be preferred in the future in larger lens-capsule wounds, particularly equatorial ones. Topical and systemic applications of antibiotics are used postoperatively as in all perforating injuries. In lens injuries, topical atropine is applied for 4 to 6 months after surgery.

In one patient, after complete perforation of the lens and fibrinogen application, good regression of the opaque areas of the lens was observed; however, the atropine treatment was discontinued too early, with resultant leaking of the capsule wound. A second fibrinogen adhesive application followed by 6 months of topical atropine treatment again resulted in regression of the lens opaque areas and a corresponding increase in visual acuity. The recommendation to use miotics in the postoperative treatment of lens injuries no longer appears to be justified.

▶ [The author of this article has been performing some fascinating studies on the intraocular use of tissue adhesive. One wonders if retinal tears could be similarly sealed?] ◀

14. Basic Sciences, Injuries and Miscellaneous

Microcomputers for the Ophthalmologist

JOHN S. READ, M.S.

Eye and Ear Infirmary
University of Illinois, Chicago

In only 10 years, desktop microcomputers have evolved from hobby kits for computer enthusiasts into business tools of formidable power. In the past 2 years, systems appropriate for use in a small ophthalmologic practice have become available in bewildering profusion and variety. Microcomputer technology continues to develop faster and faster, and systems will exist within a few years that will impact medical practice directly, such as systems for storage and retrieval of patient data as scientific records and "expert" programs capable of assisting physicians in medical decision making.

In 1984, dozens of vendors can supply complete desktop systems capable of doing an acceptable job of "computerizing" the business aspects of an ophthalmologist's practice at a cost of between $10,000 and $18,000, including the computer itself and the programs necessary to control it. However, it is important to recognize that even under the best of circumstances, the introduction of a computer playing a major role in an organization is very disruptive. It has been estimated that in terms of disruptive power, 5 computers are equal to 1 fire that completely burns down the office. Computerizing a major function like billing always means reorganizing the office, and may mean operating the new system and the old manual system simultaneously for several months—extra work for everyone. You will probably not save money in the short run because you won't be able to cut staff, even if you wanted to. So what benefits can you expect? You can expect to improve your control over the business aspects of your practice so that you always know how you stand financially; you can improve the availability of your staff to work with patients without the constant distraction of paperwork; you may improve your cash flow through more timely billing and especially by more efficient handling of insurance claims.

Microcomputer Applications in the Physician's Office

Most physicians in private practice know why they want to buy a computer. Few doctors went to medical school because they liked monotonous paperwork and record-keeping. Luckily, these business functions are just those which are most readily automated, i.e., functions such as statement preparation, recording of payments, preparation of insurance claims, and posting of adjustments and charges. A general-purpose computer can do other things as well, including word processing for preparation of correspondence, accessing remote data bases to look up literature references and facts, and for continuing education via remote teaching systems such as PLATO.

Choosing a System for Business Applications

It is essential to recognize that the choice of a computer is much less important to the physician than the choice of which program is to be used. First, the program is selected to meet your requirements. Then a computer is selected which will run the program. Sometimes the program and computer are available as a package from a single vendor. A satisfactory program is preferred over a choice of computer, since you are guaranteed that the program and computer will work correctly together and that all the right bells and whistles are attached to the computer. The problem, then, is evaluating programs. It is important to proceed systematically to avoid being overwhelmed by sales pitches. I have sketched out a protocol below, but there are good books available[1] which contain more detailed information.

PROTOCOL

Analyze your office system objectively. Since you are going to reorganize your office, you need to know in detail how it works. You also need to collect some data so that you can tell whether a particular computer system will be adequate. One approach to the analysis of an office system is to pretend that you yourself are various forms and pieces of paper—find out who handles them and how many there are per week; try to account for all the inputs and outputs of the system. Taking the role of a patient, step through all procedures with your staff. Determine volumes, i.e., patients per day, bills per month, number of insurance claims per week, and number of active records. Make a note of what procedure and diagnostic codes you use. These data determine the amounts of computer storage you need for records and how powerful the computer and programs have to be. You should expect to spend a few days doing this, and you may want to hire a consultant to help you. It can be surprisingly difficult and time-consuming to get a detailed, quantitative analysis of even your own business down on paper.

Decide what functions and reports you want the system to handle. This determines what data must be stored and what computations the system must perform. Data entry and verification are expensive and disruptive, so only the essentials should be stored. Write these items down; they become your system specification.

Armed with your written specification, see vendors and get them to show you how their system does what you want. Ignore features that are not on your specification, unless they are very impressive. Get a list of customers, preferably other ophthalmologists, who are using the vendor's system. If the vendor can't give you such a list, leave his or her store as quickly and gracefully as possible. You should consider the demonstration given by the vendor to be only a preliminary look. It is very difficult to make an effective assessment under such conditions. You can learn a bit more by trying to use the system yourself. Try to enter a patient record and some transactions. Hit keys at random to see whether the error-checking is effective. See whether the salesperson can quickly teach you to use the system, or if he or she has continually to look things up in manuals. At this demonstration, you can expect to find out whether the system meets your written specification and, in very general terms, how well it works. For example, if you plan to use the system for answering phone inquiries about account status, the system must allow you to jump back and forth easily between data entry and inquiry. Many systems do not permit this. Similarly, if you want to be able to do demand billing and insurance form preparation as patients leave your clinic, be sure that the system can do this. Many systems require that all transactions of a similar type be batched together and processed at once, and are slow and hard to use when you try to do a series of different transactions for 1 patient.

Check out the vendor's references. Make sure that the references do not have a vested interest in the system. You are unlikely to get an objective opinion from one of the codevelopers of a system.

Try the system out under conditions of your choosing. After you have narrowed your choice of systems to 2 or 3, you should invest some time and money in intensive testing. If you are buying the program and the computer separately, you can rent time on an appropriate computer at a local computer store, or possibly from the program vendor. You should reserve a couple of hours to go through a billing cycle using some of your own data. A knowledgeable representative of the vendor should be present to get you started and to answer questions. Some vendors offer a 90-day trial period during which you can return the system and get most of the purchase price refunded. Even if the trial period costs a few hundred dollars, it may be worthwhile to use it as a final selection tool.

As you go through the evaluation process, be sure to write down your thoughts about each system. You might make up a form in advance so that you can record comparable data about each system. Columns of your form could have headings like "cost," "maximal active records stored," "indexing by name or patient number?" "insurance forms handled," "trial period?" "kinds of error-checking on data entry," and so on.

Backup for your data files is extremely important. Any computer system intended for business use must have a means for making a backup copy of the data files onto some computer-readable data storage medium which can be carried away and stored in a safe location. This is extremely important for 2 reasons: (1) the large main storage disk ("hard disk"), which holds the data files when they are in use, may become defective. Repair of this drive will almost certainly mean that all of the data stored on the disk will be lost. If you have a backup system, you can easily restore the files to the status comparable to the last time you made a backup. Without a backup, all of the data would have to be reentered by hand; and (2) in case of a fire, all of your business records would be lost. Having a computer-readable backup of your records stored off-site means you can be back in business as soon as the computer is replaced and the files are restored. This "fire insurance" aspect of computerizing is a fringe benefit which is frequently not recognized. The backup storage medium is either a small, removable flexible magnetic disk ("diskette," or "floppy disk") or a magnetic tape cartridge similar to a video cassette. In systems suitable for business use, the hard disk is capable of storing some 10 million characters or more. The diskettes are usually capable of storing 100 to 300 thousand characters. If your data files become large, it can be very tedious to make a backup since it may be necessary to fill dozens of diskettes. For large files, a cartridge tape drive is much better, since 1 cartridge will hold several million characters, and can be written in a few minutes.

It is also very important that extensive help be available after you have purchased the system. Systems available through mail order houses rarely provide a sufficient level of support. Maintenance of the computer is critical. Computers, like all machines, break down eventually. Maintenance after the usual warranty period can be surprisingly expensive and unsatisfactory. The number of microcomputers in use has far outstripped the number of competent service technicians. Computer stores frequently have a difficult time providing service with a reasonable response time. Sometimes, the maintenance contract will not cover the hard disk, which is the most critical and fragile component. The reason for this is that local computer stores do not actually repair anything. Technicians are trained only to isolate defective subsystems and replace them on the spot with a used, rebuilt equivalent. The defective unit is sent back to the manufacturer to be reconditioned, and is then installed in someone else's computer. In the case of the hard disk drive, some computer stores find it unprofitable to follow this practice, since they must stock expensive spare disk drives. Be sure that you understand and agree with all of the fine print in your maintenance contract about response time and equipment coverage. If you buy a packaged system, the vendor takes responsibility for maintenance of all the hardware and for resolving any problems that might be due to either the hardware or the software. If you buy hardware and software separately, you are in a position similar to that of acting as your own general contractor for the construction of your home. It can be done, but the first time can be extremely painful.

Cost-benefit analysis is critical in making a rational business decision about computerizing, in which you and your accountant will want to assign dollar values to the costs and expected benefits of the project. The cost side is relatively easy to do, and would include such things as interest and principal payments, monthly maintenance (usually 1% to 2% of the total selling price per month), and supplies such as diskettes, printer ribbons, and forms. Figuring a dollar value for the benefits may be more difficult. If your receipts are invested, you will be able to estimate the return on an improved cash flow due to quicker turnaround on insurance claims. You can easily calculate the amount of investment tax credit from the purchase of the computer. If you are intending to expand, you may be able to estimate savings from not hiring additional staff. You should not be surprised, however, if these savings do not completely pay for the computer. It is at this point that your judgment concerning the value of the intangible benefits enters the decision. The important thing is that you should know in dollars how much the intangible benefits are going to cost. Some people object in principle to cost-benefit analysis, saying that "if Queen Isabella had insisted on a cost-benefit analysis, Columbus would never have discovered America." My guess is that Queen Isabella knew precisely what the costs and benefits were and decided that the intangibles were worth it.

A Few Words About Hardware

You should have some knowledge of the nomenclature and anatomy of the microcomputer, primarily so that you can communicate with salespeople and service technicians. The article by Toong and Gupta[2] will tell you everything you need to know on this subject. Microcomputers can be placed in several different categories, depending on the type of computer chip and the specific operating system used. The operating system is a special program that starts the running of the "application programs" according to commands you type on the keyboard and helps to control them as they run. The application programs do your work, such as printing the patient bills or adding data to files.

The manufacturer of the microcomputer uses a particular microchip (which may be built by a totally different company) and other electronics to implement the microcomputer. There are, therefore, many more kinds of microcomputers available than there are microchips. Currently, microchips come in the following popular flavors, listed more or less in increasing order of power: 8085, Z80, 6502, 8088, 68000. A large number of microcomputers were developed around the 8085 and Z80 microchips. These used the CP/M operating system but by now are beginning to be obsolete. You should avoid buying a system that uses this type of computer, since support and new products will be in declining availability. The Apple II computer was built around the 6502 chip and is likewise something of a has-been, although it is still selling well and has a large body of already-written software. The current hot item is the 8088, which is the basis of the IBM Personal Computer and its many clones. The key point here is to realize that, although the clones are advertised as being "fully IBM-compatible," it is not always true that a program developed for the IBM Personal Computer will work on a clone. The 68000 chip is the basis for the next generation of microcomputers. The Apple LISA and Macintosh systems use this chip. Most of the non-Apple 68000-based systems will use the UNIX operating system. However, relatively few programs are as yet available for 68000/UNIX microcomputers. At present, and for at least another year, the IBM system has the greatest variety of business software available that is of interest to ophthalmologists.

References

1. Spohr, M.H.: *The Physician's Guide to Desktop Computers.* Reston, VA: Reston Publishing Co., 1983.
2. Toong, H., and Gupta, A.: Personal computers. *Sci. Am.,* December 1982, pp. 87–105.

▶ ↓ There is a concentrated effort to discover the underlying pathogenic mechanisms responsible for the ocular complications of diabetes. In the following 4 articles, the authors use a wide range of experimental approaches to the problem. In the first article, studies describing the localization of aldose reductase in human retinal pericytes are described. Indeed, this work is the rationale for a clinical trial of the effects of an aldose reductase inhibitor on diabetic retinopathy. The authors of the second article have shown that inhibitors of aldose reductase will decrease sorbitol formation in lens and nerve tissue and the latter is implicated in cataracts and neuropathy. The authors of the third article have shown that vessel wall prostaglandin synthesis is modified by serum from diabetic patients, and this could presumably affect platelets. Finally, the third article contains data suggesting that aspirin may prevent cataract formation. Obviously a great deal of work remains, but we should be encouraged by the many basic and clinical studies under way. ◀

14–1 **Aldose Reductase Localization in Human Retinal Mural Cells.** The pathogenesis of diabetic retinopathy is unknown, but adverse effects from the aldose reductase-catalyzed accumulation of sorbitol may be related to the degeneration of retinal mural cells. Aldose reductase has been implicated in the pathogenesis of several diabetic complications. Y. Akagi, P. F. Kador, T. Kuwabara, and J. H. Kinosh-

---

(14–1) Invest. Ophthalmol. Vis. Sci. 24:1516–1519, November 1983.

ita (Natl. Inst. of Health) report the histochemical detection of aldose reductase in the mural cells of human retinal vessels isolated by trypsin digestion. Eleven human retinas obtained during autopsy were examined by using antibodies against purified human placental aldose reductase, produced in goats or rabbits. The retinal mural cells stained specifically for immunoreactive aldose reductase, whereas the endothelial cells did not. Enzyme was detected in the perinuclear cytoplasm of the mural cells and in some cytoplasmic processes.

This is the first direct demonstration that aldose reductase is localized in the mural cells of human retinal vessels. The findings support the proposal that aldose reductase-initiated accumulation of sorbitol may be involved in the selective degeneration of human mural cells that occurs in nonproliferative diabetic retinopathy.

14–2 **Diabetic Complications in Lens and Nerve and Their Prevention by Sulindac or Sorbinil: Two Novel Aldose Reductase Inhibitors.** Sorbitol is involved in the formation of diabetic cataracts and in neuropathy, and aldose reductase (AR) inhibition prevents sorbitol production and its pathologic sequelae in rats. Michael Jacobson, Yog Raj Sharma, Edward Cotlier, and Jan Den Hollander (Yale Univ.) compared the effects of sulindac, an inhibitor of sorbitol formation in human cataracts and the rat lens, and sorbinil, another potentially useful AR inhibitor, in studies of rat and rabbit lenses in vitro. Rabbit sciatic nerves were also used. Nuclear magnetic resonance (NMR) spectra were obtained from rabbit lenses incubated in 1-^{13}C-glucose.

Mediums containing 10 μM of either sulindac or sorbinil inhibited sorbitol formation in rat lenses incubated in a high glucose concentration. Sorbitol accumulation in rabbit sciatic nerve was also inhibited by both agents at a 100-μM concentration. Sorbinil and sulindac in the same concentration inhibited sorbitol accumulation by human cataracts by nearly 50%. Specific accumulation of sorbitol by lenses incubated in high-glucose medium was confirmed by NMR spectroscopy.

Both sulindac and sorbinil decrease sorbitol formation in cataract and nerve tissues incubated in high-glucose medium, presumably through inhibiting AR. Sulindac, widely used in antirheumatic therapy, may have clinical application in preventing diabetic complications. Testing AR inhibitors by incubating tissues in vitro appears to be a practical means of assessing the potential usefulness of such agents in target tissues.

14–3 **Prostacyclin Production by Human Endothelial Cells Cultured in Diabetic Serum.** Defective vessel wall synthesis of prostacyclin (PGI$_2$) may contribute to platelet hyper-reactivity and vascular

(14–2) Invest. Ophthalmol. Vis Sci. 24:1426–1429, October 1983.
(14–3) Diabetic Metab. 8:323–328, December 1982.

complications in patients with diabetes mellitus. To test the hypothesis that serum from diabetic patients contains factors that impair the synthesis or release of PGI_2 by the vascular endothelium and determine whether these factors are influenced by hypophysectomy, R. C. Paton, R. Guillot, P. Passa, and J. Canivet (Paris) compared PGI_2 production (PGI_2-like activity and 6-keto-$PGF_1\alpha$ levels) by human vascular endothelial cells cultured in the presence of serum from 15 insulin-dependent diabetic patients with proliferative retinopathy, 5 of whom had previously undergone hypophysectomy, and from 15 sex-matched healthy nondiabetic control individuals. When the endothelial cells had reached confluence, the cultures were stimulated with thrombin, the supernatant was examined for PGI_2-like activity on ADP-induced platelet aggregation, and 6-keto-$PGF_1\alpha$ concentrations were measured by radioimmunoassay.

The amount of PGI_2-like activity produced by endothelial cells cultured in diabetic serum was significantly less than that by cells cultured in control serum (21.9 % $\pm$ 4.8% vs. 28.3% $\pm$ 5.1%; $P < 0.05$). In addition, 6-keto-$PGF_1\alpha$ concentrations were significantly lower in cells cultured in diabetic serum than in control serum (3.15 $\pm$ 0.68 mg/dish vs. 3.94 $\pm$ 0.91 mg/dish; $P < 0.05$). A statistically significant correlation was observed between the concentration of 6-keto-$PGF_1\alpha$ and the PGI_2-like activity of the supernatants ($P < 0.001$). Serum from hypophysectomized and nonhypophysectomized diabetic patients produced similar amounts of PGI_2 and showed similar 6-keto-$PGF_1\alpha$ ratios. A statistically significant inverse correlation was observed between the 6-keto-$PGF_1\alpha$ ratios and the concentration of HbA_1 (τ $-$ 0.49; $P < 0.05$).

The findings suggest that serum from diabetic patients with proliferative retinopathy contains factors that impair the synthesis or release of PGI_2 by endothelial cells. Pituitary function does not appear to be related to this defect, although glycemic control may be involved.

14–4 **Distribution of Salicylate in Lens and Intraocular Fluids and Its Effect on Cataract Formation.** The potential therapeutic effects of salicylate on the lens depend on an adequate drug concentration after systemic or topical administration. Edward Cotlier, Yog R. Sharma, Tracy Niven, and Mary Brescia (Yale Univ.) examined the distribution of salicylate in the lens and intraocular fluids after systemic administration to rabbits and rats. Intraperitoneal injections of sodium salicylate or intravenous ^{14}C-acetylsalicylic acid in physiologic saline solution were administered, and samples of blood, aqueous humor, and vitreous humor were obtained at varying intervals. Rats with galactose-induced cataracts were given intraperitoneal injections of sodium salicylate, sulindac, and physiologic saline solution.

(14–4) Am. J. Med. 74:83–90, June 14, 1983.

Rapid penetration of labeled acetylsalicylic acid into the rabbit lens and aqueous humor was observed after intravenous injection. The production of plasma salicylate levels similar to those in human beings given 4 to 6 aspirin tablets led to accumulation of salicylate by the rabbit lens after intraperitoneal administration. Mean content of salicylate was 405 μmole/gm at 2 hours and 620 μmole/gm at 4 hours. Salicylate was cleared in 24 hours from rabbit plasma and intraocular fluids, but was retained by the lens. Penetration of salicylate into both the rabbit and rat lenses was dose dependent. Intraperitoneal injections of salicylate in a daily dose of 100 mg/kg decelerated the formation of galactose cataracts in rats. Sulindac also retarded cataract development in this model. Addition of L-tryptophan to mixtures containing glucose-6-phosphate and calf lens proteins hastened protein aggregation, but addition of sodium salicylate reduced turbidity and yellowing.

The maintenance of high levels of salicylate in the lens and aqueous humor of the rabbit depends on high plasma levels. If the lens-plasma salicylate ratio in human beings is similar to that in rabbits, significant inhibition of cataract aldose reductase could occur in persons taking four 325-mg aspirin tablets a day.

14–5 **Morphology of the Capsule-Like Portion of the Reactive Membranes on Intraocular Lens Implants** was investigated by J. Reimer Wolter (Univ. of Michigan, Ann Arbor). Examination of more than 40 intraocular lens implants removed from human eyes has given evidence of a film-like proteinaceous capsule forming part of the cellular membranes on the plastic surface of all the implants. The capsules typically are continuous and of regular thickness in clinically successful cases, and they appear to become tougher and increasingly adherent to the plastic surface over time. They are slightly eosinophilic, and usually are populated by a variety of cells, most of which arise from freely moving macrophages of the inner eye. The capsules usually are optically clear before histologic staining. The appearance of the capsule on an implant removed about a year after placement is shown in Figure 14–1. Many large, foreign body giant cells were distributed over the membranes, and numerous epithelioid cells also were present. Small fibroblast-like cells and active macrophages were distributed evenly in the interspaces.

The capsular portion probably is the most important part of the membrane that forms on the surface of an intraocular lens implant. It is similar in many respects to the lens capsule of the normal eye. The capsular formation becomes firmer and more like a glassy membrane over time. Its formation seems to be an important step in the process of an implant being accepted in the inner eye. Further studies of optically clear lens implants may provide information relevant to

(14–5) Albrecht von Graefes Arch. Klin. Exp. Ophthalmol. 220:58–65, February 1983.

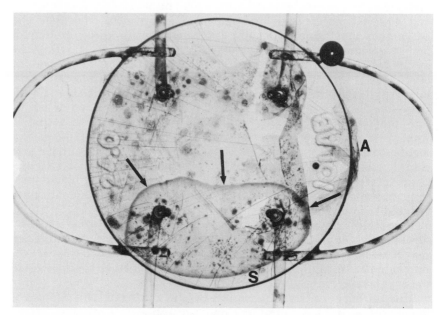

Fig 14–1.—Implant removed about 1 year after implantation. Segmental thickening of posterior capsule *(arrows)* is seen. Artificial shrinkage of posterior capsule *(S)* has exposed edge of optics below and on right. Piece of torn anterior capsule *(A)* is piled up on right. Large giant cells are seen all over implant. Black spot is caused by air bubble. Hematoxylin-eosin (lens implant cytologic technique); ×20. (Courtesy of Wolter, J.R.: Albrecht von Graefes Arch. Klin. Exp. Ophthalmol. 220:58–65, February 1983; Berlin-Heidelberg-New York: Springer.)

any setting in which a foreign substance is used to replace a normal tissue component.

▶ [Membranes evidently form on some intraocular lenses, but it is not clear if transparency is affected or what long-term effects may be.] ◀

▶ ↓ The authors of the following 2 articles discuss their experimental animal radial keratotomy studies. Repeat corneal incisions after a year apparently increase the flattening and, at least in the rabbit, the procedure is apparently safe. Unfortunately, so many human beings have already been operated on that it is probably too late to learn anything new from animal studies. The complications will be shown in our patients. ◀

14–6 **Repeat Radial Keratotomy in Monkeys.** Radial keratotomy effectively flattens the central cornea curvature, thereby eliminating or reducing the amount of myopia correction required. John W. Cowden and Brenda Weber (Wayne State Univ., Detroit) assessed the degree of change in the eye produced by a second radial keratotomy in 6 adult monkeys. The procedure consisted of 8 deep, evenly spaced, radial corneal incisions performed on the right eye 1 year after the initial procedure. All animals had previously undergone bilateral radial keratotomy consisting of 16 deep (.55 to .60 mm), evenly spaced, ra-

(14–6) Ophthalmology (Rochester) 90:251–256, March 1983.

dial corneal incisions extending from the edge of a 3-mm central optical zone to the limbus. Peripheral deepening incisions measuring .10 mm greater than the initial incisions also were made in the outer half of the incisions during the initial procedure. The 6 left eyes that were not reoperated on served as controls.

Follow-up evaluation of the 6 left control eyes 18 months after the initial procedure indicated an average change of − .32 diopters (D) in the refractive error and a further flattening of the corneal curvature of − .26 D. Six months after reoperation, the 6 right eyes showed an average change of + .50 D in refractive error and a change in the corneal curvature of − 1.33 D. Thus the average difference between the reoperated-on and control eyes was + .82 D of refractive error change and − 1.07 D of corneal curvature change. The mean keratometry values were fairly stable during the follow-up period. However, when these values were graphically displayed, eyes that were reoperated on showed considerably more individual fluctuation of the corneal curvature than did the control eyes. Two perforations occurred during the repeat procedure, but no complications were observed. Follow-up slit-lamp examination of both the right corneas and the control left corneas showed no vascularization, excessive scar formation, or epithelial irregularity, as demonstrated by fluorescein dye in the tear film. The scars in the left eyes appeared to be more prominent than those in the more recently operated-on right eyes.

It appears that a repeat radial keratotomy as performed in this study will flatten the cornea beyond the degree achieved by the initial procedure. However, the value of radial keratotomy needs to be demonstrated in human studies.

14–7 **Radial Keratotomy: Effect on Cornea and Aqueous Humor Physiology in the Rabbit.** There is concern that radial keratotomy for myopia may damage the corneal endothelium, even in the absence of perforation. David S. Hull, Steve Farkas, Keith Green, Lisa Laughter, R. David Elijah, and Karen Bowman (Med. College of Georgia, Augusta) examined the endothelial and aqueous humor changes following radial keratotomy in rabbit eyes. Eight incisions were made in the corneas of adult animals, preserving a 3.5-mm central pupillary area. The blade depth was set at .35 mm. Endothelial membrane permeability was estimated at intervals of as long as 10 weeks after the procedure, by simultaneously determining the flux of tritiated inulin and carbon-labeled dextran in isolated corneas.

No physiologically significant changes in corneal endothelial permeability to either inulin or dextran were observed at any time after radial keratotomy. Permeabilities of both inulin and dextran were increased after 9 to 10 weeks, but permeability of fluorescein, a smaller molecule, was significantly reduced, as estimated by fluorophotometry. The turnover rate of aqueous humor was significantly

(14–7) Arch. Ophthalmol. 101:479–481, March 1983.

reduced 1 week and 9 to 10 weeks after radial keratotomy, but not at 5 to 6 weeks.

These findings indicate no physiologically significant altterations in corneal endothelial barrier function or aqueous humor turnover after radial keratotomy in rabbits. It is possible that alterations might occur in other species.

14–8 **Adverse Ocular Reactions to Drugs** are reviewed by M. A. Spiteri and D. Geraint James (London). The administration of drugs for systemic effect can lead to conjunctival and corneal irritation and the Stevens–Johnson syndrome. Hypersensitivity reactions to aspirin at therapeutic dosages are common. The Stevens–Johnson syndrome has occurred with chlorpropamide, sulfonamides, some anticonvulsants, and nonsteroidal antiinflammatory agents. A progressive dry eye syndrome with corneal keratinization and ulceration has occurred with the use of practolol, but not with other β-blockers, although some of these drugs reduce tear secretion. Tranquilizers also can reduce tear production. Such drugs as hydroxychloroquine, chlorpromazine, indomethacin, and pethidine can cause corneal deposits that rarely have a permanent adverse effect on vision. Deposits also have been described with the use of the antiarrhythmic drug amiodarone.

Toxic cataract is an uncommon condition. It has been associated with the prolonged administration of oral steroids and also with some phenothiazines. Prolonged systemic steroid therapy can lead to posterior polar lens opacities in a dose-related manner. Other adverse ocular effects of drugs include retinopathy, most commonly associated with chloroquine drugs and chlorpromazine, and papilledema, occasionally seen with steroid therapy and oral contraceptive use. Inflammation of the optic nerve has been associated with several drugs, including chloramphenicol, streptomycin, isoniazid, digitalis, and oral contraceptives. Drugs with anticholinergic action have induced angle-closure glaucoma in predisposed eyes. Phenobarbital and phenytoin can alter oculomotor function. Oculogyric crisis is a feature of phenothiazine toxicity.

▶ [This is a fine review reminding us to take careful drug histories from our patients. We must also report any and all problems to the National Registry of Drug-Induced Ocular Side Effects, Department of Ophthalmology, Oregon Health Sciences University, Portland.] ◀

14–9 **Impact of Computed Tomography on Ophthalmology** is discussed by Lanning B. Kline (Univ. of Alabama, Birmingham). Computed tomography (CT) is helpful in virtually all aspects of ophthalmologic evaluation. With current scanners, multiplanar reformatted imaging permits visualization of a given area in virtually any plane of section. Other imaging methods currently under evaluation are positron emission CT and nuclear magnetic resonance imaging.

Intraocular foreign bodies may be localized by CT, and any associ-

(14–8)   Postgrad. Med. J. 59:343–349, June 1983.
(14–9)   Ala. J. Med. Sci. 20:294–301, July 1983.

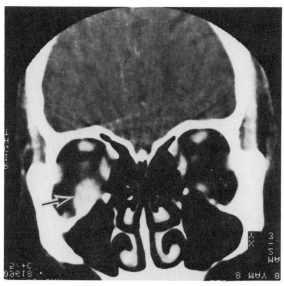

Fig 14–2.—Coronal view in patient with orbital myositis demonstrates distinct enlargement of the right inferior rectus muscle *(arrow)*. (Courtesy of Kline, L.B.: Ala. J. Med. Sci. 20:294–301, July 1983.)

ated orbital injury can be assessed. Also, CT can be used to identify extraocular extension of a malignant tumor, e.g., retinoblastoma. It is the preferred method for evaluating orbital disease, and the information obtained is helpful in planning orbital surgery. Furthermore, CT can demonstrate enlarged extraocular muscles, as shown in Figure 14–2. It delineates the extent of orbital trauma. The intraorbital part of the optic nerve is visualized by CT, and optic nerve tumors and compression can be detected. Computed tomography is helpful in the differential diagnosis of optic chiasmal compression. The cavernous sinus and the cranial nerves within it are directly visualized by CT. Close attention to the parasellar region is needed in studying data on patients with ophthalmoplegia. Visual field defects caused by abnormality of the optic tract, optic radiation, or occipital cortex can be investigated by cranial CT, and the method is sometimes helpful in evaluating patients with poor vision whose fundi appear normal.

▶ [The author of this excellent review article on x-ray computed tomography begins with the Chinese proverb, "One picture is worth a thousand words." Perhaps, because of the new non-x-ray magnetic resonance imaging machines now being installed across the country, he should have taken his introduction from Heraclitus: "There is nothing permanent except change."] ◀

14–10 **Healing of Experimentally Induced Orbital Floor Defects.** The incidence of orbital blowout fractures tends to increase with the grow-

(4–10) J. Oral Maxillofac. Surg. 41:385–388, June 1983.

ing number of traffic, sport, and work accidents, as well as acts of violence. Ferit Tovi, Nodar Pitchazade, Jack Sidi, and Trevor Winer (Ben-Gurion Univ., Beer-Sheva, Israel) tried to restore the defective orbital floor as soon as possible by supporting and stabilizing the remaining periosteum at the edges of the fracture with a Foley catheter balloon. In 63 blowout fractures, this method was used successfully. The clinical results led to a study of the healing process in 9 mongrel dogs. After anesthetizing the animals with pentobarbital, the orbital floor was fractured bilaterally in 3 dogs (group A). Bony tissue was removed, creating a defect 1 × 1.5 cm in size, the torn periosteum at the edges of the defect was preserved as much as possible. The periorbita was entered and the orbital fat exposed. The periosteal remnants were moved back almost to the original position and supported by an inflated Foley catheter balloon. In another 3 dogs (group B), the orbital floors were similarly fractured. Bony tissue, including the periosteum, was removed; the orbital fat was exposed and supported by an inflated Foley catheter balloon. In the remaining 3 dogs (group C), the procedure was similar to that in group A, but no Foley catheter balloon was used.

In group A, a membrane sealing the defect in the orbital floor was observed. Osteoblastic activity was observed in the periosteum in the histologic specimen taken at the end of the first week. In the 2-week specimens, new trabeculated bone was in continuity with the original bone at the edges of the fracture. At 3 weeks, a complete orbital floor consisting of epithelium at the maxillary antrum had formed, as well as submucosa, periosteum, and new bone. In group B, a membranous sheet was found sealing the defect at the orbital floor; the histologic picture at 1, 2, and 3 weeks consisted of dense fibrous tissue with no bone formation. Group C animals had no membrane formation at any time and the orbital floor was defective.

Blowout fractures are often complicated by entrapment of the intraorbital structures and displacement of the orbital floor, causing herniation of intraorbital soft tissues or enlargement of the orbital cavity. Visual disturbances, esthetic deformities, or depression of the eyeball may result. Late repairs do not always have satisfactory results. Early surgical treatment allows use of the periosteum at the site of injury before fibrotic changes take place. Orbital floor implants may lead to such complications as chronic draining fistulae, implant extrusion, lower lid edema, and soft tissue infarction; the use of original tissues, supported by a balloon, is a viable alternative.

▶ [The authors of this experimental animal study demonstrate that there is healing of the orbital floor over a balloon. This becomes important when one considers the many complications of repair using permanent implants.] ◀

14–11 **Custom Ocular Prosthesis With Dilating Pupil** is described by Joseph R. Cain (Univ. of Oklahoma) and Henry LaFuente and Robert

(14–11) J. Prosthet. Dent. 49:795–798, June 1983.

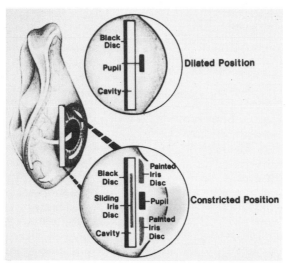

Fig 14–3.—Completed prosthesis shows component locations in constricted position. Dilated position is also diagrammed. (Courtesy of Cain, J.R., et al.: J. Prosthet. Dent. 49:795–798, June 1983.)

G. Small (Dean A. McGee Eye Inst., Oklahoma City). Although ocular prosthetics have improved, optimal esthetic results often are compromised by a fixed pupillary diameter. A method now is available to make an ocular prosthesis with 2 pupil diameters, constricted and dilated, simulating accommodation to light of high and low intensity. Pupil size is altered by the patient using a small magnet without removing the prosthesis from the orbit. The location of the components in the dilated and constricted positions is shown in Figure 14–3.

This prosthesis is indicated for the discriminating patient who desires a pupil diameter appropriate for both direct and indirect light. The need for 2 separate prostheses is eliminated. The patient must be motivated enough to accept the extra time required to fabricate the prosthesis. Although varying iris colors do not influence the fabrication procedure adversely, patients with a light-colored iris appear to show a more distinct pupillary change between extreme light intensities because of increased contrast between the iris and pupil colors. The micromagnet used to change the pupil diameter is easy to use and presents no danger to the soft tissues.

▶ [It would not be fair to some patients to dismiss the importance of their vanity. One would think a light-sensing diode with miniature circuit and solar power supply could replace the magnet and be made to adjust pupil size automatically.] ◀

▶ ↓ The authors of the following 2 articles describe the kind and incidence of ocular injuries and the assessment of special protective devices. The difficulty is in getting people to take proper precautions and wear eye shields and use seat belts. Even in modern warfare personal armor is rarely used and eye-shield compliance has been extremely poor when attempted in the field. ◀

14-12 **Ocular Injuries Sustained During Blunt Facial Trauma.** Jean Edwards Holt, G. Richard Holt, and Janet M. Blodgett (Univ. of Texas, San Antonio) determined the incidence of ocular damage in 1,436 patients seen in 1973 to 1980 with blunt maxillofacial trauma. Cases of gunshot wound injury and other penetrating wounds were excluded. All facial injuries had occurred at least 2 years before the time of review. A total of 727 patients had a formal ophthalmologic examination in the hospital.

Eye injuries were present in 29% of evaluable patients who sustained mandibular fractures, 59% of those with nasal fractures, 76% of those with midfacial fractures, and 89% of those with frontal fractures. In all, 67% of the patients assessed had eye injuries. Eighteen percent of these injuries were serious, and another 3% resulted in blindness. Temporary or minor ocular injuries frequently were multiple. Seventy percent of the patients with serious ocular or adnexal injuries had midfacial fractures. All 15 cases of blindness resulted from optic nerve injury, retinal detachment, or corneal-scleral rupture. All these patients had midfacial, supraorbital, or frontal sinus fractures.

The causes of facial fractures and the patient profiles in this series parallel those in several other series. More than 80% of the patients were men younger than age 30 years. Injuries resulted chiefly from auto accidents, fights, industrial accidents, and athletic trauma. The ocular status of patients with maxillofacial trauma should be evaluated before any treatment is administered. Two thirds of the present patients had ocular injuries. The results of ocular evaluation do not often influence the type of fracture repair, but they may dictate the timing and appropriateness of the repair. Even if there are no preoperative ocular abnormalities, corneal translucency and pupil size and reactivity should be monitored during surgery. Passive forced duction tests and intraocular pressure measurements should be performed at the end of fracture reduction, and ophthalmic monitoring should be performed as postoperative edema subsides.

14-13 **Assessment of Ocular Protection for Racquetball.** The ocular hazards from racquet sports have grown with increasing participation in recent years. Michael J. Feigelman, Joel Sugar, Norbert Jednock, John S. Read, and Peter L. Johnson (Univ. of Illinois, Chicago) assessed the ability of 11 commercially available eye guards designed specifically for use in racquet sports to prevent ocular trauma from racquetballs. Four open, lensless guards and 7 guards of the closed type were tested, as were 8 plano spectacles of various lens thicknesses and materials. A headform was used. The balls were fired at a mean velocity of 65 mph, far below speeds normally encountered at play. An effective guard did not shatter or dislodge after 10 direct blows with a racquetball, and eye contact was prevented.

(14–12) Ophthalmology (Rochester) 90:14–18, January 1983.
(14–13) JAMA 250:3305–3309, Dec. 23/30, 1983.

All the spectacles failed when either the lens or the frame shattered. The open eye guards permitted the ball to make contact with the eye, or were themselves propelled into the eye. Three of the closed guards failed when their frames broke. The other 4 guards were effective. These used polycarbonate in the lens area, and the frame was either an integral part of the unit or a housing for the lens. The support frames of the effective guards were made of polycarbonate or polyamide. None of these guards used temporal hinges.

A national standard for eye wear in racquet sports is needed to insure ocular protection. Even the most impact-resistant eye guards are ineffective if not worn, and many players report that present guards limit their peripheral vision, distort vision, fog up, and are sometimes uncomfortable. The ideal eye guard needs to be designed.

▶ ↓ In the following 2 articles the authors discuss the potential ocular hazards of light. It is evident that a great deal of work needs to be done to define the risk factors clearly. Nonetheless, light may cause damage independent of its heating effect. ◀

14–14 **Biohazards of Ultraviolet, Visible, and Infrared Radiation** are discussed by David H. Sliney (U.S. Army Environmental Hygiene Agency, Aberdeen Proving Ground, Md.). Both photochemical and thermal mechanisms are involved in radiation injuries of the ocular structures. In photochemical injury, the exposure rate-time product produces an effect that is constant over a wide range of exposure durations. Ultraviolet (UV) effects and blue-light retinal injuries are both photochemical effects showing reciprocity. Reciprocity does not hold for thermal injuries, for which it is always necessary to specify an exposure duration. Usually, "pulse duration" determines the threshold irradiance for a given wavelength and effect. As a general

Fig 14–4.—Angle of incident ultraviolet radiation at cornea is critical in assessment of ultraviolet hazard. The brow ridge shields the eye from rays coming from overhead sources (e.g., the sun at midday). Any rays striking the cornea tend to be reflected because of grazing incident angles. (Courtesy of Sliney, D.H.: J. Occup. Med. 25:203–206, March 1983.)

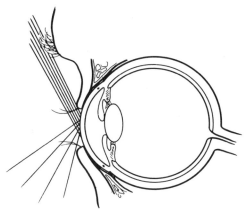

(14–14) J. Occup. Med. 25:203–206, March 1983.

rule, short-wavelength visible and UV radiation can cause photo-chemical injury even with low levels delivered across an entire shift period, whereas thermal injury is possible only from pulsed sources or for momentary exposures. With longer exposures of the retina, photochemical changes may be involved in addition to thermal mechanisms of injury. All of the effects are multistaged. The geometry of solar exposure is an important factor (Fig 14–4). The eye is relatively vulnerable in industrial settings in which welding arc or UV lasers can expose the eye directly.

Recent studies suggest that infrared radiation may be less hazardous than previously thought. Infrared lasers can produce irradiances sufficient to burn tissue, but conventional sources (e.g., molten metal and glass) appear not to produce the irradiances needed to cause either acute or chronic effects beyond the "dry eye." More unusual optical radiation sources undoubtedly will be recognized in the future. As with the laser, adequate control measures and standards should be developed before their use becomes widespread. The greatest problem with laser use today may be the fact that the risk of injury is remote, thus unprotected workers may not be injured. The only way to prevent carelessness from overconfidence is by instituting a sound educational program for workers.

14–15 **Environmental UVA Radiation and Eye Protection During PUVA Therapy.** Patients receiving photochemotherapy are at risk for the development of cataract, but probable exposure doses of ultraviolet A (UVA) radiation from environmental as well as therapeutic sources have not been estimated. Warwick L. Morison and Paul T. Strickland (Frederick, Md.) measured the UVA irradiance of various sources of visible radiation and that of a bank of psoralens-UVA (PUVA) bulbs. Sunlight, daylight, cool white fluorescent bulbs, and incandescent bulbs were assessed. The spectral power distribution and total irradiance of the UVA waveband were similar for the bank of PUVA bulbs and direct sunlight. The UVA irradiance of indirect sunlight through a window was an order of magnitude lower than that of the PUVA bulb bank. The artificial sources of illumination had UVA irradiances 3 orders of magnitude less than direct sunlight or the PUVA bulbs.

Patients must take the same precautions to protect their eyes from sunlight as they do from the UVA radiation from PUVA bulbs. Because patients often are at home or in offices with windows for hours after ingesting psoralen, they should be advised to use maximal protection for their eyes in these settings. Eye protection is much less essential under conditions of artificial illumination. Persons seldom stare directly at room lights, and the concentration of psoralen in the lens is not constant. Although window glass is an efficient filter for sunlight in the waveband of 320 to 340 nm and a plastic diffuser often

(14–15) J. Am. Acad. Dermatol. 9:522–525, October 1983.

is used to cover fluorescent bulbs to reduce their irradiance at the shorter wavelengths, the action spectrum for PUVA-induced cataractogenesis remains to be established.

14–16 **Emergency Therapy of Burns of the Eye** is outlined by Eduard Poser (Chicago). The use of water to wash out acid or alkali splashed into the eye is less reliable and effective than the use of a buffer. Prompt removal of both the dissociated and undissociated parts of the chemical is necessary whether a strong or a weak substance has entered the eye. Use of a buffer as an irrigant can rapidly neutralize the injurious chemical and restore the pH of tissue cells to a physiologic level. Water does not rapidly remove the layer of chemical adjacent to the cornea because of the adhesive nature of the surface and the lamellar flow of water over a surface. Both acid and alkali injuries are properly managed by irrigation with a buffer solution. A hypertonic buffer is helpful when ocular tissues are injured by noncorrosive, hypotonic dehydrating fat solvents such as methanol.

A useful buffer is made by dissolving 35 gm of monobasic potassium phosphate and 90 gm of dibasic sodium phosphate in 850 cc of water. The phosphate insures prompt neutralization and limits burning and resultant scarring. The pH is approximately neutral. The solution is hypertonic. Prompt irrigation of ocular burn injuries with the buffer solution is a suitable immediate treatment that can prevent denaturation of the tissues, minimize injury, and maximize final vision.

14–17 **How Do Tears Exit?** The mechanisms of tear flow, blinking, and tear drainage were studied by Michael A. Lemp and Harold H. Weiler (Georgetown Univ.) using a slit lamp fitted with a continuous 150-watt high-pressure Zenon arc light source. A 16-mm camera was attached to the slit lamp via a beam splitter, and frame speeds of up to 64 frames per second were used. Black polystyrene microspheres mixed into a suspension in an artificial tear solution were instilled into the conjunctival sac in 10 normal patients and in 3 patients with abnormal blinking patterns.

Tears were observed to be drawn into the canaliculi during the relaxation phase of blinking. Both superior and inferior puncta function as normal tear drainage routes, and the predominant direction of flow is nasally toward the punctum. Some of this flow crosses the inferior punctum, over the caruncle and up into the superior punctum. The superior punctum acts as both a normal exit pathway and also as an overflow drainage mechanism; it is sufficient to handle tear drainage. There is some regurgitation of tears from the canaliculi. An intact blink mechanism is necessary for effective tear drainage. The closure of the puncta that occurs during blinking is sufficient to effect tear exit without the lids meeting. Tear flow into the lower punctum without the lids approximating on a blink can be demonstrated, indicating

(14–16)   IMJ 164:186–187, September 1983.
(14–17)   Ophthalmol. Vis. Sci. 24:619–622, May 1983.

that the actual mechanism resides within the punctum or canaliculus and is not dependent on the actual meeting of the lid margins. To prevent tear drainage, it is necessary to occlude both the superior and the inferior puncta.

▶ [This article provides evidence that during canalicular surgery, if one of the canaliculi is normal, it should not be jeopardized by excessive manipulation with probes or plastic since it may maintain normal tear drainage on its own. Moreover, normal lid anatomy and blinking are necessary for effective tear drainage.] ◀

14–18 **Demonstration of Circulating Autoantibody Against Soluble Eye-Muscle Antigen in Graves' Ophthalmopathy.** It has been suggested that Graves' ophthalmopathy is an organ-specific autoimmune disorder in which cytotoxic antibodies or mononuclear cells are directed against putative orbital autoantigens in eye muscle, orbital connective tissue, and, possibly, lacrimal tissue. Though closely associated with Graves' hyperthyroidism, the disorder occurs in the absence of thyroid abnormality in about 10% of cases. K. Kodama, P. Bandy-Dafoe, H. Sikorska, R. Bayly, and J. R. Wall (Queen's Univ., Kingston, Ont.) describe the characteristics of mouse monoclonal antibodies against antigens in human eye muscle, orbital connective tissue, lacrimal tissue, and guinea pig Harder's gland prepared by the hybridization technique. The specificity of the derived antibodies for orbital antigens are assessed in 23 patients with active Graves' ophthalmopathy, 16 patients with Graves' disease but no eye involvement, 14 patients (all women) with Hashimoto's thyroiditis, 11 patients with subacute thyroiditis, 10 euthyroid patients (all women) with multinodular goiters, and 20 normal subjects.

More than 30 monoclonal antibodies against orbital antigens were produced from 14 fusions, of which 24 were maintained and characterized for study. These 24 monoclonal antibodies included 9 against eye muscle extract, 8 against human orbital connective tissue extract, 2 against connective tissue membranes, 2 against human lacrimal gland extract, and 3 against guinea pig Harder's gland extract. All were of the subclass IgG_1. Generally, the monoclonal antibodies against human eye muscle and lacrimal gland were species-specific and failed to fix complement. Most antibodies were organ-specific, but some cross-reacted with antigens in other tissues. Eye muscle antibodies reacted with skeletal muscle in 3 of 7 cases; both lacrimal gland antibodies reacted strongly with mucus-secreting cells in small intestine, and 1 eye muscle antibody reacted with thyroidal microsomes. Using orbital monoclonal antibodies as probes to identify orbital antigens, it was found that most antigens were in the cytosol fraction, although a few were found in cytoplasmic membranes. Circulating autoantibodies against a soluble human eye muscle antigen were found in 17 (74%) of 23 patients with active Graves' ophthalmopathy, but in only 1 of 14 patients with Hashimoto's thyroiditis

(14–18) Lancet 2:1353–1356, Dec. 18, 1982.

and in 2 of 11 patients with subacute thyroiditis. These antibodies were not detected in patients who had Graves' disease without eye involvement, nor in those with multinodular goiter.

It is likely that various autoantibodies are present in the serum of patients with Graves' ophthalmopathy. Although autoantibodies are not likely to be the cause of tissue damage in this disorder, they may be useful markers of the autoimmune process. Thus they could have clinical value in identifying patients with Graves' disease who may be prone to the development of ophthalmopathy.

▶ [Thyroid ophthalmopathy is an exceedingly difficult disease to treat and a sensitive test heralding its onset might be useful in a study of the effect of early treatment.] ◀

14–19 **Specific Reading Disability: Identification of Inherited Form Through Linkage Analysis.** Multiple etiologies are probable in the broadly defined group of individuals with reading disabilities in the absence of neurologic, intellectual, emotional, or environmental handicaps. A strongly positive family history is frequently reported. Because the available battery of genetic markers and linkage analysis provides a means of detecting a linkage, Shelley D. Smith, William J. Kimberling, Bruce F. Pennington, and Herbert A. Lubs designed a study to define 1 or more inherited types of reading disability. Minimal requirements for inclusion in the study were a proband with apparent specific reading disability, full-scale IQ greater than 90, and 1 parent or grandparent with a history of reading disability similar to that of the proband. Children were diagnosed as reading disabled if their reading level was at least 2 years below expected grade level. The Gray Oral Reading Test was used to measure reading ability, and the average of the Peabody Individual Achievement Test for mathematics and general information tests were used to determine the expected level.

Of 84 individuals tested, 50 were judged to be affected; most were males. In the linkage analysis, 21 routine genotyping markers as well as chromosomal heteromorphisms were used. Linkage analysis between specific reading disability and chromosome 15 heteromorphisms produced a lod score of 3.241 at $\theta = 0.13$ (θ is the recombination fraction). A lod score above 3.0, equivalent to prior odds of 1,000 to 1, is considered sufficient to establish linkage, thus assigning a gene for specific reading disability to chromosome 15.

▶ [Traditionally, practically the entire spectrum of the so-called reading disabilities has been left in the hands of educators. It may be that physicians should take a more active role, especially if some of the problems have a genetic basis.] ◀

14–20 **Changing Workload in Ophthalmology: Some Observations From Routine Statistics.** Most patients treated by ophthalmologists are children with squints and elderly persons with cataracts. M. J. Goldacre (Univ. of Oxford) and R. M. Ingram (Kettering, England)

(14–19) Science 219:1345–1347, March 1983.
(14–20) Br. Med. J. 286:1560–1561, May 14, 1983.

analyzed the demographic changes that occurred in England and Wales, and especially in 4 regions around Oxford, between 1968 and 1981 with special reference to the effect these changes created in the practice of ophthalmology. The total number of children younger than age 5 years in England and Wales decreased by 29% between 1968 and 1978; at the same time, the numberr of discharges in ophthalmology declined from 38/10,000 children to 35.3/10,000 children in this age group. Simultaneously, the number of individuals 65 years and older rose by 18%, and the number of discharges in ophthalmology rose from 66.4/10,000 in this age group to 71/10,000.

The Oxford region has an expanding population, thus the number of children has declined less there. From 1975 to 1981, operations on squint and cataract accounted for 50% of all hospital admissions for ophthalmologic procedures (squint, 20.3%; cataract, 30.7%). Durations of stay for cataract varied widely in the 4 districts around Oxford, but they were shortened in each district between 1975 and 1981; for instance, in district 1 the median duration of stay was 13 days in 1975 but only 8 days in 1981; in district 3, the figures were 4 and 0, respectively. In district 3, the number of operations undertaken as day cases increased from none in 1975 to 213 (99%) of 215 in 1981. By 1990, the number of persons aged 65 to 74 years is expected to rise by about 9%, and the number of those aged 75 years and older by about 30%.

Subject Index

A

Acquired immunodeficiency syndrome
  ocular manifestations of, 204
Acyclovir
  in keratitis, 251
    dendritic, with alpha-interferon, 251
    herpetic disciform, 252
Age
  carbonic anhydrase inhibitor tolerance
    and, 130
Aged
  cataract (*see* Cataract, in aged)
  macular degeneration (*see* Macula,
    degeneration, senile)
  macular disease in, and rupture of
    retinal detachment, 202
  vision disorders of, management, 65
Aging
  lens transparency and, 135
AIDS
  ocular manifestations, 204
Aldose reductase
  inhibitors, 293
  in retinal mural cells, 292
Allergic, 77
  conjunctivitis (*see* Conjunctivitis,
    allergic)
  eye disease, conjunctival eosinophils
    in, 77
Alpha-interferon
  in keratitis, dendritic, 251
Amaurosis fugax
  arteriography in, 228
Amblyopia
  Brown's syndrome and, 47
  CAM therapy with occlusion, in
    children, 50
  occlusion therapy in, binocular visual
    functions after, 52
Aminocaproic acid
  for hemorrhage after traumatic
    hyphema, 255
Analgesia
  with sedation for eyelid surgery, 273
Aneurysm
  posterior fossa, eye signs in, 231

Angiography
  in classification of central pigmentary
    retinal dystrophy, 166
  fluorescein
    accidents during, serious and fatal,
      257
    iris, and diabetic, rubeosis, 198
Anomalies
  orbit, craniofacial surgery of, 33
  vitreoretinal, ultrasound for mapping,
    172
Antibody(ies)
  autoantibody against eye-muscle
    antigen in Graves'
    ophthalmopathy, 298
  IgG-specific, in vernal conjunctivitis,
    80
Antigen(s)
  eye-muscle, in Graves'
    ophthalmopathy, autoantibody
    against, 306
  ragweed pollen, in vernal
    conjunctivitis, 80
Antiprostaglandins
  in glaucoma fistulizing surgery, 126
Aphakia, 60
  lens in
    contact, extended-wear, 60
    contact or intraocular, stereopsis
      after, 147
  rehabilitation, intraocular lens vs.
    extended-wear contact lens in, 61
  treatment, in infant, 58
Aphakic
  corneal edema, keratoplasty in, 100
  macular edema, experiences and
    concepts in, 195
  retinal detachment, prevalence, 209
Aponeurosis
  levator, in ptosis correction, 22
Aqueous humor
  after keratotomy, radial (in rabbit),
    297
  after photocoagulation, trabecular, 114
Argon (*see* Laser, argon)
Arteriography
  in amaurosis fugax, 228

Aspirin
  in vernal conjunctivitis, 81
Autoantibody
  against eye-muscle antigen in Graves'
    ophthalmopathy, 298

B

Bacterial
  corneal ulcer, treatment of, 104
Behçet's disease
  immunologic studies in, 165
Biohazards
  of UV, visible and infrared radiation,
    303
Biomicroscopy
  slit-lamp, with contact lens, 59
  of vitreous in macular breaks, 173
Bleb
  developing, and antiprostaglandins,
    126
Blepharoplasty
  eyelid, lower, by anterior approach, 23
Blinking
  mechanisms of, 305
Block (see Pupil, block)
Brown's syndrome
  amblyopia and, 47
Bullous
  keratopathy, pseudophakic, 101
Burns
  of eye, emergency therapy, 305
  laser, number of, and results in
    trabeculoplasty, 115

C

CAM therapy
  comparison with occlusion therapy, 51
  with occlusion in amblyopia, in
    children, 50
Cancer
  paranasal sinus, radiotherapy
    complications, 31
Canthus
  temporal, reconstruction, 30
Capsulectomy
  lens, during cataract surgery, in
    children, 143
Capsulotomy
  laser for, neodymium-YAG, 278
  late posterior, retinal detachment
    after, 210
Carbonic anhydrase inhibitor
  tolerance to, and age, 130

Cataract, 137
  in aged, 137
    epidemiology of, 137
    extraction, mortality after, 137
  extraction, extracapsular
    maculopathy from operating
      microscope after, 208
    planned, 143
  formation, and salicylate in lens and
    intraocular fluids, 294
  surgery
    day-case, 140
    in diabetes, neovascular glaucoma
      and vitreous hemorrhage after,
      144
    lens capsulectomy during, in
      children, 143
    trends in U. S., 149
    uveitis and, chronic, 278
    visual acuity in, interferometers for,
      139
Cell(s)
  endothelial, in diabetes, prostacyclin
    production in, 293
  retinal mural, aldose reductase in,
    292
Chalazion
  spontaneous resolution, frequency of,
    15
Chemical preparation
  of eye for surgery, 281
Children
  amblyopia, CAM therapy with
    occlusion in, 50
  cataract surgery with lens
    capsulectomy, 143
  esotropia treatment results in, 41
  infant, treatment of aphakia of, 58
  preschool, eye movements in, 53
  sarcoidosis, ocular presentation, 164
  vitrectomy in, results, 176
Chondroitin sulfate
  corneal endothelium and intraocular
    pressure after, 250
Choroid, 156
  melanoma (see Melanoma, choroid)
  neovascularization
    in macular degeneration, in aged,
      193
    photocoagulation in, 156
Computed (see Tomography, computed)
Cone and rod activity
  in retinitis pigmentosa, 221
Conjunctiva
  eosinophils in allergic ocular disease,
    77

Conjunctivitis
  allergic, 78
    decongestants in, ocular, 78
    ragweed, cromolyn sodium in, 79
  Enterovirus 70, polio-like syndrome
      after, 83
  giant papillary, due to contact lens, 81
  hemorrhagic, outbreak in Florida, 75
    clinical findings and treatment
      results, 76
  vernal
    aspirin in, 81
    IgG-specific antibodies in, 80
Contact lens, 59
  in aphakia, stereopsis after, 147
  biomicroscopy in, slit-lamp, 59
  conjunctivitis due to, giant papillary,
      81
  extended-wear, 60
    for aphakic correction, 60
    corneal swelling after, 64
    in myopia, 62
    in myopia, with Hydrocurve II soft
      lens, 63
    vs. intraocular lens in aphakia, 61
  soft, hydrophilic, philosophy of
      permanent wearing, 59
  spectacle blur with, 59
  visual acuity with, 59
Cornea
  edema, pseudophakic and aphakic,
      keratoplasty in, 100
  effects of swimming pool water on,
      106
  endothelium
    discussion of, 107
    effects of shearing intraocular lens
      on, 151
    after Healon, chondroitin sulfate and
      methylcellulose, 250
    after keratotomy, radial (in rabbit),
      297
    swelling after contact lens extended-
      wear, 64
    topographic analysis, 92
  ulcer (see Ulcer, cornea)
Corticosteroid
  intraocular inflammatory disease
      resistant to, 248
Craniofacial
  surgery, of orbital anomalies, 33
Cranium
  intracranial hypertension and oval
      pupil, 239
Cromolyn sodium
  in ragweed allergic conjunctivitis, 79

Cyclosporin A
  in intraocular inflammatory disease,
      248
Cystoid (see Edema, macular, cystoid)
Cytotoxic agents
  intraocular inflammatory disease
      resistant to, 248

D

Dacryocystitis
  acquired, management, 25
Dacryocystorhinostomy
  lacrimal duct intubation in, 26
Decongestants
  ocular, in allergic conjunctivitis, 78
Dendritic keratitis
  acyclovir and alpha-interferon in, 251
Diabetes mellitus, 143, 197, 293
  cataract surgery in, neovascular
      glaucoma and vitreous
      hemorrhage after, 144
  complications in lens and nerve, 293
  endothelial cells in, prostacyclin
      production by, 293
  hypoglycemia in, after timolol, 254
  insulin-dependent, retinopathy in, and
      normal glucose levels, 193
  intraocular lens implant in, 143
  retinopathy (see Retinopathy, diabetic)
  rubeosis, and panretinal
      photocoagulation, 198
Disciform
  degeneration in myopia, visual
      prognosis, 70
Drug(s)
  adverse ocular reactions to, 298
  cytotoxic, intraocular inflammatory
      disease resistant to, 248
  ophthalmic, topical, systemic effects of,
      249
Dry eye, 73
  discussion of, 73
  tear inserts in, 74
Dystrophy
  retina, central pigmentary,
      angiographic classification, 166

E

Ectropion
  McCord procedure in, 23
Edema
  cornea, pseudophakic or aphakic,
      keratoplasty in, 100

macular, cystoid, 195
    aphakic, experiences and concepts in,
        195
    YAG laser in, 196
Elderly (see Aged)
Electrooculography
    silicone oil in, 186
Electroretinography
    in retinitis pigmentosa, 221
    silicone oil in, 186
Endothelium
    cells of, in diabetes, prostacyclin
        production by, 293
    cornea (see Cornea, endothelial)
Enterovirus 70
    conjunctivitis, polio-like syndrome
        after, 83
Enucleation
    "no touch," in ocular melanoma, 163
    of uveal melanoma, survival after, 158
Eosinophils
    conjunctival, in allergic ocular disease,
        77
Epithelium
    retinal pigment epithelial detachment,
        202
Esotropia, 37
    accommodative
        follow-up, 40
        medical management, 37
    recurrent, after congenital esotropia
        surgery, 38
    treatment results, in early childhood,
        41
Exotropia, 42
    consecutive, after surgery, 42
    intermittent, surgical results, 43
Eye
    adverse reactions to drugs, 298
    burns, emergency therapy, 305
    chemical preparation for surgery, 281
    complications after radiotherapy of
        paranasal sinus cancer, 31
    decongestants in allergic conjunctivitis,
        78
    disease, allergic conjunctival
        eosinophils in, 77
    dry (see Dry eye)
    histoplasmosis, photocoagulation of,
        results, 191
    intraocular (see Intraocular)
    lymphoma, natural history, 219
    manifestations in AIDS, 204
    melanoma (see Melanoma, ocular)
    movement(s)
        abnormalities in internuclear
            ophthalmoplegia, 231

    in preschool children, 53
    muscle (see Muscle, eye)
    presentation of sarcoidosis, in children,
        164
    prosthesis, custom, with dilating pupil,
        300
    protection
        during PUVA, 304
        for racquetball, 302
    signs in posterior fossa aneurysms, 229
    trauma during blunt facial trauma,
        302
    20/20, in multiple sclerosis, 239
Eyelid
    lower, blepharoplasty by anterior
        approach, 23
    surgery, analgesia with sedation for,
        284

F

Face
    craniofacial surgery of orbit anomalies,
        33
    trauma, blunt, ocular injuries during,
        302
Fasanella-Servat operation
    modification, 20
FDA Report
    on intraocular lens, 148
Fluorescein (see Angiography,
        fluorescein)
Fluorouracil
    in vitreoretinopathy after vitrectomy,
        187
Forced duction test, 46
Fossa
    posterior fossa aneurysms, eye signs
        in, 229
Fracture (see Orbit, floor fracture)

G

Geriatric (see Aged)
Glaucoma
    fistulizing surgery, antiprostaglandins
        in, 126
    intraocular pressure in, and physical
        activity, 130
    neovascular
        after cataract surgery in diabetes,
            144
        panretinal photocoagulation to
            prevent, 199
        valve implant in, 128
        vitrectomy in diabetic retinopathy
            and, 185

open-angle, 118
  chronic, timolol in, 124
  iridectomy results in, 125
  photocoagulation in, argon laser, of
    trabecular meshwork, 114
  trabecular surgery in, argon laser,
    118
  trabeculoplasty in, laser, 119
  trabeculoplasty in, laser, argon,
    113
  optic disk in, 121
  optic disk and visual field correlations
    in, 129
  phakic malignant, pars plana
    vitrectomy in, 179
  retina in, 121
  simple chronic, timolol 0.25% and 0.5%
    in, 124
Glucose
  normal levels, and retinopathy in
    insulin-dependent diabetes, 197
Grating stimulation (see CAM therapy)
Graves' ophthalmopathy
  autoantibody against eye-muscle
    antigen in, 306

H

Headaches
  pupil and, 238
Healing
  of orbital floor defects (in dog), 299
Healon, 276
  corneal endothelium and intraocular
    pressure after, 250
  as emergency aid, 276
  in lens implant, intraocular, 278
Helium ion therapy
  in choroidal melanoma, 162
Hemorrhage
  after traumatic hyphema,
    aminocaproic acid in, 255
  vitreous
    after cataract surgery in diabetes,
      144
    nondiabetic, vitrectomy in, 177
Hemorrhagic
  conjunctivitis, outbreak in Florida, 75
    clinical findings and treatment
      results, 76
Herpes
  simplex keratitis, 91
  zoster ophthalmicus, complications,
    236
Herpetic disciform keratitis
  acyclovir in, 252

Histoplasmosis
  ocular, photocoagulation in, results,
    191
Hyaluronate, sodium (see Healon)
Hydrophilic
  contact lens, soft, 59
Hypertension
  intracranial, and oval pupil, 239
Hyphema
  traumatic, hemorrhage after,
    aminocaproic acid in, 255
Hypoglycemia
  in diabetes, after timolol, 254

I

IgG-specific antibodies
  in vernal conjunctivitis, 80
Imaging, nuclear magnetic resonance, of
    orbit, 17
  tumors, 19
Immunodeficiency syndrome, acquired
  ocular manifestations, 204
Immunoglobulin
  G-specific antibodies in vernal
    conjunctivitis, 80
Immunologic studies
  in Behçet's disease, 165
Implant
  intraocular lens (see Intraocular lens,
    implant)
  valve, in neovascular glaucoma, 128
Indomethacin
  in miosis after surgery prevention, 270
Infant
  aphakia of, treatment, 17
Infections
  postoperative, in ophthalmology, 283
Infrared radiation
  biohazards of, 303
Insulin
  -dependent diabetes, retinopathy in,
    and normal glucose levels, 197
Interferometers
  for visual acuity in cataract, 139
α-Interferon
  in keratitis, dendritic, 251
Internuclear ophthalmoplegia
  eye movement abnormalities in, 231
Intracranial hypertension
  oval pupil and, 239
Intraocular fluids
  salicylate in, and cataract formation,
    294
Intraocular inflammatory disease
  cyclosporin A in, 248

Intraocular lens, 145
  in aphakia, stereopsis in, 147
  FDA Report on, 148
  implant
    bilateral, 145
    capsule-like portion of reactive
      membranes on, 295
    in diabetes, 143
    lessons of first million, 152
    maculopathy from operating
      microscope after, 208
    methylcellulose instead of Healon in,
      278
    pupillary block after, 275
  shearing of, effects on corneal
    endothelium, 151
  trends in U.S., 149
  update on, 150
  vs. extended-wear contact lens in
    aphakia, 61
Intraocular pressure
  in glaucoma, and physical activity, 130
  after Healon, chondroitin sulfate and
    methylcellulose, 250
Intubation of lacrimal duct, 26
  in dacryocystorhinostomy, 26
  of nasolacrimal canal, 28
Iridectomy
  in glaucoma, results, 125
Iris
  fluorescein angiography, and diabetic
    rubeosis, 198
  neovascularization, and vitrectomy in
    diabetic retinopathy, 185
Ischemic central retinal vein occlusion
  glaucoma after, 199

K

Keratitis, 251
  dendritic, acyclovir and alpha-
    interferon in, 251
  herpes simplex, 91
  herpetic disciform, acyclovir in, 252
Keratometric results
  of radial keratotomy, 94
Keratopathy
  pseudophakic bullous, 101
Keratophakia
  update on, 93
Keratoplasty
  penetrating, results, 100
Keratoprosthesis
  review of, 103
Keratorefractive surgery
  ten caveats for, 92, 285

Keratotomy, radial, 296
  clinical study, ongoing, 95
  cornea and aqueous humor after (in
    rabbit), 297
  evaluation, prospective, 97
    design features, 97
    design rationale, 99
  experience with, 96
  repeat (in monkey), 296
  results with, visual, refractive and
    keratometric, 94
Kirisawa's uveitis, 216

L

Lacrimal duct (*see* Intubation of lacrimal
    duct)
Laser, 270 ff.
  argon
    photocoagulation (*see*
      Photocoagulation, laser, argon)
    for trabecular surgery (*see*
      Trabecular, surgery, argon laser)
    trabeculoplasty (*see* Trabeculoplasty,
      argon laser)
  neodymium-YAG
    for capsulotomy, 273
    trabeculotomy, 127
  photocoagulation (*see*
    Photocoagulation, laser)
  photodisruptors, 270
  YAG
    (*See also* neodymium-YAG *above*)
    in macular edema, cystoid, 196
Lens
  contact (*see* Contact lens)
  diabetic complications in, 293
  intraocular (*see* Intraocular lens)
  salicylate in, and cataract formation,
    294
  spectacle, artifacts due to, in
    strabismus measurement, 67
  transparency, and aging, 135
  trauma, perforating, surgery and
    postoperative care in, 289
Lensectomy
  vitrectomy in diabetic retinopathy and,
    185
Levator aponeurosis
  in ptosis correction, 22
Lid (*see* Eyelid)
Light
  -induced maculopathy from operating
    microscope, 208
Lymphoma
  intraocular, natural history, 219

M

McCord procedure
in ectropion, 23
Macula, 193 ff.
break, biomicroscopy of vitreous in,
173
degeneration, senile, 193 ff.
choroidal neovascularization in, 193
epidemiologic features, 195
disease, rupture of retinal detachment
in, in aged, 202
edema (see Edema, macular)
Maculopathy
light-induced, from operating
microscope, 208
Malignancy (see Cancer)
Medications (see Drugs)
Melanoma, 157 ff.
choroid, 161 ff.
conservative therapy, 161
helium ion therapy, 162
misdiagnosed and unsuspected, 157
ocular
metastatic, survival, 160
"no touch" enucleation in, 163
uvea, survival after enucleation, 158
Meningioma
olfactory and suprasellar, case review,
234
Metastases
of ocular melanoma, survival, 160
Methylcellulose
corneal endothelium and intraocular
pressure after, 250
for lens implant, intraocular, 278
Microscope
operating, light-induced maculopathy
after, 208
Microscopy (see Biomicroscopy)
Miosis
prevention after surgery, indomethacin
for, 270
Mortality
in cataract extraction, in aged, 137
Multiple sclerosis
20/20 eye in, 239
Muscle
eye
antigen, in Graves' ophthalmopathy,
autoantibody against, 298
palsy, surgery, 49
superior oblique (see Superior oblique
muscle)
Myopia
contact lens in, extended-wear, 62

with Hydrocurve II lens, 63
disciform degeneration in, visual
prognosis, 70

N

Nasolacrimal canal
intubation for lacrimal duct, 28
intubation of nasolacrimal canal for,
28
Necrosis
retina, acute, 216
Neodymium (see Laser, neodymium-
YAG)
Neovascular (see Glaucoma, neovascular)
Neovascularization, 192 ff.
choroid (see Choroid,
neovascularization)
idiopathic, argon laser
photocoagulation in, 192
iris, and vitrectomy in diabetic
retinopathy, 185
Nerve
diabetic complications in, 293
optic, lesions, high-resolution CT of,
233
Neuroretinitis syndrome
diffuse unilateral subacute, 213
Night
vision mobility aids, 69
NMR imaging of orbit, 17 ff.
tumors, 19
Nuclear magnetic resonance imaging of
orbit, 17 ff.
tumors, 19
Nystagmus
benign paroxysmal positional,
prospective exam, 240

O

Occlusion, 50 ff.
with CAM therapy, in amblyopia, in
children, 50
therapy
comparison with CAM therapy, 51
minimal, binocular visual functions
in amblyopia and, 52
Ocular (see Eye)
Oculomotor palsy
pupil sparing in, 231
Oculomucocutaneous syndrome
dry eye in, 74
Oculoplastic surgery
contraindications, 22

Olfactory meningioma
  case review, 234
Operating microscope
  light-induced maculopathy after, 208
Ophthalmic
  drugs, topical, systemic effects, 249
  manifestations of AIDS, 204 ff.
  prisms, measurement errors, 66
  surgery, chemical preparation of eye
    for, 281
Ophthalmodynamometry
  revisit to, 227
Ophthalmology
  CT in, impact of, 298
  infections in, postoperative, 239
  workload in, changing, 307
Ophthalmopathy
  Graves', autoantibody against eye-
    muscle antigen in, 306
Ophthalmoplegia
  internuclear, eye movement
    abnormalities in, 231
Optic disk
  in glaucoma, 121
  with visual field correlations in
    glaucoma, 129
Optic nerve
  lesions, high-resolution CT of, 233
Orbit, 16
  anomalies, craniofacial surgery of, 33
  complications after radiotherapy of
    paranasal sinus cancer, 31
  CT of, 16
  floor defects, healing of (in dog), 299
  floor fracture, 29 ff.
    surgery and timing, 29
    "trap-door," 29
  nuclear magnetic resonance imaging
    of, 17 ff.
  tumors, 19

P

Palsy
  of eye muscle, surgery, 49
  oculomotor, pupil sparing in, 231
Panretinal (see Photocoagulation,
    panretinal)
Paranasal sinus
  cancer, complications of radiotherapy,
    31
Paroxysmal positional nystagmus
  prospective exam, 240
Pars plana (see Vitrectomy, pars plana)
PERK, 97
Phakic malignant glaucoma
  vitrectomy in, anterior pars plana, 179

Photocoagulation, 114
  in choroidal neovascularization, 156
  laser, 191
    argon, 191
    argon, in neovascularization,
      idiopathic, 192
    argon, in ocular histoplasmosis,
      results, 191
    argon, of trabecular meshwork in
      open-angle glaucoma, 114
  in choroidal neovascularization in
    senile macular degeneration, 193
  panretinal, 198
    in diabetic rubeosis, 198
    to prevent neovascular glaucoma,
      199
  retinal scatter, in sickle retinopathy,
    211
  trabecular, aqueous humor after, 114
Photodisruptors
  laser, 270
Pigment
  retinal pigment epithelial detachment,
    202
Pigmentary
  retinal dystrophy, central,
    angiographic classification, 166
Polio-like syndrome
  after Enterovirus 70 conjunctivitis, 83
Posterior fossa
  aneurysms, eye signs in, 229
Posterior segment
  inflammatory disease, vitrectomy in,
    180
Prisms
  ophthalmic, measurement errors, 66
Prostacyclin
  in endothelial cells in diabetes, 293
Prosthesis
  eye, customs, with dilating pupil, 300
  keratoprosthesis, review of, 103
Pseudophakic, 100
  corneal edema, keratoplasty in, 100
  keratopathy, bullous, 101
Psychophysical measurements
  in retinitis pigmentosa, 221
Ptosis
  correction, levator aponeurosis surgery
    for, 22
Pupil, 238
  block, 274
    after intraocular lens implant, 275
    after laser capsulotomy, neodymium-
      YAG, 274
  dilating, with custom ocular prosthesis,
    300
  headaches and, 238

oval, and intracranial hypertension, 239
sparing in oculomotor palsy, 231
PUVA
eye protection during, 295

R

Racquetball
eye protection for, 302
Radial (*see* Keratotomy, radial)
Radiation
ultraviolet, visible and infrared, biohazards of, 303
Radiotherapy
of paranasal sinus cancer, complications of, 31
Ragweed
allergic conjunctivitis, cromolyn sodium in, 79
pollen antigens in vernal conjunctivitis, 80
Reading disability
specific, linkage analysis in, 307
Refraction
interobserver variation, 68
Refractive
results of radial keratotomy, 94
Reiter's syndrome
discussion of, 83
Respiratory
arrest after timolol, 254
Retina
abnormalities, ultrasound for mapping, 172
cells, mural, aldose reductase in, 292
detachment, 209
aphakic, prevalence, 209
after capsulotomy, 210
complicated, pars plana vitrectomy in, 184
pigment epithelial, in senile macular disease, 202
dystrophy, central pigmentary, angiographic classification, 166
in glaucoma, 121
necrosis, acute, 216
photocoagulation, scatter, in sickle retinopathy, 211
vitreoretinopathy after vitrectomy, fluorouracil in, 187
Retinal vein, central, 199
ischemic, occlusion, glaucoma after, 199
obstruction, differential diagnosis, 201
Retinitis pigmentosa
rod and cone activity in, 221

Retinoblastoma, 217
CT in, 217
retinocytoma as variant of, 218
Retinocytoma
as variant of retinoblastoma, 218
Retinopathy
diabetic, in insulin-dependent diabetes, and normal glucose levels, 197
diabetic, vitrectomy in, 184 ff.
early, 184
iris neovascularization and neovascular glaucoma after, 185
diabetic, vitreous surgery in, complications of, 181
sickle, retinal scatter photocoagulation in, 211
Rod and cone activity
in retinitis pigmentosa, 221
Rubeosis
diabetic, and panretinal photocoagulation, 198
Rupture
of retinal pigment epithelial detachment, 202
Rye grass
antibodies to, in vernal conjunctivitis, 80

S

Salicylate
in lens and intraocular fluids, and cataract formation, 294
Sarcoidosis
ocular presentation, in children, 164
Scatter photocoagulation
retinal, in sickle retinopathy, 211
Sclerosis
multiple, 20/20 eye in, 239
Sedation
with analgesia for eyelid surgery, 284
Senile (*see* Aged)
Shearing
of intraocular lens, corneal endothelium after, 151
Sickle retinopathy
retinal scatter photocoagulation in, 211
Silicone oil
in electroretinography and electrooculography, 186
Sinus
paranasal, cancer, complications of radiotherapy, 31
Sodium hyaluronate (*see* Healon)
Sorbinil
for diabetic complications in lens and nerve, 293

Spectacle blur
with contact lens, 59
Spectacle lens
artifacts due to, in strabismus
measurement, 67
Stereopsis
in aphakia after contact or intraocular
lens, 147
Strabismus
artifacts due to spectacle lens in
measurement of, 67
Subconjunctival
treatment of bacterial corneal ulcer,
104
Sulindac
for diabetic complications in lens and
nerve, 293
Superior oblique muscle recession, 45
measured graduated, 45
vs. tenotomy, 45
Suprasellar meningioma
case review, 234
Swelling
cornea, after extended-wear contact
lens, 64
Swimming pool water
effects on cornea, 106

T

Tear, 73
deficiency, discussion of, 73
drainage, mechanism of, 305
flow, mechanisms of, 305
inserts in dry eyes, 74
Tenotomy
vs. superior oblique recession, 45
Timolol, 123, 254
follow-up study, 123
in glaucoma, chronic
open-angle, 124
0.25% and 0.5% in, 124
hypoglycemia in diabetes after, 254
respiratory arrest after, 254
Tolosa-Hunt syndrome
discussion of, 232
Tomography, computed
high-resolution, of optic nerve lesions,
233
in ophthalmology, impact of, 298
of orbit, 16
in retinoblastoma, 217
Trabecular, 114
meshwork, photocoagulation of, in
open-angle glaucoma, 114
photocoagulation, aqueous humor
after, 114

surgery, argon laser, in glaucoma,
open-angle, 120
uncontrolled, 118
Trabeculoplasty, 115
argon laser
case review, 117
in glaucoma, open-angle, 113
number of laser burns and results,
115
laser, in open-angle glaucoma, 119
low-dose, 116
Trabeculotomy
laser, neodymium-YAG, 127
Trauma
eye, during blunt facial trauma, 302
face, blunt, ocular injuries during, 302
lens, perforating, surgery and
postoperative care in, 285
Traumatic hyphema
hemorrhage after, aminocaproic acid
in, 255
Tumors
orbit, NMR imaging of, 19

U

Ulcer, cornea, 104
bacterial, treatment, 104
demographic and predisposing factors,
105
Ultrasound
for vitreoretinal abnormality mapping,
172
Ultraviolet
A radiation, environmental, 304
biohazards of, 303
Uvea
melanoma, survival after enucleation,
156
Uveitis
chronic, and cataract, 278
factors in initiation and recurrence,
155
Kirisawa's, 216

V

Valve
implant in neovascular glaucoma, 128
Vein
retinal (see Retinal vein)
Vernal (see Conjunctivitis, vernal)
Virus(es)
Enterovirus 70 conjunctivitis, polio-
like syndrome after, 83
herpes (see Herpes)

Vision
  disorders, management in aged, 65
  night, mobility aids, 69
Visual
  acuity
    in cataract, interferometers in, 139
    with contact lens, 59
    measurement, interobserver
      variation, 69
  field with optic disk correlations in
    glaucoma, 129
  functions, binocular, in amblyopia, 52
  loss, functional, 241
  prognosis in myopia with disciform
    degeneration, 70
  results of radial keratotomy, 94
Vitrectomy, 174
  in diabetic retinopathy (see
    Retinopathy, diabetic, vitrectomy
    in)
  in inflammatory disease of posterior
    segment, 180
  pars plana, 174
    anterior, in phakic malignant
      glaucoma, 179
    prognostic parameters in, 175
    results, 174
    results, in children, 176
    in retinal detachment, complicated,
      183
  vitreoretinopathy after, fluorouracil in,
    187

in vitreous hemorrhage, nondiabetic,
    177
Vitreoretinopathy
  after vitrectomy, fluorouracil for, 187
Vitreous, 171
  abnormalities, ultrasound for mapping,
    172
  floaters, 171
  hemorrhage (see Hemorrhage, vitreous)
  in macular breaks, biomicroscopy of,
    173
  surgery in diabetic retinopathy,
    complications, 181

W

Water
  swimming pool, effects on cornea, 106
Workload
  changing, in ophthalmology, 307

Y

YAG laser (see Laser, YAG)

Z

Zoster ophthalmicus
  herpes, complications, 236
Zovirax (see Acyclovir)

Index to Authors

A

Abelson, M. B., 77, 81
Adams, H. P., Jr., 228
Aiello, L. M., 144
Akagi, Y., 292
Akeo, K., 216
Albert, D. M., 158
Anand, V., 209
Anderson, A., 195
Anderson, D. H., 175
Anderson, D. R., 121
Apt, L., 281, 282
Arden, G. B., 221
Arentsen, J. J., 97
Aron, J. -J., 278
Aron-Rosa, D., 278
Arrigg, P. G., 217
Arrowsmith, P. N., 94
Aslin, R. N., 53
Atlas, B. F., 101
Auer, C., 183
Avila, M. P., 171, 173, 193
Azen, S. P., 151

B

Baert, A. L., 16
Ballow, M., 80
Baloh, R. W., 231
Bandy-Dafoe, P., 304
Banerjee, D., 140
Banks, M. S., 53
Barba, D., 239
Barnes, R. W., 148
Barnham, J. J., 103
Barricks, M., 162
Barza, M., 104
Bath, P. E., 148
Baum, J., 104
Bayly, R., 306
Becker, B., 128
Bedi, M., 151
Belcher, C. D., III, 270
Benson, W. E., 179
Berlin, L. A., 172
Bernstein, J., 151
Bernth-Petersen, P., 61
Besson, P., 283
Betharia, S. M., 20
Biglan, A. W., 79
Binder, P. S., 63
Binder, S., 180
Bird, A. C., 70

B (continued)

Blase, W. P., 177
Blodgett, J. M., 302
Bosanquet, R. C., 15
Bouquety, C., 278
Bourque, L. B., 97, 99
Bowers, S. A., 239
Bowman, K., 297
Brant-Zawadski, M., 17
Braunstein, R. A., 213
Bravo, J., 210
Brescia, M., 294
Brown, D. W. C., 148
Brown, G. C., 176, 211
Brown, M. H., 67
Brubaker, R. F., 114
Buckley, E. G., 45
Burd, E. M., 254
Buschmann, W., 285
Butrus, S. I., 81
Buxton, J. N., 148
Buzney, S. M., 270

C

Cain, J. R., 300
Calhoun, J. H., 38
Callahan, A., 33
Campbell, C. J., 195
Canell, K., 251
Canivet, J., 293
Carliner, N. H., 254
Caronni, E. P., 33
Carr, R. E., 239
Carter, R. M., 195
Castro, J. R., 162
Cavanagh, H. D., 100
Centifanto-Fitzgerald, Y. M., 91
Chan, C. -C., 248
Chapman, L., 42
Char, D. H., 162, 217
Chen, G. T. Y., 162
Christopher, S., 83
Ciuffreda, K. J., 53
Clancy, J., 241
Clark, S. W., 76
Clarke, W. N., 47
Clayman, H. M., 145
Clover, G. M., 221
Cohn, H. C., 278
Collier, M., 162
Collins, J. W., 23
Collum, L. M. T., 252
Corbett, J. J., 228, 241

C (continued)

Cotlier, E., 293, 294
Cottrell, D. G., 15
Cowden, J. W., 296
Cox, T. A., 241
Crane, T. B., 231
Crawford, J. B., 162
Cruess, A. F., 211
Culbertson, W. W., 76

D

Dangel, M. E., 278
Dannemiller, J. L., 53
Darin, J. J., 96
Das, S. K., 209
Davidorf, F. H., 157
Deckert, T., 197
deFaller, J. M., 78
de Koning, E. W. J., 251
DeMets, D., 68
Dieckhues, B., 165
Doesburg, W. H., 59
Donshik, P. C., 78
Dortzbach, R. K., 23, 29
Douglas, W. H. G., 114
Drews, R. C., 152

E

Edelhauser, H. F., 250
Edmund, J., 177
Elander, R., 96
Elijah, R. D., 297
Erickson, P. A., 184
Ernst, W. J. K., 221

F

Fagadau, W., 273
Farkas, S., 297
Fawcett, I. M., 15
Feigelman, M. J., 302
Felman, Y. M., 79
Ferber, I., 114
Ferris, F. L., III, 195
Fine, S. L., 156
Fiscella, R. G., 250
Fisher, S., 148
Fisher, S. K., 187
Fleischman, J. A., 196
Flynn, J. T., 45
Folk, E. R., 42
Folk, J. C., 198

321

Foos, R. Y., 204
Fornander, M., 51
Forster, R. K., 75, 76
François, J., 174
Freeley, D. A., 38
Frenkel, M., 255
Freyler, H., 180
Friday, G. A., 79
Friedland, G. H., 205
Friedlander, M. H., 93
Friedman, A. H., 207
Frost-Larsen, K., 197

G

Gass, J. D. M., 213
Gelender, H., 97, 99
Gieser, R. G., 106
Giombini, S., 234
Gola, R., 29
Goldacre, M. J., 307
Goldberg, M. F., 255
Goodrich, G. L., 69
Görne, M., 120
Gottlieb, M. S., 204
Grabner, G., 107
Granet, N., 93
Green, K., 297
Green, W. R., 219
Grover, A. K., 20
Guerin, C. J., 187
Guillaumet, L., 283
Guillot, R., 293
Gulati, A. K., 83
Gupta, S., 83
Gutman, F. A., 172
Guyton, D. L., 66, 67

H

Haag, J. R., 106
Hahn, H., 41
Halliday, B. L., 139
Hampton, G. R., 70
Harris, C. A., 205
Harris, W. S., 142
Hartmann, E. E., 53
Haskin, M. E., 233
Hatch, M. H., 75
Hawes, M. J., 29
Hawkes, R. C., 19
Hayashi, H., 179
Hayreh, S. S., 129
Hedges, T. R., III, 217
Hepler, R. S., 231
Herman, P., 238
Hermsen, V. M., 198
Hershey, B. L., 233
Hervouet, F., 283
Hess, F., 147
Hess, K., 240
Hiatt, R. L., 37
Hidayat, A., 218

Hiles, D. A., 79
Hilton, G. F., 162
Hirsch, R. P., 137
Hitchings, R., 126
Hofbauer, J. D., 96
Hoffer, K. J., 96
Hogg, C. R., 221
Holden, B. A., 64
Holladay, J. T., 148
Holland, G. N., 19, 204
Holland, J. E., 162
Hollander, J. D., 293
Holt, G. R., 302
Holt, J. E., 302
Hoover, E. D. 233
Horsten, G. P. M., 46
Howell, E. R., 52
Huber, C., 147
Hull, D. S., 297
Hurt, A., 151
Hurwitz, J. J., 25
Hyndiuk, R. A., 250

I

Iijima, H., 166
Ingram, R. M., 140, 307
Irvine, A. R., 162, 208
Isenberg, S., 281, 282

J

Jacobs, M. E., 148
Jacobson, M., 293
Jaffe, M. S., 145
Jaffe, N. S., 145
Jalkh, A. E., 171, 173, 193
Jallut, Y., 29
James, D. G., 298
Jampol, L. M., 255
Jansen, J. T. G., 270
Jednock, N., 302
John, T. J., 83
Johnson, P. L., 302
Juster, R., 115

K

Kador, P. F., 292
Kaiser, F. E., 254
Kalra, B. R., 20
Kaminski, A., 162
Kaminski, R. M., 75
Kapetansky, F. M., 127
Karakousis, C. P., 160
Karesh, J. W., 95
Kataria, S., 164
Kataria, Y. P., 164
Kathol, R. G., 241
Katiyar, B. C., 83
Katzen, L. E., 95, 196
Kaufman, H. E., 91, 93
Kaufman, P., 118

Kean, D. M., 19
Kearns, T. P., 201
Keates, R. H., 127
Keith, C. G., 52
Kellen, R. I., 114
Keulen-de Vos, H. C. J., 270
Keys, H., 31
Kimberling, W. J., 307
Kimura, C., 216
Kinoshita, J. H., 292
Kirkham, T. H., 227
Klein, B. E. K., 68
Klein, R., 68
Klein, R. S., 205
Kline, L. B., 298
Kodama, K., 306
Kohen, D., 70
Kopelman, J., 118, 218
Kowler, E., 53
Kracher, G. P., 60
Kraff, M., 274
Kreis-Gosselin, F., 59
Krogh, E., 175
Krupin, T., 128
Kupersmith, M. J., 239
Kuwabara, T., 292

L

Laatikainen, L., 199, 202
LaFuente, H., 300
Laibson, P. R., 99
Lakhanpal, V., 95
Lamberts, D. W., 73
Lamer, L., 62
Langford, M. P., 76
Lanier, B. Q., 78
Lao, C. -S., 148
Laughter, L., 297
Lauritzen, T., 197
Lavin, P. T., 158
Lehto, I., 119
Lemmens, W. A. J. G., 59
Lemp, M. A., 305
Lennerstrand, G., 50
Lerman, S., 135
Leske, M. C., 137, 148
Letson, A. D., 157
Levenson, J. E., 96
Levine, E., 157
Lewis, G. P., 187
Lewis, R. A., 129
Liang, G., 144
Lichter, P. R., 117
Liesegang, T. J., 114, 236
Lindstrom, R. L., 97, 99
Liotet, S., 283
Logen, P., 252
Lonn, L. I., 162
Lubs, H. A., 307
Luscombe, S. M., 145
Lyman, J. T., 162
Lyness, A. L., 221

M

McDonald, H. R., 208
McDonald, M. B., 93
McGetrick, J. J., 255
McGhee, E. T., 148
McKinna, A. J., 229
Maclure, G. M., 124
McMeel, J. W., 193
McNally, J. J., 64
McPherson, A. R., 210
Mac Rae, S. M., 250
Madiwale, N., 77
Magargal, L. E., 211
Maguire, M. G., 185
Mainster, M. A., 270
Mandell, A. I., 128
Mann, R. B., 219
Margo, C., 218
Markowitz, S., 123
Marks, R. G., 94
Marmor, M. F., 69
Marshall, L. F., 239
Martin, N. F., 60
Martins, A. J., 53
Maumenee, A. E., 60, 150, 273
Meier, U., 147
Mendelsohn, G., 219
Mendelson, L., 80
Merin, S., 130
Mertz, G. W., 64
Metz, H. S., 49
Meyer, R. F., 105
Michels, R. G., 177, 181, 183, 185, 278
Migdal, C., 126, 161
Miller, D. L., 79
Miller, M. T., 42
Mills, C., 17
Mills, K. B., 124
Misra, S., 83
Mitchell, D. E., 52
Mitchell, P. G., 274
Moffitt, S. D., 97, 99
Momirov, D., 186
Momoeda, S., 179
Montague, P. R., 198
Moore, R., 160
Moore, W. S., 19
Morello, G., 234
Morens, D. M., 75
Morin, J. D., 123
Morison, W. L., 304
Morrissette, D. L., 69
Moseley, I., 17
Moss, S. E., 68
Mullie, M. A., 227
Murakami, K., 171, 173
Murphey, S. M., 79
Murphy, R. P., 156
Murray, G. C., 137, 149
Musch, D. C., 105
Myers, W. D., 97, 99

N

Nadeau, S. E., 231
Nagahara, K., 216
Nakissa, N., 20
Neill, R. S., 284
Nelson, J. I., 239
Nelson, L. B., 38
Nerini, A., 29
Neubauer, H., 276
Neuhann, T., 81
Nikitas, J. A., 83
Nirankari, V. S., 95
Niven, T., 294
Noel, L. P., 47
Nussenblatt, R. B., 248
Nyman, K. G., 51

O

Obstbaum, S. A., 97, 99
O'Connor, G. R., 155
O'Donnell, J. J., 187
Oei, T. H., 46
Okajima, O., 166
Okamoto, M., 166
Older, J. J., 22
O'Malley, R. E., 210
Onorato, I. M., 75, 76
Opremcek, E. M., 127
Oshima, K., 179
Oyakawa, R. T., 177, 181
Ozawa, H., 216

P

Palestine, A. G., 248
Papacz, P., 80
Parks, M. M., 43, 143
Passa, P., 293
Paton, R. C., 293
Patriarca, P. A., 75, 76
Pavan, P. R., 198
Pennington, B. F., 307
Pepose, J. S., 204
Percival, S. P. B., 209
Pettit, T. H., 96, 204
Peyster, R. C., 233
Phelps, C. D., 129
Pinckers, A. J. L. G., 59
Pitchazade, N., 299
Podos, S. M., 128
Pollack, I. P., 113
Poser, E., 305
Powell, D. J., 221
Prince, D. S., 254
Punt, H., 59
Putman, S. F., 228

Q

Qualman, S. J., 219
Quinlan, M. P., 221
Quivey, J. M., 161

R

Raitta, C., 119
Rajpal, S., 160
Rand, S., 79
Rast, A., 240
Ratner, C. M., 183
Ravencroft, T., 252
Read, J. S., 302
Reinecke, R. D., 148
Reinig, J., 151
Renardel de Lavalette, J. C. G., 270
Rice, E. F., 185
Rice, T. A., 181, 183, 185
Richard, G., 165
Richard, J. M., 43
Richards, R. D., 95
Ritch, R., 128
Rizk, S., 19
Robin, A. L., 113
Robinson, N., 158
Rodgers, K. J. A., 25
Roholt, P., 45
Romanchuk, K. G., 101
Romano, P., 45
Roper-Hall, M. J., 103
Rosenberg, P. R., 205
Ross, J. E., 139
Rothbach, C., 79
Rouwen, A. J. P., 59
Rowsey, J. J., 92, 97, 99, 285
Rubin, P., 31
Ruderman, J., 115
Ruderman, J. M., 274
Ruprecht, K. W., 26
Rydberg, A., 51

S

Safir, A., 93, 97, 99
Saga, U., 216
Samuelsson, B., 50
Sanders, D. R., 94
Sandyk, R., 232
Saunders, W., 162
Scattergood, K. D., 67
Schachat, A. P., 181
Schanzlin, D., 97
Schanzlin, D. J., 97
Schepens, C. L., 171, 173, 193
Scherfig, E., 175
Schonberger, L. B., 75
Schultz, R. O., 250
Schuman, J. S., 207
Schwartz, A., 162
Schwartz, A. L., 118
Schwartz, B., 137
Sebestyen, J. G., 143
Seddon, J. M., 158
Seiple, W. H., 239
Selvin, B. L., 249
Shapiro, A., 130

Sharma, Y. R., 293, 294
Shea, M., 184
Shipp, M. D., 150
Shrader, C. E., 130
Sidi, J., 299
Sikorska, H., 306
Simmons, R. J., 130
Singh, A. K., 83
Singh, G., 51
Singh, R. B., 83
Sires, B. P., 228
Sklar, V. E. F., 75, 76
Sliney, D. H., 270, 303
Small, C. B., 205
Small, R. G., 300
Smith, J. P., 78
Smith, R. E., 151
Smith, S. D., 307
Smits, J., 16
Solero, C. L., 234
Sørensen, T., 61
Soshi, S., 216
Sourdille, P., 283
Sparks, K., 80
Sperduto, R. D., 137
Spiteri, M. A., 298
Stark, W. J., 60, 148, 149, 150, 273, 278
Steel, D., 151
Steinkogler, F. J., 30
Stephens, B. R., 53
Stephens, R. F., 211
Stern, A. L., 101
Stern, W. H., 187
Stone, R. D., 162
Straatsma, B. R., 162
Strickland, P. T., 304
Strohl, R., 31
Stur, M., 107
Sugar, A., 105
Sugar, J., 302
Sulit, H., 162
Swan, K. C., 40
Szymanski, C., 127

T

Taglioni, M., 283
Talbott, M. W., 148

Talmant, J. C., 28
Tanino, T., 166
Tasman, W. S., 176
Taylor, D. M., 101
Taylor, D. S. I., 58
Terry, A. C., 273
Terry, S. A., 128
Thomas, J. V., 130
Thomas, N. E., 148
Thompson, H. S., 228, 241
Thompson, J. T., 66
Thompson, R. K., 140
Tinning, S., 175
Toole, B. M., 239
Tovi, F., 299
Traynar, M. J., 144
Tremblay, N., 78
Trempe, C. L., 171, 173, 193
Trevathan, G. E., 164
Trobe, J. D., 231
Trokel, S., 196

U

Uemura, Y., 216
Uliss, A. E., 205
Utermann, D., 120

V

van Bijsterveld, O. P., 251
Van Buskirk, E. M., 275
Vanhulst, L., 174
van Lith, G. H. M., 186
Van Rij, G., 270
Varnell, E. D., 91
Velde, T. M., 254
Verbraeken, H., 174
Verhagen, W. I. M., 46
Vogel, R., 74
v't Pad Bosch, A. A. I., 59

W

Wafai, M. Z., 143
Wall, J. R., 306

Wand, M., 143
Waring, G. O., III, 97, 98, 100
Watzke, R. C., 198
Weber, B., 296
Weber, P. A., 127
Weder, W., 125
Weiler, H. H., 305
Weingeist, T. A., 198
Weinreb, R. N., 115, 116
Weinstock, F. J., 65
Weiss, E. T., 157
Weiss, P. A., 239
Welch, S. N., 100
Wesley, R. E., 23
Weston, J. H., 77, 79
Wieser, D., 41
Wilensky, J. T., 115, 116
Wilms, G., 116
Wilson, J., 151
Wilson, L. A., 100
Wilson, R. S., 163
Winer, T., 299
Wolf, E., 130
Wolter, J. R., 295
Womack, L. W., 236
Worthen, D. M., 148, 149
Worthington, B. S., 19
Wright, P., 72

Y

Yee, R. D., 204, 231
Yoshimuri, R., 281, 282

Z

Zakov, Z. N., 172
Zeidler, M., 125
Zimmerman, L. E., 218
Živojnović, R., 186
Zografos, L., 257